QUANTITATIVE METHODS FOR HEALTH MANAGEMENT

Robert McGrath, PhD, is a professor in the Department of Health Management and Policy at the University of New Hampshire. He was the founding director of programs in Health Data Science as well as the founding director of graduate analytics and data science for the university. His research spans health policy, data science, and public health, with numerous peer-reviewed publications and funded research projects. He is also the coauthor of three textbooks on health policy, analytics, quantitative methods, and healthcare administration. Dr. McGrath has held leadership roles in health analytics education and has been a featured speaker at national and international conferences. He holds a PhD and MS from The Heller School at Brandeis University, an MS from The Harvard University School of Public Health, and a BS from the University of New Hampshire.

Esmaeil Bahalkeh, PhD, MS, is an assistant professor in the Department of Health Management and Policy at the University of New Hampshire. His research focuses on health data science and healthcare operations management, with an emphasis on improving quality, efficiency, and effectiveness within healthcare settings. As an educator, Dr. Bahalkeh teaches a range of interdisciplinary courses across multiple programs, equipping students with essential analytical and operational skills. His courses include Machine Learning in Healthcare, Healthcare Operations Management, Quality and Process Improvement in Healthcare, and Statistics for Health Professionals. Dr. Bahalkeh holds a PhD in Industrial Engineering from Purdue University, an MS in Industrial and Systems Engineering from Ohio University, and a BS in Industrial Engineering from Sharif University of Technology.

Lee F. Seidel, PhD, is professor emeritus of Health Management and Policy at the University of New Hampshire (UNH). His teaching also includes being a visiting professor in the executive MBA in Health Administration Program at the University of Colorado, Denver. He is the founding director of the UNH Center for Excellence in Teaching and Learning and he has authored four books and numerous articles on health administration, health administration education, and effective college teaching. He holds MPA and PhD degrees in community systems planning and development, with an emphasis on health administration, from the Pennsylvania State University.

Joanna Gyory, PhD, MS, is a lecturer in the Department of Health Management and Policy at the University of New Hampshire. She teaches undergraduate and graduate courses in data science methods, data visualization, statistics, and computer programming. Dr. Gyory has mentored dozens of masters students in practicum projects that apply data science methods to real-world problems. She holds a PhD from the Massachusetts Institute of Technology, an MS from the University of New Hampshire, another MS from the State University of New York at Stony Brook, and a BA from Cornell University.

QUANTITATIVE METHODS FOR HEALTH MANAGEMENT

Robert McGrath, PhD

Esmaeil Bahalkeh, PhD, MS

Lee F. Seidel, PhD

Joanna Gyory, PhD, MS

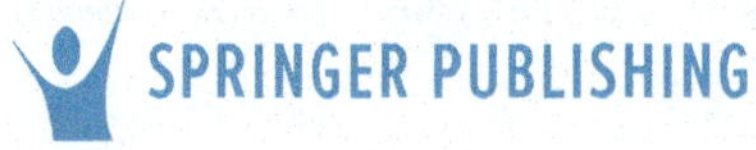

Springer Publishing Company, LLC
902 Carnegie Center/Suite 140, Princeton, NJ 08540
www.springerpub.com
connect.springerpub.com

Acquisitions Editor: David D'Addona
Content Development Manager: Lucia Gunzel
Production Editor: Susan White
Compositor: Transforma

ISBN: 978-0-8261-5352-4
eBook ISBN: 978-0-8261-5353-1
DOI: 10.1891/9780826153531

SUPPLEMENTS:

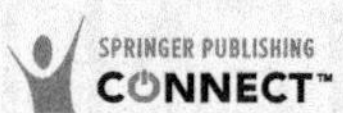

A robust set of instructor resources designed to supplement this text is located at **http://connect.springerpub.com/content/book/978-0-8261-5353-1**. Qualifying instructors may request access by emailing **textbook@springerpub.com**.

Instructor Materials:
LMS Common Cartridge With All Instructor Resources ISBN: 978-0-8261-5357-9
Instructor's Manual ISBN: 978-0-8261-5354-8
Instructor Test Bank ISBN: 978-0-8261-4546-8
Instructor Chapter PowerPoints ISBN: 978-0-8261-5355-5
Instructor Sample Syllabus ISBN: 978-0-8261-9005-5

Student Materials:
Data Sets ISBN: 978-0-8261-5159-9
Tutorial Videos with Transcripts ISBN: 978-0-8261-5987-8

25 26 27 28 / 5 4 3 2 1

Library of Congress Cataloging-in-Publication Data
Names: McGrath, Robert, 1967- author | Bahalkeh, Esmaeil author |
 Seidel, Lee F. author | Gyory, Joanna, author
Title: Quantitative methods for health management / Robert McGrath, Esmaeil
 Bahalkeh, Lee F. Seidel, Joanna Gyory.
Description: New York : Springer Publishing, [2026] | Includes
 bibliographical references and index. | Summary: "Quantitative Methods
 for Health Management is a practical, application-oriented textbook
 designed to equip healthcare students and professionals with the
 analytical skills needed for data-driven decision-making in a complex
 healthcare environment. Drawing on extensive experience in
 AUPHA-certified programs and related fields, the book emphasizes the
 use of quantitative methods–such as statistical modeling, forecasting,
 and financial analysis–to solve real-world challenges in areas like
 patient flow, cost control, and strategic planning. Structured in six
 progressive sections, it covers foundational data principles through to
 advanced topics like predictive analytics and project management, all
 aligned with current AUPHA domains. Enhanced with real-life case
 studies and 28 tutorial videos, the text prepares readers to become
 data-literate leaders capable of navigating modern healthcare systems
 shaped by rapid technological and policy changes"—Provided by
 publisher.
Identifiers: LCCN 2025025859 | ISBN 9780826153524 paperback | ISBN
 9780826153531 ebook
Subjects: LCSH: Health services administration—Data processing | Health
 services administration—Statistical methods | Quantitative research
Classification: LCC RA971.6 .M37 2026
LC record available at https://lccn.loc.gov/2025025859

Contact sales@springerpub.com to receive discount rates on bulk purchases.

Printed in the United States of America.

CONTENTS

PREFACE

In the ever-evolving landscape of healthcare management, the ability to make informed, data-driven decisions is more critical than ever. From hospital administrators to health system analysts, professionals must navigate an increasingly complex environment that demands both efficiency and effectiveness in service delivery. This text, *Quantitative Methods for Health Management*, serves as a foundational resource for students and professionals seeking to develop the analytic skills necessary to excel in today's data-driven healthcare sector or in their programs of study.

Grounded in decades of teaching experience within Association of University Programs in Health Administration (AUPHA)-certified programs, as well as the fields of data science, engineering, and public health, the authors bring a wealth of practical expertise to the study of quantitative methods and analytic decision-making. Their collective experience has shaped this book into a practical, application-oriented guide.

At its core, this text emphasizes quantitative methods as a critical decision-making tool, empowering healthcare managers to apply systems thinking, statistical modeling, forecasting techniques, and data-driven analysis to solve complex organizational challenges. The book is structured to provide a progressive learning experience, beginning with fundamental data management principles before advancing to more sophisticated predictive modeling and financial analysis techniques. Throughout, real-world examples and case studies illustrate the application of these methods to issues such as patient flow, cost management, quality improvement, and strategic planning. In addition, 27 tutorial videos have been created for this edition as a key tool for skill building.

A distinctive feature of this book is its alignment with the current AUPHA body of knowledge domains model, ensuring that students are developing the key skills required for success in certified health administration programs and accredited healthcare management or public health programs. These domains—ranging from analytical thinking and financial management to leadership and systems evaluation—are central to preparing future healthcare managers for the challenges ahead.

The book is structured into six sections, each progressively expanding on core quantitative concepts. Section I lays the groundwork by introducing data sources, statistical foundations, and techniques for data visualization and interpretation. Section II focuses on internal efficiency, guiding readers through process analysis, decision modeling, and capacity evaluation. Section III shifts toward balancing demand and supply, covering simulation techniques, queueing theory, and supply chain management.

Advancing into predictive analytics, Section IV delves into forecasting techniques, including time series analysis, regression modeling, and seasonality adjustments, equipping health managers with essential forecasting tools. Section V introduces financial analysis, explaining key economic concepts such as the time value of money, cost-benefit analysis, and investment evaluation. Section VI rounds out the discussion by applying quantitative methods to project management and strategic decision-making in healthcare settings.

This text is designed not only to provide students with a robust analytic tool kit but also to instill critical thinking skills that will enable them to adapt to the rapid technological advancements and policy shifts that define modern healthcare in the era of artificial intelligence and automated processes. As the field continues to evolve, the need for competent, data-literate managers will only grow. We hope that this book serves as a valuable resource in that journey, equipping students with the quantitative expertise necessary to lead in the healthcare sector.

Robert McGrath
Esmaeil Bahalkeh
Lee F. Seidel
Joanna Gyory

STUDENT RESOURCES

- **Data Sets**
- **Tutorial Videos With Transcripts**
- **Quizzes**
- **Discussion Questions**
- **Flashcards**

INSTRUCTOR RESOURCES

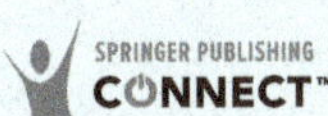

A robust set of instructor resources designed to supplement this text is located at **http://connect.springerpub.com/content/book/978-0-8261-5353-1**. Qualifying instructors may request access by emailing **textbook@springerpub.com**.

Available resources include:
- LMS Common Cartridge With All Instructor Resources
- Instructor's Manual
- Instructor Test Bank
- Instructor Chapter PowerPoints
- Instructor Sample Syllabus

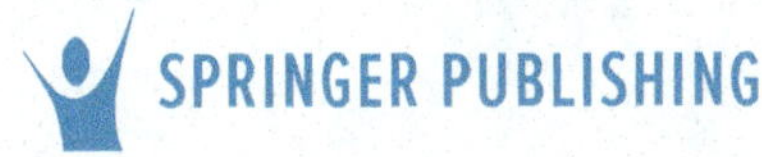

Visit https://connect.springerpub.com/ and look for the **"Show Supplementary"** button on the book homepage.

DATA, ANALYSIS, AND TRANSLATION TO ACTION

CHAPTER 1

USING QUANTITATIVE AND ANALYTIC METHODS FOR MANAGING HEALTHCARE SERVICES

LEARNING OBJECTIVES

1.1. Describe how quantitative methods inform the management of health services organizations and systems.

1.2. Use quantitative methods to gain a broader model of decision-making.

1.3. Differentiate between efficiency and effectiveness as they relate to supply and demand.

1.4. Recognize how quantitative methods stem from and are reliant upon systems of data collection, storage, upkeep, and dissemination.

LEARNING OBJECTIVE 1.1: DESCRIBE HOW QUANTITATIVE METHODS INFORM THE MANAGEMENT OF HEALTH SERVICES ORGANIZATIONS AND SYSTEMS

Health services administration, as a profession, deals with the management of human, fiscal, and physical data and information resources to meet the goals and objectives of healthcare organizations and systems. Survival of healthcare entities in a competitive environment involves multiple factors, including the ability of managers to effectively monitor complex systems, sometimes in real time, and to make a myriad of decisions. One of the challenges is that many of those decisions exist in ever greater environments of uncertainty. It is therefore imperative that the healthcare manager be equipped with a robust set of tools for making decisions in responsive but also reasoned and informed ways.

Being a competent manager in a healthcare environment can mean quite different things depending upon one's role expectations, perspective, and the decision circumstance. Healthcare managers are often assigned different functions, each within different departments and divisions and often with different expectations for scope and competency. Managers in the human resources department of a hospital face different management challenges than the managers in the hospital's marketing department, or still a director of home care services for a care-at-home organization. In addition, diverse types of healthcare organizations often require different sets of managerial skill sets.

Healthcare organizations also may shift their definition of desired or needed management competencies because of a shift in their objectives, the characteristics of the environment, or both.

The changes that have affected the health system because of the COVID-19 pandemic are a good case in point. The entire health system was forced, in a short amount of time, to rework the core nature of their missions and then integrate those core missions within their service lines for the optimal outcomes of patient health and survival. What followed was a realignment of where, how, and how many services were offered. While acute, the implications of the COVID-19 disruption are still being felt today.

Underpinning all the variability and change in the current health services landscape is the exponential growth of technology. Modern technologies continue to challenge the very nature of how health services are defined and where and how they are provided. In one setting, a manager may be charged with analyzing the daily patient and payor mix from a financial and predictive perspective, while in another, a manager may be charged with assessing how to develop "hospital-at-home" capabilities in a cost-effective way.

Decisions are made in organizations every day, typically on subsets of data. Sometimes, these data are for the analytical purpose at hand—did the patient show up for an appointment?—but often they are not. For example, can we examine the likelihood of future high-cost patients based on current panels of patients who may develop other conditions?

These types of decisions are often made under varying degrees of uncertainty, and they beg thoughtful questions such as:

- What data are we using and how was it generated and populated into our database or file?
- How representative of the current (or future) environment is the decision?
- Can it answer the question we are asking, or how closely can it?
- Can we retrieve it and has it already been manipulated?
- How quickly can we pull it together into an analytic file?
- What types of models are possible and at what level of confidence?
- How will we use these analyses?

It is, therefore, imperative that the next generation of analytically enabled healthcare managers understand not only the methods for analysis but also the limitations and parameters of those methods and the decisions they affect.

LEARNING OBJECTIVE 1.2: USE QUANTITATIVE METHODS TO GAIN A BROADER MODEL OF DECISION-MAKING

Quantitative Methods and the Systems Model

Management, as a profession and field, has long used various methods to assist decision-makers with the analysis, design, and implementation of system and process change as organizations strive to enhance their efficiency and effectiveness. Some methods, still in use today, trace their birth to the era of scientific management and the needs of large-scale production lines designed to efficiently produce physical products such as automobiles. In this prior era, the complex organization was conceptualized as a machine with the pieces of the organization thought of as cogs in the greater machine. Workers were considered cogs. Equipment was considered cogs. Managers were trained and utilized to design systems and use the organization's resources in the most efficient way possible.

The thinking in this era emphasized that more efficient machines were more desirable than less efficient machines, that workers were merely extensions of the machine, and that science or engineering could be used to analyze operations and design or redesign work processes. Some of the quantitative methods used today by health administrators trace their conceptual roots to this era.

Techniques drawn from industrial engineering, operations research, and operations management emphasize the production characteristics of the organization. Although the era of managers looking to classical bureaucratic theory and the principles of simple scientific management is over, many new analytic and technology-driven quantitative techniques are available for health administrators to use to analyze, design, and then implement.

FIGURE 1.1 The general systems model.

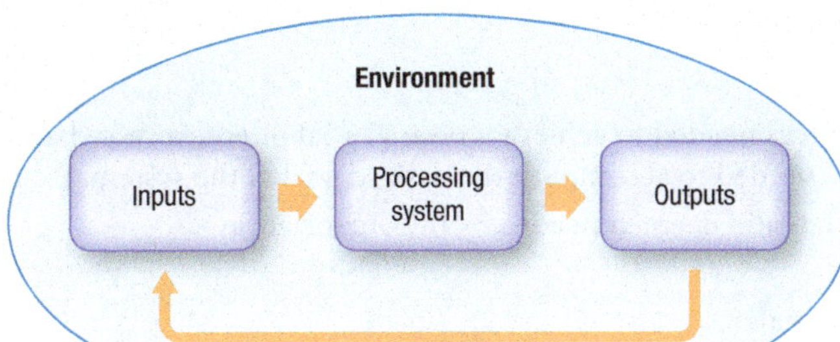

This book uses the modified common systems approach. The general systems model presented in **Figure 1.1** is the framework used to integrate many of the perspectives presented here and is based upon the recognition that managers need tools to assist in the analysis, design, and implementation of decisions within systems of resources and then monitor and modify those decisions while thinking about potential future factors and outcomes. This theory suggests that healthcare organizations are one example of goal-directed systems with identifiable inputs, work processes that convert inputs into outputs, identifiable outputs, and feedback loops that serve to direct and control the system.

In this model, resources are applied to a given process to produce a given outcome. Those outcomes are assessed against what was expected or optimal, and then the resources and/or process can be adjusted and the system modified to improve the outcome. This system's flow falls against the backdrop of the environment the implementing organization exists in and the effects of that outcome, as well as any expectation of future potential.

To understand the complexity of activity within any organization, the general systems model provides the ability to assign activities or features of the organization to one of four categories: inputs or resources, conversion processes (i.e., what is done with the inputs), outcomes (i.e., what is desired), and feedback.

Organizations are considered open systems that are influenced by events and circumstances external to the organization. As open systems, organizations draw resources from their dynamic environment and provide back to their environment some valued product or service. Despite this fundamental change in the way managers think about organizations and management, quantitative methods originally developed during the era of emerging efficiency are still used and considered central in the repertoire of methods that defines the unique abilities of the manager.

Elements of the General Systems Model

Using the systems model to improve the efficiency and effectiveness of the healthcare organization requires appreciation of the defining elements of the systems model.

Organizational Goals

Any system strives to attain its goals by accumulating sufficient resources and converting these resources into desired products or services. Goals express the intent of the system. Organizations, however, have multiple and sometimes conflicting goals. For example, maximizing organizational profit and providing services to anyone regardless of their ability to pay are potentially conflicting goals for any healthcare entity. Therefore, the use of the general systems model may be limited by the type and degree of goal ambiguity or conflict that exists in the healthcare organization.

The first and most important analytical challenge faced in our quest for improved efficiency and effectiveness is to identify system goals.

Inputs Are Resources

Inputs are the resources needed to achieve a desired goal often expressed as a desired output or outcome. Inputs are needed to accomplish the desired goal of the system. Examples include:

- People, each with a skill deemed needed by the organization
- Time
- Supplies and materials
- Capital assets, such as buildings and equipment
- Information and data

Based on this definition, it is reasonable to expect that different types of healthcare organizations, because of their different goals, have different input resources. For example, the input resources needed by a nursing home are different from the input resources needed by an acute care hospital or by a clinic. An organization's wealth may also determine its inputs.

Because most inputs can be purchased, the amount and type of input resources held by the organization may be a product of the financial position of the organization. As they are used, most input resources are counted. Financial accounting counts expenses and revenues by category. Other processes count the number and type of workers employed and the number of hours worked. Still other systems count the supplies used or the information storage used or needed.

Conversion Processes Add Value

Conversion processes convert inputs into outcomes. A surgical procedure is a conversion process. It takes a specific array of inputs (e.g., people such as a surgeon and nurses plus capital assets and equipment, not to mention patients and insurance) and converts them into a desired outcome, such as the removal of a diseased gallbladder. Data analysis is a conversion process. Data are converted from raw inputs to translated outputs that can be used to alter decision-making. Conversion adds value. Working with clinicians, health administrators strive for efficient and effective conversion processes.

Outcomes and Outputs

Outcomes or outputs are the results created by the system. It is hoped that these results are the desired, intended, or expected goals of the system (or subsystem). If results match expectations, the system is accomplishing its goals. If results do not match expectations, change may be required. Examples of outcomes include the improved health status of the population, the organization's financial position, the number and type of hospital patient days or discharges, the anticipated mix of patients by reimbursement or diagnosis type, the variability of patient flow in the emergency department, the number of readmissions, the general prevalence of disease in the population catchment area, or even the number of meals served. Outcomes or outputs are the units of service produced by the organization. Many outcomes or outputs are counted by the organizations. Outcomes involving the worth of an organization are counted using financial accounting. Others are captured in an organization's key performance indicators (KPIs), which are simply metrics that help manage those key functions that relate to some desired outcome. These can include the average daily census, capacity measures of a system, wait times, transfers out of the system, and others. These are often reported in static, time series, or sometimes real-time dashboards.

Subsystems and Suboptimization

For analysis, design, and implementation, large complex systems are usually conceptualized as having multiple layers or subsystems. For example, a human body as a system has one subsystem for circulation and another to control its nerve function. Subsystems serve systems. For example, dietary, imaging, medical information, and patient process subsystems in a hospital serve the acute care system, called a hospital, created by the interplay of numerous subsystems.

Within the hierarchical and interdependent arrangement created by subsystems within a system, suboptimization is expected. Suboptimization is the recognition that the ultimate goal of any subsystem is to meet the requirements of its larger system and that meeting these larger and more important system requirements may mean that any individual subsystem may need to operate at less than its highest level of efficiency. Suboptimization occurs when subsystems are either not correctly identified and modeled or are performing below their expected potential so that the overall organization as a system meets its goals and objectives. In some instances, managers design subsystems to perform below their potential. In other words, suboptimization can be a design parameter used in designing subsystems.

Feedback and Analysis

Feedback is typically information that the organization generates to adjust inputs and/or conversion processes to change the desired outcome or make the actual outcome. Feedback can take many forms and be utilized in varying time increments from yearly (year-end reports) to real time (patient flow, lab, and radiology reporting).

Healthcare organizations produce multiple forms of feedback. Patient outcomes are feedback. Patient opinions about their service encounters are feedback. Market share is feedback. The balance sheet and statement of income and expense are feedback, just as conversation between employees is a form of feedback. Feedback is system or subsystem output information used to monitor, evaluate, adjust, or change the system or subsystem so that the organization can better achieve its stated goals and objectives.

Internal and External System Modifiers Can Influence a System

System modifiers influence inputs and conversion processes. Examples of modifiers include need, demand, want, social values, and physical climate. A system modifier is something that influences a conversion process but is outside the direct control of the system. For example, how a hospital converts resources into patient days is influenced by the "need" for medical care. As "need" changes, such as with the advent of HIV infections, conversion processes are changed (e.g., blood is transfused using different procedures/universal precautions). Laws, regulations, and scientific advances modify and influence conversion processes.

System modifiers can be as bold as a fundamental change in reimbursement policies or as subtle as a specific health profession striving for the autonomy, status, and income historically reserved for the physician. A system modifier also can be the cultural attributes of the specific organization when these attributes either cannot or will not be changed. These modifiers can often be monitored using statistical control methods examining variation over time, both anticipated and unanticipated for signals of change, or simulated when an expected change may be forthcoming, such as a proposed change in regulation that would impact aspects of the organization.

Future Considerations and the Role of Uncertainty

The world continues to evolve at an exponential pace. The daily flow and amount of information at our fingertips continues to grow as does the ability of technology and artificial intelligence (AI) to augment, automate, and supplement human experience and our roles. Intel's Gordon Moore, in 1965, developed Moore's Law, which states that technology tends to double in capacity every 24 months, an estimate he later said is waning due to the cresting of traditional computer chip speeds and cost, but one that could also be reconsidered as quantum technologies grows (Takahashi, 2015). Both organizations and societies in the form of governments and policy attempt to place guideposts and guardrails on that growth to better ensure the flourishing of people, societies, and their organizations. These are, however, guesses about the future. Organizations are also always vulnerable to the unknown. For example, it was well posited through the late 1900s and early 2000s that a pandemic was likely; however, it was inefficient to fully plan for one given the uncertainty of the event. Yet, in 2020, the pandemic did occur and then fundamentally changed how organizations and society operated.

Uncertainty is a strategic variable that affects the scope and precision of future estimation. This becomes a statistical exercise in what is often called confidence, margin of error, or what economists call a level of sensitivity. It is also the foundations of simulation. Creating what-if scenarios and being given some level of statistical likelihood of some set of outcomes is quickly making its way into the strategic lexicon of health services operations and management.

As such, systems flow and current decision-making will necessarily have to have some adjustment for future state-of-the-world factors. These final two components—internal and external modifiers and future considerations and uncertainty—bear in multiple directions in a more dynamic systems model, and all should be considered when making important organizational decisions.

The general systems model provides the framework for our examination of specific quantitative methods. This model focuses our attention on inputs; conversion process; outputs; feedback loops; and modifiers, both internal and future. It is sufficiently robust to capture the essence of all types of healthcare organizations and tells managers to analyze and design healthcare organizations as systems and subsystems. Efficiency and effectiveness are the two primary performance measures used in healthcare organizations. To be an effective healthcare manager requires the ability to view the healthcare organization as a system and to make the organization perform better on both performance measures. Quantitative methods exist to assist managers to analyze and design systems and facilitate implementation of change within the organization, not as ends but as means to enhance organizational effectiveness and efficiency.

A quantitative method is a specific tool, technique, or model that can be used by managers to help address specific situations or problems. Frequently, quantitative methods involve collecting information (or using information collected by others) and manipulating the information using mathematics and statistics. Examples include economic analysis, queuing theory, Program Evaluation Review Technique (PERT), and general systems flowcharting. Many quantitative methods involve using specific mathematical models to analyze systems. Some methods have specific applications and specific rules governing their application. Methods included in this work have been drawn from many fields, including industrial engineering, operations research, and general management. Selected methods can help managers analyze systems, design or redesign systems, and implement desired changes in systems.

Another way to explain quantitative methods for health services managers involves application. To be considered a quantitative method in this context, the tool, technique, or model must have broad application in the healthcare organization and serve the needs of managers. The method must be in the repertoire of any health administrator working in the hospital, nursing home, or ambulatory clinic. Not all quantitative methods have applications in health services management. Not all statistics are quantitative methods used by health services managers. Also, some quantitative methods are not purely mathematical. For example, in statistics, students might learn the rudiments of testing a hypothesis using a t and f test. These tests are statistical methods used under specific conditions to test a hypothesis based upon a sample. In contrast, often in the same statistics course, students learn basic linear regression. As taught in statistics, the t or f test is not a quantitative method for health services management; it is a statistical method. Its use in health services management situations is limited. In contrast, linear regression is a professionally recognized technique used often by health services managers in forecasting. General systems flowcharting is a specific method used to analyze systems. It is not mathematical or statistical; however, it meets the criterion of being used in certain situations by health services managers.

For these reasons, it is important for the manager to fully understand the nature of the operational question being asked and bridge that to the analysis needed. For example, let us consider the use of expanded telehealth services. The organization must not only consider the proliferation of enabled devices among the patient population but also the reimbursement for services. If it is anticipated that future reimbursement would be affected by the payers at some future date, that could alter the implementation of the current telehealth program.

Inherent at each of these stages is the need for analysis. The ability to analyze data, processes, and outcomes as a core managerial competency relates to the core functions of data use and decision-making. Those functions are as follows:

- *Description:* Understanding what a current process, system, or landscape currently looks like. This can mean individual aspects of a system or comparisons within or between other variables or systems.
- *Prediction:* This is the ability to estimate future occurrences or impacts given levels of certainty or probability. Typically, this involves some form of modeling estimation.
- *Prescription and simulation:* This is the ability to develop what-if scenarios and attempt to derive optimal system function now and into the future.

Some of these methods are purely quantitative, and others can require some level of qualitative assessment.

For example, process or flow design (patients or information) as a managerial competency often involves engineering because it encompasses the ability to break down desired capabilities, such as an organization's goals and objectives, into requisite components or parts and then model those parts into an operational system with its own inputs, throughputs, and outputs. If the organization desires a new service or function, it is an analyst's or manager's responsibility to design the service by first determining the different mix of human, fiscal, physical, and information resources needed to provide the service and then specifying exactly how much of each will be needed to provide the service as well as the adaptability of the function or service to changes in the environment, such as days of the week, hours of the day, or unexpected demand increases or decreases. Design of new work processes, or the redesign of existing ones, involves developing detailed plans so that when the plans are executed, the desired capability has been incorporated into the organization. Design also involves developing these detailed plans as to what is needed and how the needed resources should be used or optimized by end users.

Implementation as a core management competency is the ability to change organizational processes. The process of implementation may require the manager to change the behavior of employees, clients, or patients. It also may involve the manager's ability to accumulate and operationalize the resources necessary to achieve desired goals. Whereas design may be the management competency that determines what is needed, implementation is the management competency that installs new or revised elements in the organization. Thus, the manager's repertoire needs to include both quantitative and qualitative methods to assist implementing change within the organization.

In the chapters that follow, we break down these analytic tools by function and provide examples of how each might be used and deployed for a given set of questions.

LEARNING OBJECTIVE 1.3: DIFFERENTIATE BETWEEN EFFICIENCY AND EFFECTIVENESS AS THEY RELATE TO SUPPLY AND DEMAND

A healthcare organization is any organization that provides health and/or medical services to patients; residents; and clients, such as an acute care or specialty hospital, a nursing home, or an ambulatory care organization, such as a university health services, public health clinic, a home care agency, and many others. The defining characteristic in this definition of a healthcare organization is patient care, or care provided by physicians, nurses, ancillary providers, technicians, and therapists to prevent and treat disease or infirmity. The mission of these organizations serves to distinguish them as healthcare organizations.

Services provided to patients could include a surgical procedure, diagnostic examination, specialized treatment, or disease prevention or screening programs. These services also could be an appropriate meal, a safe and comfortable environment, or an accurate and timely bill for service. All healthcare organizations provide a range of services and specialize in providing individual patients with an array of services based upon a patient's needs. The central and defining element of all healthcare organizations is the provision of personal and personalized experience and high-quality health or medical service. As such, a central expectation shared by all health administrators is the expectation that management practice will lead to the efficient provision of effective services to people in need of service. This means meeting the demand for services with an adequate supply of services at a given price and within the mission of the organization or entity.

Effectiveness Versus Efficiency

Effectiveness as a Clinical Interest

The interests of managers, the interests of clinicians, and the interests of the healthcare organizations that employ both are often difficult to distinguish and can "sometimes" seem at odds. Clinical interests stress the needs of individual patients and the identification of appropriate service interventions (e.g., gathering as much information and performing whatever diagnostic tests or treatments that may be able to aid or assist the patient). Decisions made by clinicians are based upon what they consider to be effective approaches—interventions that have some probability of clinical or medical success. The physician, nurse, therapist, or other provider has been educated and trained to select and apply current knowledge to assist patients, more recently with the assistance of best practices or AI-driven tools. Clinical interests and perspectives are focused on the effectiveness of a service—the ability of a service to accomplish its predetermined objective—but not necessarily on doing so at the lowest resource cost. Effectiveness often considers the demand side of the equation but not always the supply or resource element. This is a bit of an oversimplification, but it is useful for understanding the different perspectives.

Healthcare organizations and health administrators rely upon physicians, nurses, therapists, and other providers to determine or diagnose the needs of a patient or group of individuals accurately and to plan and execute interventions or treatment that have some probability of success in maintaining or improving overall health status. Although clinicians are not necessarily oblivious or insensitive to efficiency, their unique role and function stem from their commitment to providing effective service to patients. They alone have the expertise to determine a patient's needs (i.e., diagnosis) and to meet them (i.e., treatment) and are judged by their peers, specific systems, and patients based upon their ability to provide an effective, but not necessarily an efficient, service.

Efficiency as a Management Interest

Efficiency is a ratio measure of output divided by input. High efficiency is achieved when a service is rendered at an optimal outcome using the fewest resources. Inefficient clinical practice, such as requiring more clinical tests than necessary to make an accurate diagnosis or prescribing contraindicated drugs due to imperfect personal health information, can lead to highly inefficient outcomes. Using more or fewer staff than dictated by patient flow is another example of operational inefficiency. If a postanesthesia care unit staffs with too few nurses, then care and patient safety could be seriously undermined. However, too many nurses could make care unclear or handoffs confusing or there would be idle staff waiting for but not caring for patients, which are all suboptimal outcomes.

Unlike operational effectiveness, which is in the clinician's province, operational efficiency lies within the dual province of clinicians and managers.

Inefficient work processes waste scarce resources. Efficient work processes provide services that maximize the opportunities created by the mix of resources used to produce the service. Managers and analysts are employed by organizations to ensure that desired levels of efficiency are attained, not by accident but by design. Being interested in efficiency differentiates the health services manager from the health service clinician. Striving for maximum appropriate efficiency is a management value that requires a specific repertoire of skills—the ability to analyze current levels of efficiency, the ability to design and redesign services to achieve desired levels of efficiency, the ability to implement new or revised services, and the ability to predict demand and the flow of patients.

Effectiveness as a Management Interest

Effectiveness means the ability to accomplish a defined task, objective, or goal. For example, if a specific drug can cure a specific infection, it can be considered effective. If a specific medical procedure or therapy can cure or alleviate a specific disease or infirmity, then the procedure is effective. To be effective, the procedure or drug must accomplish its intended purpose. Multiple factors may influence the effectiveness of planned intervention or treatment. For example, some patients may respond differently to the same drug. Sometimes, the effectiveness of a procedure or treatment is influenced by the behavior of the patient, something not controlled by the clinician.

Effectiveness is not always guaranteed 100% of the time. Most treatments are those treatments that have some probability of success <100% but hopefully >0%. These probabilities may be 5%, 50%, or 95%, depending upon any number of factors from the state of clinical and scientific knowledge, the existing health status of the patient, or other variables in the broader environment.

Healthcare organizations rely upon clinically trained professionals—and more recently, assistive predictive modeling—to select the appropriate clinical services or treatments for specific patients from the array of services offered by the organization. If the services are not available in the healthcare organization, another organization can provide the services via a referral. In the healthcare organization, managers are not empowered to override or veto clinical judgments involving a patient's diagnosis or treatment if the manager is not themselves a medical professional. Many organizations now utilize medical providers as administrative leaders, and so the distinction of where the onus for decision-making lays can be convoluted.

It is at the strategic level of organizational decision-making that managerial interests involving organizational effectiveness emerge. For example, the costs and benefits of investing in modern technology must be identified and examined from both a clinical and organizational perspective before the decision is made by the organization to acquire and implement it. Even though modern technology may enhance the effectiveness of the clinicians affiliated with the organization and thereby increase the organization's effectiveness, its acquisition and/or operational cost to the organization may prevent the organization from acquiring it.

One such example is pursuing extended telehealth or even "hospital-at-home" services. Costs such as technology deployment, the availability of traveling providers, or even the uncertainty of the reimbursement and regulatory environment can offset against the demand for more convenient, patient-centered care.

Efficiency and Managerial Competence

Just as clinical operational effectiveness is the responsibility of the clinical professional, operational and organizational efficiency is the primary responsibility of the health administrator. As stated, efficiency means providing a needed service using no more resources than necessary; it is a ratio measure of output and input. Health administrators are employed, in part, to ensure that any service provided by the healthcare organization is supplied in an efficient manner. Determining current efficiency levels is an example of analytic proficiency as a managerial competency. Being able to design or redesign how the organization does something to enhance efficiency is an example of design as a managerial competency. Being able to change how the organization provides a service to enhance operational efficiency is an example of implementation as a managerial competency.

Striving to make the healthcare organization efficient is a dominating, unique, and defining value associated with management and managers and the field of health administration, whereas the credit for effective clinical practice must be given to the clinical sciences and professions and the technologies they use.

LEARNING OBJECTIVE 1.4: RECOGNIZE HOW QUANTITATIVE METHODS STEM FROM AND ARE RELIANT UPON SYSTEMS OF DATA COLLECTION, STORAGE, UPKEEP, AND DISSEMINATION

The landscape of data and our ability to analyze it has exponentially grown in recent years and will continue to do so. Advances in computing power and the lessening cost of data storage combined with automated and code-based analytical tools mean that even moderately sized organizations have new tools at their disposal for a wide variety of purposes. Earlier, we mentioned the three primary uses of data: description, prediction, and prescription (or simulation). However, what constitutes that data has similarly changed in recent years.

In **Figure 1.2**, we can easily overlay the three functions of data into each of the boxes: description and prediction in the first and partially in the second while prescription aligns in the third. And it is here that many organizations have struggled to attempt to right size their efforts or to balance what skills to employ in house and which to contract for. The answers are not easy and are dependent upon several factors, such as the size of the organization, the types of questions they must answer, and their internal data capabilities. All this also rests upon the backdrop of ever-changing technologies and end-user automation tools, as well as privacy and security issues—both internal and stemming from governmental policy requirements.

Most analytic questions still reside in the first box and specifically within the scope of description. Performance dashboards using KPIs and metrics and a host of other systematic reports reside here and are crucial to the ongoing monitoring of the organization and its processes. Some dashboards can have prediction or simulation functions, but their core is for descriptive purposes. It is also important for the analyst/manager to understand the relationship between their organization's information systems and technology functions and their analytic functions.

This relationship differs widely by organization, yet the two functions remain integrally linked. **Figure 1.3** shows the general data use cycle for an organization. Data procurement refers to how

FIGURE 1.2 Evolution of data.

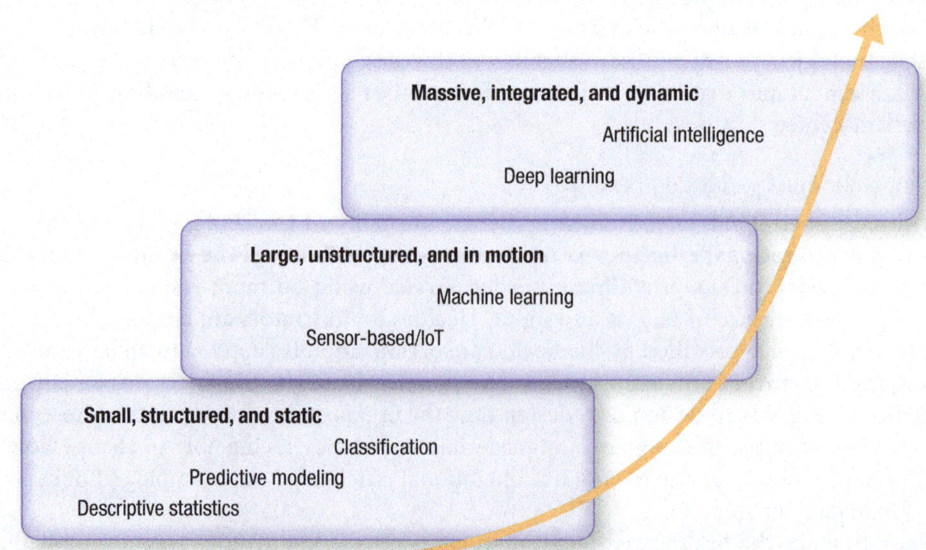

Source: Adapted from Priestley, J., & McGrath, R. (2021). *Closing the analytics talent gap: An executive's guide to working with universities*. CRC Press.

FIGURE 1.3 General data use cycle.

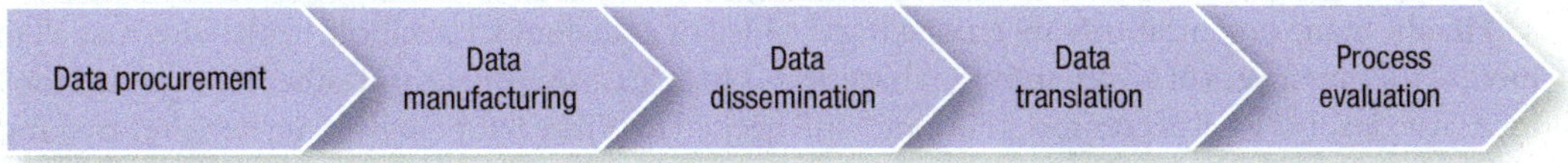

data are populated, how often, and with what parameters and metadata—or the meaning of each data element. Data manufacturing refers to data that have been manipulated in some way, such as calculated fields and metrics, for example, the average length of stay. Data dissemination and translation refer to reports, dashboards, and, most importantly, who has access to the data. Process evaluation represents the feedback loop within the general systems model. The analyst and manager might have interaction with any number of these steps depending on the organization, but as one moves from left to right, the role of the decision-maker is augmented.

There are a whole host of data storage capabilities, from enterprise warehouse systems and mainframes to data lakes, analytic use environments, and cloud-based storage solutions that may or may not allow access depending on hosting rules that organizations use in their data ecosystems. Similarly, analytic tools may vary depending on the analyst and organization. Many organizations employ data engineers and data scientists whose job is to populate and ensure robust data environments and perform complex analyses. The end analyst or manager would use these individuals to assess end-user capabilities. For example, for a complex simulation, an elevated level of base coding may be needed to build some models. Those models can then be deployed into a data or information production environment. These are further explored in Chapter 2, "Data, Data Sources, Data Quality, and Foundations."

These foundational systems continue to evolve as do the roles related to each of them. Depending on the organization, one might find themselves occupying roles such as:

- Departmental or general data-enabled manager
- General analyst/specialized analyst
- Chief data officer
- Chief analytic officer
- Chief technology officer
- Data governance specialist
- Data engineer
- Data scientist
- Security and privacy officer
- Electronic medicare record (EMR) analyst/superuser

This is only a brief list as the number of titles and functions of those roles change regularly. Additionally, organizations can have either centralized, decentralized, or a hybrid mix of data and analytic functions. In a centralized model, data and core analysis rest in one department or organization and the data products needed for management are pushed out to the end users and units. In a decentralized model, the analysts are function specific (for example, financial analysts or systems analysts) and have more direct ability to manipulate and access the organization's data relative to that function. Each has pros and cons but can affect the type of questions to be answered and the flexibility the manager/analyst has.

Increasingly, many organizations have begun migrating to hybrid structures, where core data are held in secure environments and access is granted based on role and need. Often, subsets of tables might be created for end users that meet most of the ongoing reporting needs of the organization. This is more present in healthcare than in many other industries as regulation dictates the level of necessary security, privacy, and data transfer allowed. Added to this is the constant need to guard against hacking and data hostage holding that can cripple organizations if not prepared. These types of concerns are often easier to manage with a centralized core layer of security.

Finally, many organizations are embracing the idea of data democratization, or the idea that all or most of the employees of an organization have access to at least some data and either have guided tools for its use or some level of comfortability and skill needed to utilize it for data-driven decision-making.

This text provides some of those basic tools to support those either beginning this journey or augmenting their current skill sets.

AN OVERVIEW OF THIS TEXT

Health administrators have unique repertoires and skills as managers employed by a healthcare organization need to know (as part of their defining repertoire), such as how to design efficient systems of health and medical care and how to improve the efficiency of existing systems of care. In other words, efficiency is important to health service managers. Tools, techniques, and models used to improve the efficiency of health and medical care systems are essential elements in the repertoire of health services managers. Most methods are related to "efficiency." However, this should not be misinterpreted to mean that health services management is only interested in or trained to improve "efficiency." Efficiency and effectiveness are central values for the professional manager of health services.

Management, like many other fields, can be thought of as reasoned judgment. In applying reasoned judgment, managers need formal methods to assist them to define and resolve problems. Just as master chefs need and create recipes to govern their culinary creations, health services managers need formal methods to analyze and improve complex systems. Using quantitative methods, however, does not absolve the manager from the broader responsibility of being a manager; quantitative methods and tools merely aid the manager in making reasoned judgments.

This book expands a health services manager's abilities to analyze, design, and implement. It provides methods to analyze systems and complex work processes. It also provides methods to design and implement new or revised work processes or subsystems in healthcare organizations.

This book is ordered into functional sections that mimic both the foundational skills needed to perform managerial analyses and the flow by type of analysis, from internal (descriptive and comparative) to external and strategic (predictive and prescriptive).

Section I, "Data, Analysis, and Translation to Action," provides basic skills needed to understand data and the mathematical and statistical foundations for using data. These are utilized in later chapters. For some, it will be a well-known material. For others, it provides a needed review. The foundation competencies include Chapter 2, "Data, Data Sources, Data Quality, and Foundations"; Chapter 3, "Statistical and Analytical Foundations"; and Chapter 4, "Data Display."

Section II, "Internal Efficiency," examines the analysis of existing organizational processes. Chapter 5 looks at process flow and quality improvements. Chapter 6 delves into quantitative decision analysis modeling and Chapter 7 examines capacity analysis.

Section III, "Matching Demand and Supply," begins to examine flow-based measurement and some prediction. Chapters 8 and 9 examine simulation and simulated modeling. Chapter 10 examines queueing and other scheduling, and Chapter 11 addresses the topics of inventory and supply chain management.

Section IV, "Forecasting and Prediction," addresses many approaches that can be used to forecast. Chapter 12, "Foundations of Forecasting," points out that although many aspects of forecasting are quantitative in nature, subjective and qualitative factors are also critical to the process. Chapter 13, "Time Series Forecasting Techniques," covers specific mathematical models to detect and extend trends for purposes of forecasting that are time dependent. Chapter 14, "Linear Regression Forecasting," covers the application of this statistical model to forecasting and Chapter 15, "Seasonality and Other Model Considerations," examines the structural and unanticipated issues that affect many of the other forecasting methods and provides methods to detect and correct for them. Overall, this section establishes the health services manager's ability to understand and use basic analytical forecasting to construct logical and reasoned forecasts. Forecasting is presented as a core competency associated with the health services manager's role. Basic algebraic and statistical competencies are needed to complete this section of the book.

Section V, "Financial Analysis," provides a foundational overview into financing as it relates to organizational or process efficiency. Chapter 16 covers the time value of money and the nature of compounding and discounting, as well as weighing the real and future costs of investments in programs and processes. It further includes specific methods related to the cost of capital and project risk. Chapter 17 uses economic analysis as its foundation to look at concepts of rate of return, adjusted return rates, and net present value of investment opportunities.

Section VI, "Projects and Strategy," includes Chapter 18, "Project Management," which covers several applied quantitative methods related to projects. A project is defined as a one-time activity or significant modification to an existing service. Here, we examine tools such as flowcharting, PERT, and other techniques to define new projects and to establish an appropriate time schedule and project implementation control system. The final chapter reflects on the integration of quantitative methods with strategic considerations and reflects on the text as a useful set of tools for the health manager or analyst. The chapter presents a framework for organizing and evaluating the external environment of a healthcare organization and the various strategic lenses needed to do so depending on the organization's goals and mission.

This book expands the health services manager's analytic repertoire to analyze complex systems and to be able to design and implement changes in those systems. Applications are drawn from hospitals, nursing homes, ambulatory care clinics, public health, and other health-related organizations and functions.

This text provides a necessary foundation with the understanding that more advanced analytical management applications are reserved for more advanced presentations. Application is of paramount importance. Throughout the book, repeated reference is made to the importance associated with the ability to effectively communicate results. No matter how perfect or insightful the analysis or design, if it cannot or is not effectively communicated to decision-makers in the healthcare organization, the health services manager has failed. Quantitative methods are a robust tool in the repertoire of the health services manager and must be used skillfully.

END-OF-CHAPTER RESOURCES

DISCUSSION QUESTIONS

1. How might a systems perspective be useful when starting a new line of service in a hospital or clinic?

2. List some services commonly found in health settings that are best evaluated for their effectiveness but not necessarily efficiency.

3. List some services commonly found in health settings that are best evaluated by efficiency standards.

4. How might data be better leveraged to understand the top drivers of utilization in a practice, clinic, or hospital unit? What are the barriers to collecting all data required for a more complete assessment?

LEARNING ACTIVITIES

CourseConnect ➤

To access self-assessment questions and interactive, competency-based learning activities for this chapter, visit www.springerpub.com/courseconnect. See inside front cover and tear-out card for CourseConnect details.

REFERENCE

Takahashi, D. (2015, May 11). Intel's Gordon Moore speculates on the future of tech and the end of Moore's Law. *Venture Beat*. https://venturebeat.com/mobile/intels-gordon-moore-speculates-on-the-future-and-the-end-of-moores-law

CHAPTER 2

DATA, DATA SOURCES, DATA QUALITY, AND FOUNDATIONS

LEARNING OBJECTIVES

2.1. Examine the drivers for health data and explore common components of health data systems.

2.2. Classify types of data elements and their measurement features.

2.3. Examine common models of data quality, their uses, and potential data gaps and their implications.

LEARNING OBJECTIVE 2.1: EXAMINE THE DRIVERS FOR HEALTH DATA AND EXPLORE COMMON COMPONENTS OF HEALTH DATA SYSTEMS

The evolution of health data systems, driven by technology, regulations, and the digital age, has accelerated an explosion in the size, or the raw amount of data. Many organizations take data for granted, but it is important to understand the evolution of data and data systems as the pace of change is not uniform across the industry and also not slowing. **Figure 2.1** shows this. Early adopters of the digital age leverage the latest technological developments, while industry laggards still utilize paper and fax machines. Healthcare organizations operating for over 10 years will have to manage the operation and transition from older legacy systems built on operating systems that require manual maintenance all while moving toward new systems with ever-increasing automation.

Every aspect of healthcare, whether it is public health or personalized medicine, requires the study of a significant amount of data about many people over many years. The vast majority of healthcare data is comprised of services rendered by providers like hospitals, doctors, clinics, and pharmacies; a host of ancillary providers; and the administrative processes necessary to pay for these services. The evolution of health systems and data, conceptualized in **Figure 2.1,** has been aided by a number of historical advancements or policy prompts. A few notable ones were as follows:

- **1970s:** The digitization of health records and computer images
- **1980s:** The rise of personal computers and local area networks drives healthcare software innovation.
- **1990s:** The internet and Health Insurance Portability and Accountability Act (HIPAA) trigger a material push for electronic health records (EHR; U.S. Department of Health and Human Services, n.d.).
- **2000s:** The Office of the National Coordinator for Health Information Technology (ONC) is established, and Health Information Technology for Economic and Clinical Health (HITECH) Act is passed (Assistant Secretary for Technology Policy [ASTP], n.d.-b).

FIGURE 2.1 Evolution of healthcare systems and data.

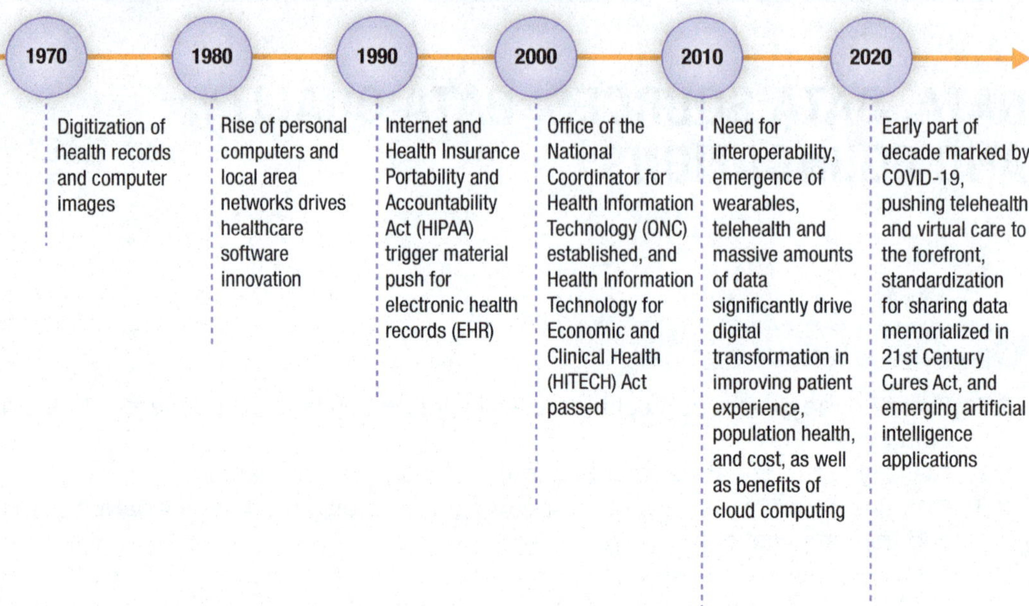

- **2010s:** A greater awareness of the need for interoperability (the ability of data sources to link and connect), along with the emergence of wearables, telehealth, and massive amounts of data, significantly influences digital transformation in improving patient experience, population health, and cost, as well as benefits of cloud computing.

- **2020s:** The early part of the decade was marked by COVID-19 pushing telehealth and virtual care into widespread adoption; the standardization of data sharing, as memorialized in the 21st Century Cures Act (ASTP, n.d.-c); and emerging artificial intelligence (AI) applications.

If you went to see a doctor in the 1980s or 1990s, it is likely that your medical records were largely collected and written on paper; filed away in folders with a patient number for privacy; and stored in large filing cabinets, open bookshelves, or perhaps off-site data storage centers. When patient data had to be transferred from doctor to doctor, charts were copied and sent by carrier or through the mail. This occurred even though the first EHR was invented in the 1960s (Hunt et al., 2005). While hospitals and doctors were slow to adopt technology, what did evolve during this time were computer systems that performed administrative tasks such as processing medical claims and making appointments.

In 2004, the federal government formed the ONC to promote the adoption of EHRs (ASTP, n.d.-a). This was a pivotal moment in the transition to digital healthcare at a national level. Shortly thereafter, in 2009, with the passing of the HITECH Act, hospitals and physicians were financially incentivized to adopt and meaningfully use certified EHR technology. This was a significant development in health data systems because data in digital form allows for collection and analysis at a scale previously unavailable and unattainable.

Simultaneously occurring in the 2010s were advancements in data collection and storage and the "big data" era, AI, and cloud computing. HITECH inadvertently increased the adoption of cloud computing services because it allowed providers and healthcare organizations to meet HITECH objectives without incurring the cost for expensive infrastructure needed for data management, security, and computing resources. Storing data in the cloud also allowed for easier sharing and connectivity with other data sources such as mobile devices and wearable technology.

Data engineering, data integration, data preparation, and data analysis can all occur seamlessly in one place without having to move or copy data from one system to another.

More recently, data has become a critical asset for improving patient care, operational efficiency, organizational performance, and decision-making processes. Enabled by technological improvements and cloud computing, healthcare organizations are continuously improving and adopting sophisticated data management systems to harness the power of their vast information repositories. These systems span across various layers, from data storage and processing to integration and user interfaces, creating a comprehensive data and information ecosystem that supports the needs of the healthcare industry. Health services administrators must have a fundamental understanding of how these systems handle source data in order to effectively use that data to monitor and improve care processes.

Types of Data Systems

Enterprise data warehouses (EDWs; **Figure 2.2**) serve as the backbone of healthcare data management, providing a centralized repository for vast amounts of clinical, operational, and financial data. These systems bring together information from diverse sources within an organization, such as EHRs, laboratory and pharmacy systems, enterprise resource planning (ERP) tools, patient surveys, customer relationship management (CRM) platforms, and third-party data sets acquired from outside the organization. In order to consistently use and leverage their data, organizations must consolidate otherwise fragmented, or siloed data, into a single source of "truth" for comprehensive analytics and reporting at given points in time. The term "truth" is often used in health settings, but it is important to note that most "truth" is sensitive to elements of both timing and data quality, which is covered later in this chapter. Suffice to say that many data elements constantly evolve and are being updated, so at minimum, a point in time for all estimates is important to reflect. Integrated data allows health services managers and healthcare administrators to examine historical data for extended periods, monitor trends in patient outcomes, and examine operational efficiencies and the effectiveness of interventions. To achieve large-scale integration of multiple systems and to consolidate and manage data to support complex queries, EDWs need to store data in an organized, structured manner with defined schemas (comprised of tables, fields,

FIGURE 2.2 Data management systems: Enterprise data warehouse.

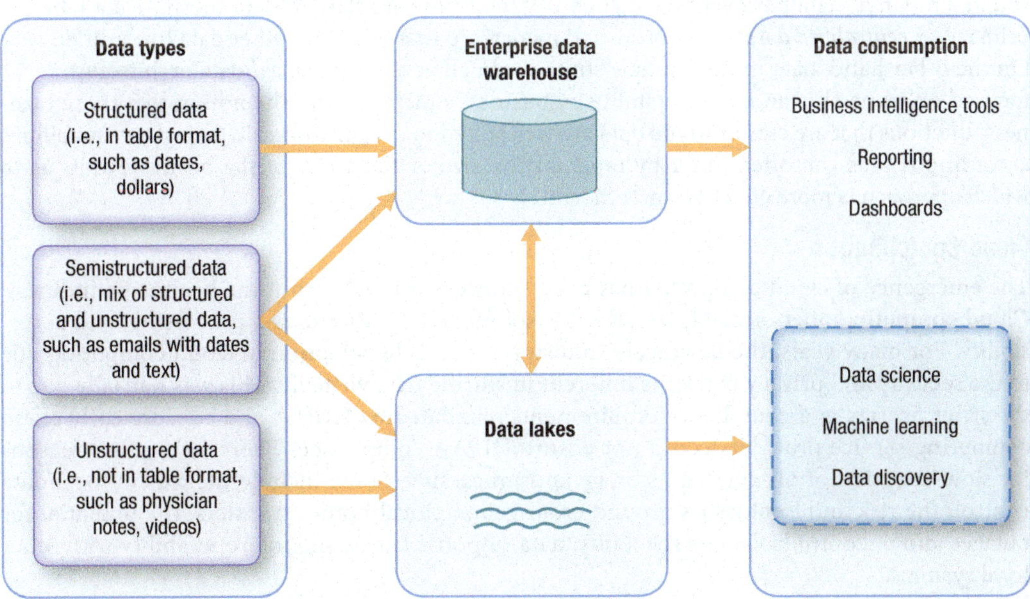

and relationships between data elements), libraries (collections of data), and governance (set of rules or policies to ensure quality and compliance). This requires extensive upfront planning and design and necessitates longer development and implementation periods. In return, EDWs provide highly curated, standardized, and consistent data suitable for business analysts that develop batch reporting, business intelligence, dashboards, and visualizations. The term "business" is used here to reflect common technology and job description nomenclature.

Data Management and Data Lakes

With the increasing digitization of healthcare data, diverse data types need to be stored and managed, beyond structured data. To handle data without a set structure or format, such as videos and text, a new system or repository, referred to as data lakes, was designed to store structured, unstructured, and semistructured data, which are a combination of structured and unstructured formats such as emails.

Data lakes, which can be part of an overall data architecture, allow for the loading of large amounts of unstructured data, such as doctor's notes, medical images, or sensor readings from wearable devices, for storage, access, and analysis. Unlike EDWs, data lakes can house data without standardization or modification as they do not require a structured schema to follow. Massive amounts of raw data can be stored in mixed format, providing greater flexibility to accommodate diverse types of data at lower costs. By landing data in raw form, researchers and data scientists can perform data analysis and discovery on preprocessed data and avoid biases that might have been introduced through an EDW data curation process. For example, some data warehouses will not contain the hour that patients are discharged from a hospital, only the discharge date. Researchers looking to analyze the time of discharge will not be able to use the data in the data warehouse but will need to procure the raw claim record. In addition to data discovery tasks, data lakes provide a platform suitable for advanced analytics, such as machine learning, predictive modeling, and prescriptive modeling. With the wide variety of applications enabled by data lakes, healthcare organizations have implemented more complex data architectures that include data lakes and EDWs in their enterprise data strategies.

Data management systems will continue to evolve to include additional forms of data processing and handling. Due to the large volumes of data being generated every day, integrating and reusing data without having to move and store it more than once has become more common. Architectures like data fabrics and data meshes offer more flexibility, reusability, and access, making them more conducive to business function-specific rules and applications. While the names sound similar, a "data fabric" has a slightly different purpose than a "data mesh." Data fabric is primarily a *centralized* data architecture and ownership that brings together data in a unified way. On the other hand, data mesh is a new strategy aimed at a *decentralized* data architecture more focused on ownership and accountability by business functions with the notion that those business functions that are closest to the data are well suited to design and scale their data capabilities accordingly. This can often differ by organization size or the scope of the business units as to which approach is more effective and efficient.

Cloud Computing

The emergence of cloud computing has been transformational within the healthcare industry. Cloud computing offers scalable and flexible solutions for data storage, processing, and accessibility. For many years, the healthcare industry avoided the adoption of cloud computing due to the security and privacy concerns inherent in storing data virtually. This was partially due to the strict privacy and compliance requirements mandated by HIPAA and because early cloud computing service providers could not ensure HIPAA compliance. There were other reasons for slow adoption of off-site data storage and processing. Some include the loss of local data control, the risk and legal issues around cross-geographical border transfers, the potential for outages and uncontrollable data reliability, data response times, and interoperability with other local systems.

While many of these issues proved addressable, ensuring security continues to be an ongoing game of cat and mouse. The number of data breaches and ransom demands at large and small hospital systems and claims processing centers continue to increase every year, which gives the industry reason to both fear for its data security and seek ongoing and evolving solutions for it. Even localized hardware systems are subject to attacks because integration with external systems are unavoidable and often required in all aspects of the enterprise. Many software solutions today only offer cloud-based applications.

Despite concerns over privacy and data breaches, adoption of cloud technology in healthcare is growing rapidly due to the advantages it provides, such as system interoperability and data sharing. For example, cloud computing has led to accelerated clinical analyses, automated data processing, improved care collaboration across providers for patients, and improved operational efficiencies.

Data Integration, Processing, and Staging

While cloud computing greatly enables the ability to share data and integrate systems, actual data integration remains a challenge for the industry at large. Health data is exponentially more valuable when combined together in ways that support the strategic intentions of the organization. To bring healthcare data together to bring value, organizations must have a deliberate and evolving data architecture and strategy for data staging. Data staging simply refers to a set of processes used to convert raw data into ready-to-use data.

Common across the various data architectures are the stages or layers of data processing and integration. Generally, there are three stages that include data storage, data integration or transformation, and data analytics. Recent developments stemming from data lakes refer to the three stages as a "medallion architecture" (Databricks, 2024). Bronze, silver, and gold are used to describe the respective layers as stages in the data transformation process and have been extended to various data management systems, beyond data lakes (**Figure 2.3**).

The first foundational stage data storage where data processing begins with raw data from various sources. Data is input or imported—sometimes also termed "ingested"—and stored in its unprocessed form. This layer retains the original structure of the data as it comes in from the source, including any relevant metadata (data about the data—such as time stamps, field identifiers, and process identifiers). The main purpose for this layer is to preserve the data for historical retention and use for processing and reprocessing without having to go back to the source. For example, researchers looking to analyze chronic diseases will collect historical data over time. Once data is stored, researchers can use it repeatedly, or use it for other research purposes, without having to retrieve and ingest it again. In a medallion architecture, this function resides in the bronze layer.

FIGURE 2.3 The three data stages.

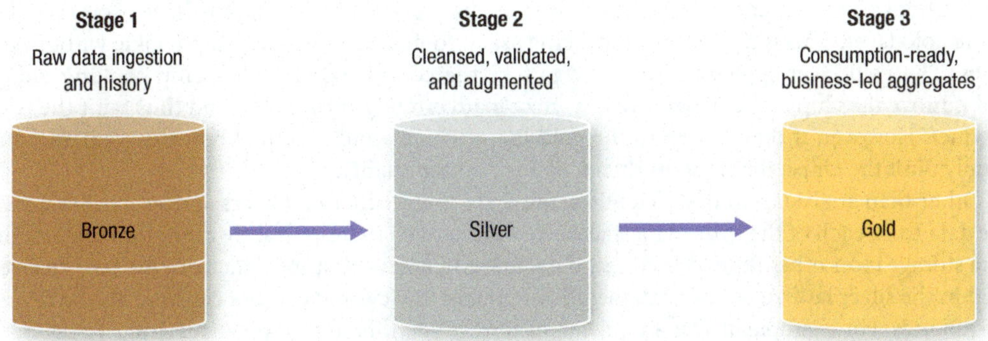

The second layer, the silver layer, represents data that has been integrated and transformed. Combining healthcare data from many sources is common practice. Examples include reference data for the mapping of codes or locations or geocoding which is the process of converting a physical address into geographic longitude and latitude coordinates. Doing so might be necessary to calculate geographic distances or to define population areas for study. The transformation layer prepares the data by converting it into a consistent format, thereby eliminating siloes and maintaining quality standards. Proper data hygiene and data governance are important practices in this layer, both of which are part of the ongoing processes to ensure the cleanliness and accuracy of the data. Proper data hygiene practices ultimately help to remove errors; remove unnecessary duplicated records; and provide standardizations to the data such as ensuring consistent naming conventions, like choosing between state names or two-letter abbreviations. While some data hygiene practices are fundamental to all data used in an organization, such as removing errors, other more specific process requirements are based on how data will be used for a certain unit or practice, thereby adding to the list of standardizations performed. Keeping track of all these transformations is important for data quality and consistency. The formation of a data governance program, with dedicated people in decision-making roles, can greatly help establish a complete set of data definitions, handling rules and criteria needed when data are used and explored by analysts and data scientists, and before being delivered to end users, often known as being put in "production."

The third and final stage is the gold or analytics layer. Data preparation in the analytics layer is typically optimized to serve specific operations or subject areas. As the name implies, the gold layer is this highest level of quality and enrichment, where the data is consumption-ready for downstream applications and use. Depending on the different uses for refined and aggregated data, multiple data models may be required in this layer. For example, analysis based on populations may require a patient-centered data model, whereas an analysis based on adverse reactions from medications may require a data model centered around drugs.

Data Consumption: Users and Interfaces

At the center of the long journey data take to become useful and provide valuable insights is the end user. The end user is the person or team that drives what the data will be used for and who will be using it. Use cases, or the purposes for using data, for an operational analyst will be different from that of a clinical researcher. The data prepared through each of the three stages will have to address a variety of use cases presented. This means that data can be consumed by an end user, such as a data scientist, or interfaced with a system, such as a business intelligence tool, at any of the three data stages that is most appropriate based on the use case.

Analysts and data scientists will want to use cleansed and transformed data from the silver layer if they are looking to build their own assumptions and aggregations. Ad hoc reporting and analysis that is not available from data in the gold layer—because it has been overly curated or limited for other purposes—should utilize the silver layer, where it has been augmented just enough for quality and format. Analysts and data scientists will want to use data from the silver layer so as to not introduce any bias added from business rules and aggregations that may have been included in the gold layer. This is akin to one day being asked to make a chocolate chip cookie without the chips. The gold layer approach would be to take the completed chocolate chip cooking dough and remove the chips. The baker (analyst) may inadvertently miss a chip and thus taint the final product. However, if they return to the gold layer, which would be the known ingredients, and simply omit the chips, the final product will be of better quality.

Other than analysts and data scientists, there are many other end users and systems that may use data from each of the three data stages. However, given there are rarely other functions to the data storage layer other than to hold raw data, few end users consume data from the bronze layer. Within the silver layer, use cases can include interfaces to view and explore data and also to run ad hoc queries. For example, if you are unsure of how to identify and find cancer drugs in the data, you would want to run the appropriate queries to find the cancer drug codes. This stage plays a

FIGURE 2.4 Table transformation example.

Patient	Condition
A	X
B	Y
C	X
D	Z

Patient	Condition X	Condition Y	Condition Z
A	1	0	0
B	0	1	0
C	1	0	0
D	0	0	1

critical role in providing users their first look and access to clean and standardized data. It is common to spend a lot of time and resources in this layer to fully understand the data and properly design the gold layer. Those with a knack for data quality, data "wrangling," or data development will enjoy their time in this stage. Data engineers will also interface directly with this data layer, using programming languages such as structured query language (SQL), Scala, R, and Python to create analysis, business rules, and data sets for the gold layer. Once prepared for analytic capabilities, the gold or analytic layer enables users to access preaggregated data. Users can create those key metrics and in-depth analysis that are vital to strategic organizational decision-making and objectives. Executive dashboards can be delivered through interfaces with business intelligence applications such as Excel, Tableau, or Microsoft Power BI. Further, applications with large language model capabilities can allow users to ask natural language questions that translate into queries on the gold layer for customized insights. For example, users can get a visual graph by simply asking "what is the total cost of care for members with coronary artery disease by state in the Southwest region last year?" These types of applications will no doubt continue to proliferate as AI tools become more sophisticated and are integrated into the gold layer.

In some cases, the gold layer may be specifically built for predictive modeling purposes. Data models can be optimized to deliver relevant features and calculated fields needed for machine learning applications. For example, data may need to be transposed from rows to columns or reformatted to be a binary value as a feature in a model. A simple example of this is shown in Figure 2.4 where data stored in an original diagnosis table is converted to a second table format.

Application Programming Interfaces

One significant advancement in interfaces in the early 2000s was the emergence of application programming interfaces (APIs). APIs are a set of protocols and definitions that serve as an intermediary between software components. In the case of data systems, APIs make it possible for the data layers to communicate and exchange data with software applications. This increases the value of the gold layer as the reach of innovative insights can be easily and effectively shared more broadly. As an example, hospitals discharging patients to a skilled nursing facility or home with home health services can seamlessly send patient records directly to other providers outside their organization using standardized APIs, avoiding costly point-to-point system integrations.

LEARNING OBJECTIVE 2.2: CLASSIFY TYPES OF DATA ELEMENTS AND THEIR MEASUREMENT FEATURES

What is "data"? We used to think of data as those elements that would populate the ever-present spreadsheet. They were usually numbers or sometimes words or "strings" in columns with headings that (sometimes) referenced what they were or represented. More often than not, however, we needed yet another table—a lookup table—to tell us what all the numbers or codes meant. So, if we saw a 2, 3, 4, 5, or 6 in a cell under the heading (variable name) of INSUR, we could look up what that meant. We may find that INSUR is short for INSURANCE TYPE and that the field of values were the numbers 0 to 99, where 0 = "Uninsured," 1 = "Medicare," 2 = "Medicaid" … 99 = "Missing," and so forth.

These types of data still exist and are still a large part of the world of data we have today. We call this standard data in that it can be placed in the cells of a spreadsheet. Many of the tools we have discussed and continue to discuss relate to standard data types. Yet, it is important to know that over the past 20 years, nonstandard forms of data have begun to flood data storage centers worldwide. These come in the form of images, video, text, and audio files. Many of these are captured in data lakes as mentioned earlier.

Historically, these types of data were first prompted by the proliferation of new data capture tools (smartphones) but then surpassed by automated tools such as remote cameras and sensors. New tools such as image recognition and OpenAI tools have also begun to generate enormous amounts of data. Add this to advances in computing power and storage ability and we begin to see a fundamental change in the data landscape. Many have related this change to the four Vs: **V**olume, **V**ariety, **V**elocity, and **V**eracity (Laney, 2001). Volume relates to the sheer amount of data being collected. Variety is the issue of data types being standard and now increasingly nonstandard. Velocity refers to data that can be collected in shorter increments or in near real time. Think about temperature as a simple example or stock price changes. If one were to watch these changes, they would have to be recorded by the second or even millisecond. Each of those observations needs to be time stamped and then stored for later display or analysis. Veracity then relates to the accuracy and completeness of data. Think of images collected at a toll booth via camera. If one does not pay the toll, the license plate is identified and the driver charged. There needs to be a certain level of accuracy lest the wrong plate be tagged. Now, think about this when using AI and algorithms to detect likely pathology or cancer cells from imaging. These are issues well beyond the scope of this text but the idea of the four Vs extends through most organizations. These issues have also been linked to the idea that many organizations are "data rich but information poor," meaning they do not know how to or have the ability to glean actionable information from the data they collect.

Recall Figure 1.2 from the previous chapter that depicts the evolution of data. For the most part, data used for health systems management is structured. And even within this one data type, there are a number of analyses and considerations needed, depending on what is being managed, measured, or analyzed. Before jumping into any form of analysis, however, it is imperative to explore the foundations of data types, how they are measured, and then the limits on what analysis can be done with each. We explore this and other analysis concepts in Chapter 3, "Statistical Foundations." Next, you should explore some common sources of data, both public and private. Data sources are continually in flux and have a wide myriad of origination points. **Box 2.1** shows a few of the publicly available sources, although this is by no means an exhaustive list. **Box 2.2** shows a few of the source types of other forms of healthcare data.

LEARNING OBJECTIVE 2.3: EXAMINE COMMON MODELS OF DATA QUALITY, THEIR USES, AND POTENTIAL DATA GAPS AND THEIR IMPLICATIONS

While diverse data sources and advanced technologies help bring data together to create more comprehensive and accurate insights in healthcare, the most important, and often most under-developed area for many health entities and data stewards, is data quality. Unlike data collected from a controlled scientific lab, real-world data is naturally biased by factors as varied as people and their behaviors, DNA, and preferences. Other factors affecting data quality can come from administrative processes and workflows where data are missing or contain simple input and clerical errors. For example, if understanding the efficacy of a particular drug is dependent on the time the drug was administered but no time stamp is available, then it could affect the result of the analysis. Another might be if an input form or survey subtly changes the wording of a question, for example, when inquiring about education level, asking the number of years of education is different than asking the highest level of education completed.

Box 2.1 Public Sources of Healthcare Data

data.cms.gov
healthdata.gov
www.nlm.nih.gov/oet/ed/stats/03-000.html
www.nlm.nih.gov/NIHbmic/domain_specific_repositories.html
cqls.oregonstate.edu/hdi/data-sources
www.ahrq.gov/data/hcup/index.html
data.cdc.gov
www.cdc.gov/nchs/index.html
open.fda.gov
databrowser.researchallofus.org
www.healthdata.org/research-analysis/gbd-research-library
datatopics.worldbank.org/health
www.dhhs.nh.gov/programs-services/population-health/health-statistics-informatics
archive.ics.uci.edu
bphc.hrsa.gov/data-reporting
hrsdata.isr.umich.edu/data-products

Box 2.2 Examples of Commonly Collected Healthcare Data

Electronic Health Record/Electronic Medical Records

Electronic health records (EHRs) and electronic medical records (EMRs) are often used interchangeably. Both refer to patient health information recorded and gathered at the time of service. However, there is a difference between medical records and health records in that EMRs focus on data from a single practice, like a doctor's office or radiology center. An EHR encapsulates a broader view that is maintained by multiple providers across multiple settings, such as a large integrated health system with hospitals and physicians, and contains more comprehensive patient data. As such, EHRs are used for direct patient care, as well as quality improvement, population health management, and clinical research.

Sample List of Data Elements	Sample List of Metrics Using EHR Data
Patient demographics Progress notes Vital signs Medical histories Diagnoses Medications Immunization dates Laboratory results Radiology images Payment amounts—billed charges, allowed amounts, and paid amounts	• Daily census for inpatient facilities—how many beds are occupied on any given day • Admissions/discharges per month—number of people arriving and leaving a facility each month (this could be in days, weeks, or years) • Clinical quality measures—measures how well providers deliver evidence-based care for preventive screenings and chronic conditions like hypertension and diabetes • Provider workflow efficiency—evaluates tasks performed and time spent on various activities, including documentation and treatment duration or total time of patient visit • Facility-acquired infections—identification and reporting of infections that patients get while at the facility which were not present at admission; these can often be expensive if followed by a readmission which is not reimbursed at the same level • Readmission rate—the number of discharged operative patients that are subsequently readmitted due to some complication of infection from the initial procedure

EHR, electronic health record.

(continued)

Claims Data

Insurance claims data is another vital source of healthcare information. This data is transaction based and used to facilitate payment between healthcare providers and insurance companies. Claims data is widely used in areas like policy decision-making and pricing and provides valuable insights into healthcare utilization and costs. Insurance claims data typically include the following:

Sample List of Data Elements	Sample List of Metrics Using Claims Data
Member demographics Claim ID Dates of service Service provider data High-level clinical information: diagnosis codes and procedure codes such at CPT or DRG codes Payment information: billed charges, allowed amounts and paid amounts	• Admissions/1,000: number of inpatient admissions for every 1,000 population in a given time period (e.g., per month or per year) • ALOS: the average number of days between admit and discharge dates for a set of admissions or for a group of patients • Outpatient visits/1,000: The number of outpatient visits for 1,000 population in a given time period (e.g., ED visits) • Total cost of care: The amount of dollars spent on health services • Cost per service: Dollar amount for every service performed • Dollars PMPM: PMPM is a unit of measure used by insurance companies to calculate average monthly costs for each member in a coverage plan. • Disease prevalence rates: Count of diagnoses codes for a particular disease, such as diabetes and cancer, to see how many people in that population have that disease • Provider practice patterns: Referring provider is identified on a claim, and by looking at services performed, physician referral patterns can be analyzed and modeled. • Claims denial rates: For instances where claims were submitted but denied payment, analysis of denial reasons and rates provides insight ways to improve financial performance. • Hospital readmission rates: Hospitals are measured, and financially penalized, on how many times patients discharged from a hospital return to any hospital within 30 days of discharge.

ALOS, average length of stay; CPT, current procedure terminology; DRG, diagnosis-related groups; PMPM, per member per month.

Other Forms

There are several other important types of data collected for healthcare. Here is a sample of common ones and their associated uses.

Prescription Data From Retail Pharmacies

- Prescriptions (scripts) per person, adherence to prescriptions (can only measure if medications were filled and picked up but not if the person is actually taking them), off-label use rates

Personal Devices Such As Fitbit and Other Sensor Devices

- Steps per day, average heart rate, changes in weight

(continued)

Patient surveys

- Patient satisfaction data are critical to provider performance measures.

Enrollment and Census Trends

- Enrollment is when a member joins a health plan, whether it is an employer-sponsored plan or a federal program such as Medicaid or Medicare.

- Census includes demographic information such as addresses, age, gender, and ethnicity.

Clinical Trials

- Data collected by pharmaceutical companies for the effectiveness of their drugs going through the clinical trial period

Health Information Exchanges

- Health information exchanges (HIEs) are organizations that have been established to increase interoperability between EHRs/EMRs.

- Common data exchanged are admits, discharges, and transfers (ADT), where notifications can be sent to providers or care teams for care coordination.

Lab Results and Diagnostic Reports

- Results from lab cultures are important in antimicrobial stewardship programs to manage overprescribing antibiotics.

There are many different factors to consider when preparing data, many requiring upfront consideration before any time is spent on the analysis. There is nothing more disappointing than putting in hours of work into analyzing data only to find the results are incorrect or biased due to poor data quality. In fact, the amount of time a data scientist or analyst spends on data cleansing and exploration, to truly understand how well the data is established and prepared, is likely to take up the majority of their time. Data quality directly impacts data usability and value, and poor data quality contributes to inaccurate or wrong results. This is a critical aspect of healthcare data management, where the stakes on data-driven decisions are high and can have life-altering consequences.

Data Quality Models

To ensure the appropriate levels of data quality from diverse sources, healthcare organizations may choose to leverage one of many established frameworks to employ various strategies and measures. Data quality models provide general guidelines for assessing and improving the quality of data.

While there are many models of data quality, we have synthesized a few of the major ones, specifically the Wang and Strong model (Wang & Strong, 1996), the Data Management Body of Knowledge (DAMA-DMBOK) model (DAMA International, n.d.), the International Organization for Standardization (ISO)/International Electrotechnical Commission (IEC) 25012 model, and the AIM Quality (AIMQ) model, into domain themes and functions. Some models reference six data quality dimensions, yet others cite as many as 15. The right number of dimensions each organization or individual uses needs to consider the answer to questions such as:

- What will the data be used for?

- What are the risks of having poor quality data?

- How will we assess how strategic data quality is to the organization? (Yang et al., 2002; ISO, 2008)

- What priority will data quality take?
- What dimensions of quality are to be captured at baseline?

Once these questions are considered, the analyst or data governance group must decide what the error tolerances or target acceptance criteria will be. For instance, claims data will have errors for many different reasons, such as if there are too many errors found in birthdays and precise age is a critical data element. If so, then the organization would want to measure this data element throughout the data preparation stages to ensure precision.

Overall, there may be multiple measures across different quality dimensions to put in place, but the majority focus on six major domains. They are accuracy, completeness, consistency, timeliness, validity, and uniqueness. While these quality dimensions may sound very similar, each has their own definitional function.

- **Accuracy** describes how well the data represents what occurred in the practice. For example, is this the correct patient name or the correct dosage of medication. This is highly important for things like reducing errors and correct coding for billing.

- **Completeness** describes whether data is present, such as ensuring all required fields in vaccination records are filled in. An example here would be how many secondary diagnosis fields there are or if the zip code for patients has been left blank.

- **Consistency** describes how similar data formats are across originating data sources or how uniform they are throughout the stages. Here, one may pay close attention to data elements that include leading zeros as they are easy to drop and hard to notice (e.g., if one element has six instead of seven zeros which would cause it to be eliminated from a query). A common example of problems arising here are when organizations develop homegrown codes or special codes that slightly alter the original and then cannot later be reintegrated or analyzed correctly.

- **Timeliness** describes how up-to-date or real-time data is and how available it is when needed. Claims data is very lagged because it takes a long time to get through the billing process, whereas data collected in an EHR is often real time. Many other data are batched daily. Still, other data, like surveys or the census, may be conducted yearly or biyearly.

- **Validity** describes the degree to which the data adheres to predefined business rules or formats. For example, dates are very important in healthcare, from birthdates to dates of service. If dates are presented in the wrong order or as a date range, then the data may not be valid if the system requires a specific format.

- **Uniqueness** measures whether there is one single recorded instance of that data or data set. Before doing any analyses, always check for duplicates first. This is by far the easiest and most important step toward data quality. With healthcare data so widely distributed, merging files can sometimes introduce duplicate records, usually inadvertently.

SUMMARY

The healthcare data landscape is constantly evolving. The past 20 years have seen marked advancements in data collection, data storage, data processing, and data dissemination, often to the point where many healthcare leaders believe they are "data rich" but "information poor." But while the sources of data and the tools for storage and analysis will continue to change, the savvy analyst, data scientist, and manager will focus more on the structure of those processes and in ensuring data quality, security, and privacy. Most of you will have heard the often-used adage, "garbage in, garbage out." With data becoming the functional lifeblood of many organizations, this has never been truer. Further, the future will hold important discussion relative to AI, large language models, automation, and open versus closed data, sometimes also known as data democratization. As more care moves from inpatient to outpatient and even into the home, organizations and individuals will both be supplying data that will ultimately guide health outcomes.

END-OF-CHAPTER RESOURCES

DISCUSSION QUESTIONS

1. How is the evolution of data collection and data types affecting healthcare today?

2. How might artificial intelligence adoption in healthcare pose potential benefits and problems?

3. Discuss how using data warehouses versus cloud data storage presents issues for operations in health settings and those analyzing the data.

4. List some of the challenges in getting data ready for analysis that are commonly encountered. What might these lead to if not addressed?

5. Discuss how "data savvy" end users need to be and the trade-offs of ensuring that occurs in health settings. For example, how much data quality do nurses or physicians need to know? Why?

6. If you could develop an application that all nurses could use in a hospital to make care more efficient, what would that look like? What data would you need? How often would it need to be updated? How would you ensure its quality?

LEARNING ACTIVITIES

CourseConnect ▸

To access self-assessment questions and interactive, competency-based learning activities for this chapter, visit www.springerpub.com/courseconnect. See inside front cover and tear-out card for CourseConnect details.

REFERENCES

Assistant Secretary for Technology Policy. (n.d.-a). About ASTP. https://www.healthit.gov/topic/about-astp

Assistant Secretary for Technology Policy. (n.d.-b). *Health IT legislation.* Retrieved December 1, 2024, from https://www.healthit.gov/topic/laws-regulation-and-policy

Assistant Secretary for Technology Policy. (n.d.-c). *ONC's Cures Act Final Rule.* Retrieved December 1, 2024, from https://www.healthit.gov/topic/oncs-cures-act-final-rule

Databricks. (2024). *What is a medallion architecture?* Databricks. https://www.databricks.com/glossary/medallion-architecture

DAMA International. (n.d.). *DAMA˚ Data Management Body of Knowledge (DAMA-DMBOK˚).* https://www.dama.org/cpages/body-of-knowledge

Hunt, S. A., Abraham, W. T., Chin, M. H., Feldman, A. M., Francis, G. S., Ganiats, T. G., Jessup, M., Konstam, M. A., Mancini, D. M., Michl, K., Oates, J. A., Rahko, P. S., Silver, M. A., Stevenson, L. W., Yancy, C. W., Antman, E. M., Smith Jr, S. C., Adams, C. D., Anderson, J. L., … Riegel B. (2005). ACC/AHA 2005 Guideline Update for the Diagnosis and Management of Chronic Heart Failure in the Adult: A report of the American College of Cardiology/American Heart Association Task Force on Practice Guidelines (Writing Committee to Update the 2001 Guidelines for the Evaluation and Management of Heart Failure): Developed in collaboration with the American College of Chest Physicians and the International Society for Heart and Lung Transplantation: Endorsed by the Heart Rhythm Society. *Circulation, 112*(12), e154–e235. https://doi.org/10.1161/CIRCULATIONAHA.105.167586

International Organization for Standardization. (2008). *ISO/IEC 25012:2008*. https://www.iso.org/standard/35736.html

Laney, D. (2001). 3D data management: Controlling data volume, velocity and variety. *META Group Research Note*, 6(70), 1.

U.S. Department of Health and Human Services. (n.d.). *Health information privacy*. Retrieved December 1, 2024, from https://www.hhs.gov/hipaa

Wang, R. Y., & Strong, D. M. (1996). Beyond accuracy: What data quality means to data consumers. *Journal of Management Information Systems, 12*(4), 5–33. https://doi.org/10.1080/07421222.1996.11518099

Yang, L., Strong, D. M., Kahn, B. K., & Wang, R. Y. (2002). AIMQ: A methodology for information quality assessment. *Information & Management, 40*(2), 133–146. https://doi.org/10.1016/S0378-7206(02)00043-5

CHAPTER 3

STATISTICAL AND ANALYTIC FOUNDATIONS

LEARNING OBJECTIVES

3.1. Understand the primary functions of analysis.
3.2. Calculate descriptive statistics.
3.3. Compare different types of data using statistical inference and hypothesis testing.

REAL-WORLD SCENARIO

James Walden is the chief executive officer (CEO) of Port City Hospital, a medium-sized hospital located in a moderately populated seacoast region in New England. It services a community of approximately 230,000 people but has four competitor hospitals within a 30-mile radius. Over the past 10 years, civic development leaders have been transforming a closed Air Force base into a trade center and have been slowly attracting corporate entities to the area. In the past year, two major employers have relocated their corporate offices and/or large manufacturing centers to the trade center, adding an estimated 30,000 new persons to the area. In addition, a large insurance company has doubled its workforce in the same town as Port City Hospital, creating an additional 4,000 jobs, at least two thirds of which they anticipate filling from outside the area. Within the hospital, Mr. Walden has been hearing increased concerns from physician and nursing leadership about workload increases. In looking at utilization data, Mr. Walden is curious if the hospital is realizing a growth pattern that is both different than previous years and different than other hospitals in the area. Knowing this might facilitate his decision to expand certain services or the hospital itself.

Numbers are a form of language. For managers, they facilitate the way we communicate about the functioning of organizations. They allow us to count, describe, compare, and predict. Mathematics and statistics—the calculation and manipulation of numbers—are the primary tools that facilitate these numerical "conversations."

Numbers and analysis also provide justification for action (or sometimes inaction), and when used properly and transparently, they allow those interpreting their analysis to make reasoned and informed decisions. Health services managers utilize numbers extensively in their work because most of what is done in any organization must be quantified. As the adage goes, "If you can't measure it, you can't manage it."

This chapter reviews the basic forms of mathematical and statistical analysis used in health services administration, including various descriptive and inferential statistics. The chapter concludes with basic guidelines and examples of how to best present data in tabular and graphical form.

LEARNING OBJECTIVE 3.1: UNDERSTAND THE PRIMARY FUNCTIONS OF ANALYSIS

In Chapter 2, "Data, Data Sources, Data Quality, and Foundations," we learned that data can be static, systematically collected, and structured—sometimes even small and manageable. But data also can be nonstandard, unstructured, and sometimes massive and collected in real time.

Selecting what analysis to perform and what statistical methods to employ can be a daunting chore for students. This chapter provides general tools to help students focus their analyses.

Prior to conducting any analysis, it is important to first think about why the analysis is being conducted. These purposes need to be explicit and well understood. This may appear to be counterintuitive for some. For years, we have seen students who get lost in "analysis paralysis" and/or develop long and winding presentations with much analytical depth but little significance to the work at hand. Taking a strategic question approach will aid in avoiding these two major pitfalls.

To do this, one simply need to ask:

What question am I trying to answer and how does it fit with the needs of this project, program, unit, department, or organization?

There are four questions for conducting any strategic inquiry. These four questions can be used when starting almost any new project, when trying to demonstrate how a process runs, or when evaluating the effectiveness or efficiency of a project or function. We elaborate on a few of these in other chapters, but they come from the literature on strategic planning and are as follows:

1. Where are we now?

2. Where do we want to go?

3. How do we want to get there?

4. How will we know we are there?

Answering these questions can employ many quantitative tools and methods, but some tools are better served for some questions more than others. To better understand this, let us now superimpose the basic functions of data, which are also presented in a short and general framework. The basic analytical functions are as follows:

1. To describe something

2. To compare something

3. To predict something—including simulating something with changing future parameters

Sometimes, these are listed as the analytic functions of description, prediction, and prescription. Here, we break out comparison (No. 2) as its own function because the analytical tools used to compare two things comprise a specific set of statistical functions that students should be familiar with. Similarly, we combine prediction and prescription as they are both forms of prediction, albeit with different statistical methods. We address a few of these in detail and others as an introduction.

Now, we can update our earlier figure to include both the question and the analytical function, as shown in **Table 3.1**. Taking each in turn, here are some examples of how you might find yourself using these functions for each type of question.

Example 1: Your organization is concerned about the number of new urgent care clinics and microhospitals moving into the area. They would like to examine how their own urgent care unit might be impacted. To answer this question, one first needs to assess: "Where are we now?" This could be measuring several things, including the number of urgent care visits, the type of visits,

TABLE 3.1 Types of Analytic Functions

Strategic Questions	ANALYTIC FUNCTIONS		
	Description	**Comparison**	**Prediction**
Where are we now?	X	X	
Where do we want to go?	X	X	X
How will we get there?	X	X	X
How will we know we are there?	X	X	

the timeframe for them, the number that require follow-up care versus no follow-up, the number that require a specialty referral, and so forth.

Most of these are simple descriptions. In the next section, we get into the specific analysis one might use, but suffice it to say that description primarily involves counting and displaying those counts over time, when appropriate.

A second answer to this question may involve comparison. For example, how do our visit volumes vary by day of the week or by month? Or, if we have multiple urgent care centers, how does one compare to the other? Are volumes increasing or decreasing? Answering these types of questions is imperative to forming options for further decision-making.

Example 2: Payment rules concerning telehealth are changing and we wish to take advantage of this potential market. What is the best path forward? This would be the second type of question: Where do we want to go? It also touches on the question—how do we want to get there? To answer these requires both quantitative and qualitative methods. In this case, even if we have identified different approaches to starting a telehealth practice or program, we are not guaranteed visit volume. This requires some form of description (who our patients are and what our current capabilities are) as well as our future needs (i.e., what we want things to look like in the future) and possibly some prescription (what if our foundational assumptions change?). Doing this will require making either static estimates of future demand or allow for some computer modeling to provide a range of probable future outcomes given our current assumptions or understanding.

Example 3: We ran a program to reduce the percentage of our patient population who identify as patients with diabetes in order to improve our diabetes management and quality measures and to also lower the indicators for diabetes within our patient population through our path to a wellness diabetes program. Specifically, we examined patients' blood glucose levels (i.e., H1c), weight, the number of medications they use, and their quality of life via a validated survey instrument. We operated the pilot program for 1 year and are considering our decision options of expanding the program to all potential patients, altering the program, or eliminating the program. These types of questions require an evaluation of the current programs after a defined amount of time, thereby determining whether they are successful and answering the question, "How do we know when we are there?" Here, we would first describe our patients, but it is more likely we would then compare our patients in a pre-/posttest manner, measuring them at intake and then at points in time and/or at the program's completion.

Once the strategic nature of our question and the analytic functions are defined, we need to perform the analyses. In the next sections, we take each analytic function in turn and describe the statistical tools that can be used depending on the type of data points one is examining.

LEARNING OBJECTIVE 3.2: CALCULATE DESCRIPTIVE STATISTICS

 ## VIDEOS FOR LEARNING OBJECTIVE 3.2

- Video 3.1 Creating Summaries of Categorical Variables
- Video 3.2 Calculating Descriptive Statistics
- Video 3.3 Creating a 95% Confidence Interval

Statistics uses mathematical relationships between data to allow making decisions about both the data itself and about the likelihood that sampled data represent a broader and more generalized trend or population. For managers, some simple categorizing of techniques can help focus statistical analysis in ways that are easily understood and applied.

Managerial statistics have the same three primary functions mentioned earlier: description, comparison, and prediction. Before describing statistical functions, however, a discussion about the nature of structured data is needed. Structured data can be recorded or coded into an analytical file, typically a spreadsheet. These data are simply numbers within a context. For example, green, although a nice color, is only an adjective by itself. If, however, we record the eye color of a room of 20 people and record that in a spreadsheet and were to then count the number of people with green eyes, we have performed a statistical function—the calculation of a descriptive statistic. We could summarize this variable by counting the number of recorded values equaling "green" or by reporting the relative percentage of our data set that reported green out of the total. We could also create a graph from this data.

Many different types of analyses can be performed on structured data. Yet, when it comes time to conduct these analyses, students are often unclear on what analysis to do on what data points or data sets. Imagine, for example, that you find yourself in a new position and have been asked by your supervisor, Mr. Walden, to look at some utilization trends using data from the organization's data warehouse. You pull up the corresponding data files and find there are 30 variables (columns on a spreadsheet) and tens of thousands of records (rows on a spreadsheet representing individual patient visits). In the middle is a sea of numbers of various sorts that continue as you scroll down the screen. In some organizations, there may be millions of data records in thousands of tables, which is intimidating to be sure. However, a data file with 10,000 rows and one with 20 rows are not particularly different. Each can be described in similar ways. What is important is the data itself. Understanding what the numbers represent (the context) and how they were created will lead you down certain analytic paths and not others, allowing you to put some statistical methods aside for some types of data. Next, we discuss the characteristics and uses of data by type, understanding, of course, that all data contexts, what is known as metadata, need to be fully understood. For example, if the provider table has a variable called provider type, and in those cells are numbers that range from 1 to 99, it is important to have a source to understand what these codes mean in order to translate them into usable information. These are typically found in the files themselves or in "look-up tables," often called a data dictionary.

Structured Data Types

Structured data come in four varieties. Students of introductory statistics will recall the terms nominal, ordinal, interval, and ratio types of data. All refer to the measurement or ability to measure certain data variables. Variables are data that can take on different values, depending on what is being measured. In the earlier example, the color of 20 people's eyes was recorded, thus creating the variable "eye color." In this instance, it is a variable that is measured nominally, often also called categorically. Nominal refers to data that exist in nonoverlapping categories. They have no ranking and are mutually exclusive, for example, eye color, insurance type, gender, and ethnicity. There are two special subsets of nominal, or categorical, variables. One are those with only two categories, such as "yes" and "no." These are called dichotomous variables. The other are ordinal variables. Ordinal variables are slightly different in that the categories have a ranking. An example of this would be satisfaction scales, where responses such as *somewhat satisfied* might be followed by *very satisfied* and so forth. These are common in health surveys. The final two types are often taken together as interval/ratio variables. These are often termed *continuously measured variables*; examples include time and currency. Interval variables are those where the distance between the categories is equal. Think of a time scale as derived in seconds—1 second, 2 seconds, and so forth. We could derive smaller increments if we so wished, creating fractions of seconds as is often done in Olympic time trials and racing. The increments do not matter, however. What does matter is that the distance between them is equal. This allows mathematical calculations on these forms of data.

At this point, some might realize that there are distinct features of all variables—those that have equal distances between measurement points and those that do not. Often, these distinctions are recognized by labeling nominal and ordinal data as categorical and interval/ratio data as continuous. We, too, follow this convention. But the main point is that it is important to understand

TABLE 3.2 Types of Data Structures

DATA TYPE	CHARACTERISTIC
Nominal	Unordered categories
Ordinal	Ordered categories
Interval/Ratio	Continuous
	(Categories of equal size)

the type of data being used because different types of data are analyzed differently using different techniques. **Table 3.2** summarizes data by type.

Describing One Variable (Univariate)

Descriptive statistics include categorical data and either nominal or ordinal data measurements. **Tables 3.3A** and **3.3B** provide data of a sample of patients both by count and percentage, recording their insurance type. Insurance type is a categorical variable that is of the nominal type. The categories are not ranked, nor is there any relationship among them. Patients usually claim a type of primary insurance (or lack thereof) upon visit. To describe this and any nominal (and much ordinal) data, we are limited to only a handful of techniques. The first is to simply count. Here, we can count the total number of patients or the number of patients by the type of insurance, as we have done in **Table 3.3A,** column 3.

The second summary statistic we can create first requires basic mathematics. To do this, we calculate the percentages for the number of people falling into each category. A percentage is the number of persons in a category divided by the total number of persons in the sample or population under study, multiplied by 100. Not multiplying by 100 is also correct, although this provides a decimal fraction and not a percentage. For example, we may wish to know how many people reported having United as their insurer. One way to summarize this would be to count, which amounts to 883 individuals in **Table 3.3B**. To calculate a percentage, we would divide that 883 by the total of 3,541 (i.e., the total number in the study), which gives us 0.25 (rounded to the nearest whole person) or 25% of patients.

TABLE 3.3A Counts of Patients by Insurance Type

CODE	INSURANCE TYPE	NO. OF PATIENTS
1	Cigna	973
2	Medicare	394
3	Medicaid	156
4	Tri Care	98
5	Aetna	330
6	United	883
7	Kaiser	123
8	Humana	17
9	CVS Health	567

TABLE 3.3B Percentage of Patients by Insurance Type

CODE	INSURANCE TYPE	NO. OF PATIENTS	% OF PATIENTS
1	Cigna	973	27%
2	Medicare	394	11%
3	Medicaid	156	4%
4	Tri care	98	3%
5	Aetna	330	9%
6	United	883	25%
7	Kaiser	123	3%
8	Humana	17	0%
9	CVS Health	567	16%
Total		3,541	100%

Percentages and fractions provide more information than do counts. Inherent in them is the context of the whole. If we tell you 883 patients had United insurance, you may question whether that is a high or modest amount; but if we say 25% of patients had United, you now have some sense of the entire group of patients, even though we have not provided the total. Here, providing the total in addition to the percentage provides both the count and the total, creating a more complete picture of the data being described. Listing counts and percentages of categorical data is also called creating frequencies from the data. From a descriptive standpoint, this is the limit of analyzing a singular categorical variable. We also discuss the best practices for determining which information to include in visual displays and how to display data in Chapter 4, "Data Display."

Continuous data are the other data type you will encounter. Again, these are actually categorical data in nature, but the categories are of equal size. Examples include variables such as time, money, or height. Video 3.1 shows how to summarize categorical variables in Excel. The equal distances between categories are what allow for mathematical analysis of these data. So, for example, adding one dollar to two dollars adds the same amount as adding one dollar to 10 dollars. This allows us to calculate several descriptive measures that examine the centrality of the data and its spread, which are both useful for our purposes. We first examine measures of centrality, or what is called *central tendency*.

Measures of Central Tendency: Mean, Median, and Mode

Data collected across many observations vary from observation to observation; thus, they are termed *variables*. Some may have high values, some low, and some may have the same values. It is completely possible that two people can have the same height, for example. Graphing these data reveals both the spread (how high and low individual values might be) and the clustering of individual observations (how close together or spread apart they are). An example is given in **Figure 3.1**.

From the data in **Figure 3.1**, we can see that the number of charts pulled appear to be centered between 10 and 30 per day, with a few days of higher volume and one with lower volume. What would be helpful for analytic purposes would be to have a set of summary statistics to describe the data; thus, we find the mean, median, and mode. Video 3.2 shows how to create descriptive statistics in Excel.

The statistic that is the mathematical center of a data set is the average or mean. It is the foundation for many other statistical concepts as well. To calculate the mean, simply add up all the values of the variable and divide by *n*, which is simply the total number of observations. We can also find the median, which is the center of the numerical distribution of data when all the observations are arranged from lowest to highest (or highest to lowest). The mode is the most

FIGURE 3.1 Graph of charts filed by day.

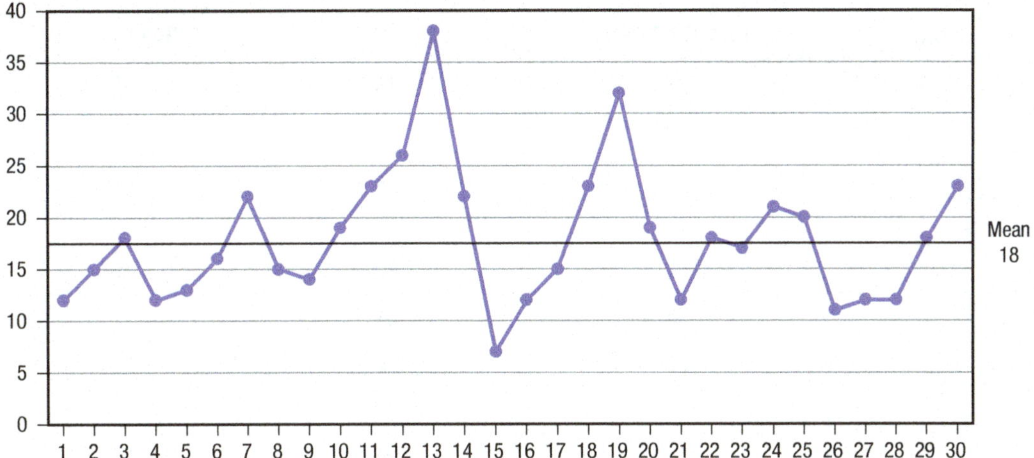

frequently reported data value. **Table 3.4** shows these measures of central tendency for a sample of patient chart pulls.

In this instance, the median and mean number of charts pulled are the same value, 18. The mode is 12 or the most frequently reported value. This indicates that the average number of charts pulled per day was 18. Similarly, if we were to order the days by fewest charts pulled to greatest across all 30 days, the middle of that list would also be 18 charts pulled.

Had the mean been higher than the median, it would indicate that there were some high values of the data that were pulling the mean upward. Instead, say we are looking at the quarterly household income of a small sample of people and we get the following range of income values: $13,000, $25,000, $33,000, $42,000, and $56,000. The mean of these data is $33,800. The median is $33,000. If, however, we replace the value of $56,000 with $120,000, notice what happens. The median is still $33,000, yet the mean increases to $46,600. This is because the median is not dependent on all other values in the list or distribution. It is what we call a *robust measure*, or one that is resistant to other values. The mean is not robust, as we demonstrated. When examining data distributions, it is appropriate to look at both the mean and the median. Doing so can indicate the presence of outlying values and the spread of the data.

Measures of Spread

Although the mean, median, and mode describe the middle or centrality of the data, we may also be interested in how varied and spread out the data are. This is helpful both to understand the range of data values and to examine the possibility of outlier values that might be affecting our measures of central tendency. Examine the data again in **Table 3.4**. We know that the mean of these data is 18 charts filed. We also know that there are many days when the number of charts filed exceeds 18 per day and also falls short of 18 per day. The maximum and minimum values tell us this and are important measures for summarizing our data. In **Table 3.4,** they are 38 and 7, respectively. The difference, or 31 (38 – 7), is what we call the *range*. Examining the range in addition to other measures of central tendency allows a clearer picture of the data distribution (even without a graph).

There is one final measure of spread that should be considered. If we were to draw a line at the mean on a graph of the data from **Table 3.4**, as shown in **Figure 3.1**, it would show that approximately half of the data points were clustered above and half below. Here, we see that some points lie closer to the mean than others, whereas some lie on the mean. Thus, each point of observation lies some distance from the mean, whether positive or negative. What would be interesting is to know how far from the mean are the data on average. The final summary measure of spread does this, which is the standard deviation. Simply put, the standard deviation is the average distance

TABLE 3.4 Charts Filed by Day

DAY	CHARTS FILED	DAY	CHARTS FILED
1	12	16	12
2	15	17	15
3	18	18	23
4	12	19	32
5	13	20	19
6	16	21	12
7	22	22	18
8	15	23	17
9	14	24	21
10	19	25	20
11	23	26	11
12	26	27	12
13	38	28	12
14	22	29	18
15	7	30	23
Mean	**18**		
Median	**18**		
Mode	**12**		

of a given data point (i.e., measurement) to its mean. In the chart filing example, we are asking: On average, how far do the data points diverge from their mean? To do this, we could start by measuring the distance of each point to the mean and then simply dividing by n (the total number of points) to get the average. Because the mean is the mathematical average of all the points, the distances when summed will always total zero in real terms. Therefore, to counter this problem, the negative distances must be eliminated by squaring them all. This eliminates our zero total problem but also converts all our original distances into squared distances. When we add them up and divide by n, we obtain the average squared distance, also known as the variance. In this case, this creates a measure interpreted as the number of charts pulled squared. This also creates an interpretive problem in that we no longer have the same units with which we started. Returning to our original units requires that we eliminate the squared term by taking its square root, thus providing the standard deviation. Also, it is important to note that when working with samples, we do have to make adjustments. As we discuss in the next section, samples are more variable than if we had all the data in the world on a variable or what is known as a population. In this instance, we divide the final variance not by n but by $n - 1$ to adjust for this. If we had all the data for a population, we would simply use n.

Working With Samples

The calculation within **Table 3.5** provides the standard deviation for a specific set of sample data. If those data constitute a complete set of observations and generalization to some larger population

TABLE 3.5 Summary Statistics for Charts Filed by Day

DAY	CHARTS FILED	DISTANCE FROM THE MEAN	SQUARED DISTANCE FROM THE MEAN
1	12	−6	34.81
2	15	−3	8.41
3	18	0	0.01
4	12	−6	34.81
5	13	−5	24.01
6	16	−2	3.61
7	22	4	16.81
8	15	−3	8.41
9	14	−4	15.21
10	19	1	1.21
11	23	5	26.01
12	26	8	65.61
13	38	20	404.01
14	22	4	16.81
15	7	−11	118.81
16	12	−6	34.81
17	15	−3	8.41
18	23	5	26.01
19	32	14	198.81
20	19	1	1.21
21	12	−6	34.81
22	18	0	0.01
23	17	−1	0.81
24	21	3	9.61
25	20	2	4.41
26	11	−7	47.61
27	12	−6	34.81
28	12	−6	34.81
29	18	0	0.01
30	23	5	26.01
Mean	18		
Total		0	1241
Total / $(n-1)$		Not possible	42.78
Square root			6.541

6.54 is the standard deviation of this sample of data.

Note: We divide by $n-1$ because it is a sample.

is not being made, then the standard deviation should be calculated in this way. However, if we are using a sample value, which is known, to say something about a population value, which usually cannot be known, we must make an adjustment. Samples are inherently more variable than populations. We are simply more likely to get data points further away from the "true" population means in a sample than were we to continue to collect more data. Because of this variability, when calculating our standard deviation, we divide by $n - 1$.

When dealing with sample data, caution must be used. **Table 3.5** is a sample of data for 1 month of chart filings. If we are only interested in that month, we can treat the data as a population statistic. However, if we want to treat this 1 month as representative of all months, adjustment is required. The mean of the data in **Table 3.5** was 18 chart filings. If we were to resample these data over another time period, what is the likelihood that 18 would again be the mean? If we designate 18 as a sample value representative of the "truth," we are in fact saying that it is and always will be 18. This is quite unlikely. However, it is often not possible for us to know the "truth" for all present and future data. Instead, we can create an interval that we can say with some level of confidence contains the "true" population mean. Since it is impossible to report the actual true mean of any population using a sample, confidence in a sample mean can be supported by also calculating a numerical range for the true value. Equation 3.1 calculates the 95% confidence interval for the actual mean value estimated by a sample statistic:

Equation 3.1

$$\text{Mean} \pm (1.96 \times \text{standard error})$$

where the standard error = standard deviation × square root (n).

The value of 1.96 is the value that cuts off the upper and lower 2.5% of the standard normal distribution (discussed briefly later in this chapter), and the use of the standard error rather than the standard deviation is to adjust for the fact that we are using a sample (with greater variability) to represent a population. The reporting of confidence intervals should be included with any mean that has been derived from sample data. Video 3.3 exemplifies how to create a 95% confidence interval using Excel.

LEARNING OBJECTIVE 3.3: COMPARE DIFFERENT TYPES OF DATA USING STATISTICAL INFERENCE AND HYPOTHESIS TESTING

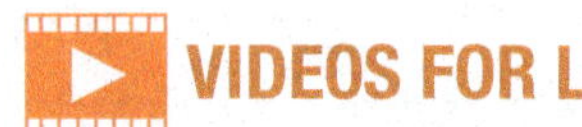 **VIDEOS FOR LEARNING OBJECTIVE 3.3**

- Video 3.4 Correlation Test Using Excel Functions and Data Analysis Tools
- Video 3.5 *t* Test for Unequal Variances

Bivariate Analysis

The second primary function of managerial statistics is to compare two or more variables. This can mean comparing a variable measured at two points in time, such as the number of births from 1 year to the next, or in two locations, such as comparing births between hospitals. It can also mean comparing two distinct types of data, such as the number of ED visits over a time period with the number of lab tests performed during that same period. Each type of analysis again requires knowing what types of data you are comparing. Like descriptive statistics, there are certain types of analyses you will perform and others you can set aside, depending on how the data are measured. Before doing so, however, we first need to review the need for hypothesis development and testing.

Hypothesis Testing

Students may recall from an introductory statistics course that comparisons of variables are best tested using hypotheses. These are simply statements of association that are first stated and then, using analysis, either supported or refuted. The reason for doing this is that most data are simply representations of phenomena that exist in real life. The problem is that it is usually unrealistic or impossible to measure all phenomena completely. Think about measuring an entire population. We may want to know the actual number of people in the United States, but our ability to measure this is limited. Realistically, we cannot find and count everyone in the United States without missing some people, and the number of people changes hourly because of births and deaths, so by the time we were done measuring, the "real" answer would have already changed. Yet, we also know that for a given point in time, there is a "real" measurement, even if we are unable to observe it. We can, however, estimate, within some level of certainty, whether the measurement we observe or the data comparison we make is likely to be representative of what is "real" at that point in time.

This is why we create hypotheses (e.g., a premise) and then use statistical tests to either support or refute them. Two primary types of hypotheses are used in statistical analysis. The first is the null hypothesis, which is always the hypothesis of no association or difference. The second is the alternative hypothesis, which is most often the converse of the null but can also be directional, such as two data elements having a positive or negative association.

Managers in healthcare settings are often assessing data for comparative purposes, and often, they use samples of data taken at a point in time. The question managers need to be concerned with is not only whether there is an observable difference or association in the data but also with what level of confidence they can believe it to be true and not because of mere chance. Otherwise stated, if the manager collected another sample of data, would the association or difference reverse itself or would the data be reflecting the same pattern? These are the foundational questions behind hypothesis testing. Consider a manager who collected data on the number of safety protocol violations within two hospital units. In summarizing these violations, they find the mean number of violations of unit A to be 21 over a 1-year period and 27 in unit B over the same period. In real terms, unit B does report more violations than unit A. The question is whether this trend is an authentic trend or a result of pure chance. Thus, the question we ask is how likely are we to record or see a difference in the next year as big as we have this year, or is the real difference actually zero? Again, the term *real* is a generalization. We are essentially making educated guesses, using probability theory and methods to inform those guesses, or in practice, management decisions. It is important to note that what we are attempting to understand is very important to the interpretation, as is understanding the need for the level of specificity in our results. These concepts continue to be debated in the scientific literature, as are the effectiveness of some analysis and quantitative tests, such as confidence intervals, in practice (Morey et al., 2016).

Students often say that the stating of hypotheses is unduly confusing. In fact, it is quite simple. The null hypothesis always states that there is no difference or association between the two things (i.e., data variables). For example, we could hypothesize that the mean number of violations in unit A is no different than the mean number of violations at unit B "in reality," if we were to continue to measure over time.

The alternative is that there is a real difference between the two observations. But here, we have an option. We can say that historically, the mean number of violations at unit B has been different than unit A, whether that is higher or lower. When direction does not matter, we are conducting a two-tailed hypothesis test. Our second alternative is to say that one is higher than the other or lower than the other. In this case, we might say the alternative hypothesis is that the mean number of violations at unit B is higher than the mean number of violations at unit A. In this case, we are conducting a one-tailed hypothesis test. The difference occurs primarily with respect to interpretation of the tests and is explored later in the chapter. The stated null hypothesis, abbreviated H_0, or that of no difference, for this example would be:

H_0: There is no difference in the mean number of safety violations between unit A and unit B over the 1-year period.

The stated alternative hypothesis, abbreviated H_a, is the converse of this and, assuming a two-tailed test, would be:

H_a: There is a difference in the mean number of safety violations between units A and B over the 1-year period.

The analysis we perform will allow us to either reject or fail to reject our null hypothesis at some value of alpha, or a predetermined cutoff of some level of probability, most usually at .05, which would be a 95% level of probability. The rule here is that one never completely accepts a hypothesis. Why? Because we can never be 100% certain what the relationship between two things is "in reality" at a given point in time, for reasons stated earlier in this section. Instead, we use hypothesis testing and statistics to make probabilistic inference into the relationship between two sets of measured data or observations. Interpreting our hypotheses now requires the use of statistics and a brief introduction to theoretical probability distributions, otherwise thought of as why we can be certain we are at least partially certain.

When performing analyses to test hypotheses, it is useful to have a common framework, regardless of the type of variables one is working with or the type of distribution used. Here, we present them as steps that can be followed easily.

- **Step 1:** State the null (H_0) and alternative (H_a) hypotheses for the analysis being conducted or the question being addressed.

- **Step 2:** Determine the appropriate test statistic. These will vary but **Figure 3.2** presents a summary guide for determining which to use given the variables being examined. Some common ones are z, t, F, and chi-square. We discuss some of these later in this chapter.

- **Step 3:** Determine your decision rule for rejecting H_0. This can be stated as "If test statistic calculated $\geq$ test statistic critical value, reject H_0."

FIGURE 3.2 Statistical analysis quick guide.

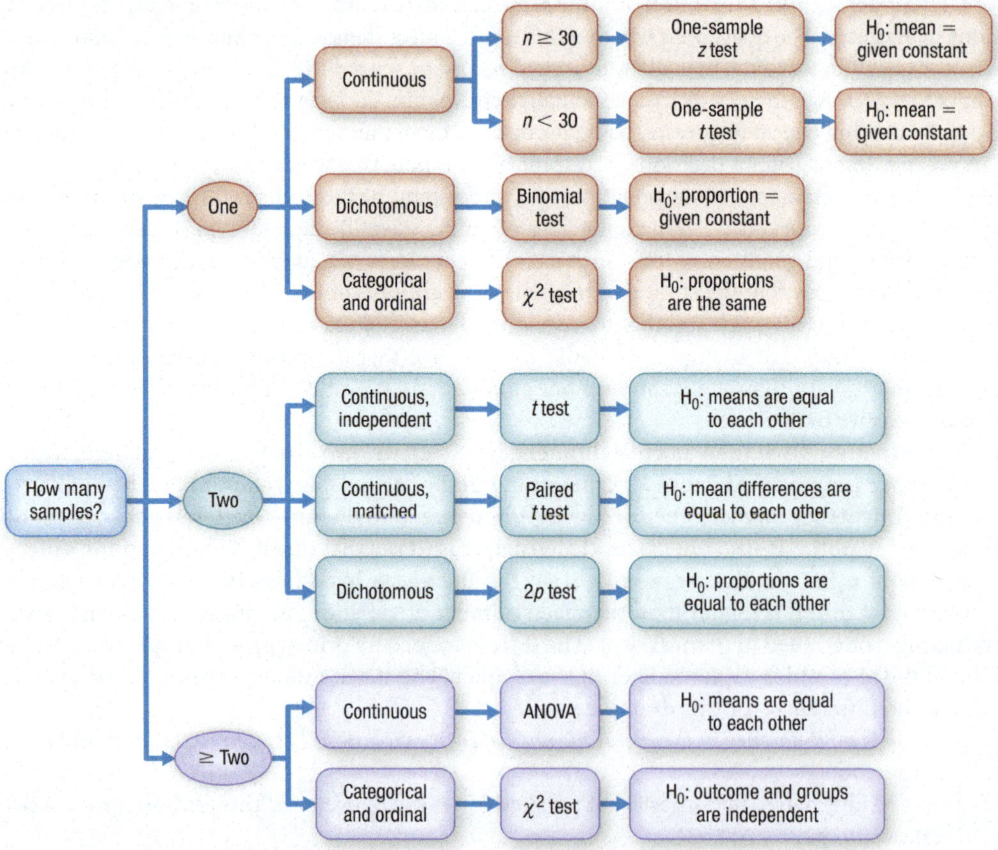

ANOVA, Analysis of Variance.

- **Step 4:** Calculate the test statistic.
- **Step 5:** Make conclusions relative to your hypotheses. This usually starts with a rejection of H_0 or a failure to reject and then some reference to the variables being analyzed. This may also reflect some probability value.

Probability Distributions

If someone were to ask you what the probability of flipping a normal coin and having it come up heads, you would no doubt say that it is a 50/50 chance, or 50% of the time. Yet, you would also likely agree that it is quite possible that you could flip a coin and heads would come up three times in a row. How can this be? There are two reasons: First, each coin flip is not dependent on the previous one. There are two sides of the coin, so you only have two possible outcomes. Each time you flip, they are equally likely to come up (if the coin is balanced and not a trick coin). Second, we know that if you continue to flip repeatedly, the number of heads and tails will start to equal out. In statistical language, we would say the probability of heads grows closer to .5 as your n (number of flips) increases. Suffice it to say that flipping a coin has a known probability. Could we observe 37 heads in a row? Sure, but it is highly unlikely.

Most phenomena in the world have a distribution of measurement, whether height, weight, income, hair length, or other attributes. Consider height. There are a range of heights of individuals throughout the world. Some are quite tall, and others are not. If, for example, we see someone who is 8 feet tall, we might think that it is unusual but not impossible. But how do we test this statistically?

Comparing Two Variables

Two Continuously Measured Variables

There are different analytic techniques for comparing a continuous data variable measured at different points in time or across locations, and for comparing two different continuous variables to one another. First, let us examine comparing two different continuously measured variables, such as lab tests and ED visits, using the correlation function.

Correlation

In this instance, we look to statistics to provide a measure of association between two differently measured and occurring phenomena. Because they are measured in increments of equal distance, respectively, we can assess how unit changes in one variable are correlated to unit changes in the other. This becomes an algebraic relationship, in which if we label one variable x and the other y, we can express y as being some function of x. A note of caution here: We can compare any two continuous variables and calculate their relationship; however, this does not mean that a causal relationship actually exists. The computer will give us a value, but it is important for the student to know whether it has any practical use. For example, we could compare the number of pieces of gum chewed in Duluth, Minnesota, over a year and correlate that to the number of births in Guatemala and we would get a statistical likelihood. Whether these two variables are actually related is very highly unlikely.

Table 3.6 measures the number of ED visits and lab tests for a sample period in September. If they were perfectly correlated, these variables would have a one-to-one relationship. In this example, a perfectly positive correlation would mean each additional ED visit would result in the same additional number of lab tests. Similarly, if there was a perfectly negative relationship, for every ED visit, lab tests would consistently decrease by a set amount. To do this, we calculate the linear correlation coefficient (r), which will indicate the associative, but not causal, relationship between the number of ED visits and the number of lab tests performed per day. The correlation coefficient will also indicate the strength of the linear association between the two variables.

TABLE 3.6 Correlation of ED Visits and Lab Tests Performed

DATE	ED VISITS	LAB TESTS
15-Sep	55	67
16-Sep	78	88
17-Sep	87	91
18-Sep	111	100
19-Sep	143	204
20-Sep	45	66
21-Sep	57	72
22-Sep	81	142
23-Sep	76	93
24-Sep	100	158
25-Sep	97	145
26-Sep	69	84
27-Sep	59	78
28-Sep	88	101

Statistics indicates that a correlation coefficient (r) of 1.00 (100%) indicates a perfectly positive correlation (an increase in x is always associated with a parallel increase in y) and that a negative correlation coefficient of 1.00 indicates a perfectly negative correlation. By definition, correlation coefficients can only range from -1.00 to 1.00. For the data in **Table 3.6**, the correlation coefficient is .855, which indicates a strong positive correlation between ED visits and lab tests. Although this seems to be an indication of a powerful correlation, the association cannot yet be said to be statistically significant or not one because of random chance.

Here, we have collected a sample of data based on 14 days of observation. The question we must ask is whether the observed phenomenon could be owing simply to chance rather than some real association. Stating our hypotheses is helpful in doing this. Here, our null and alternative hypotheses are as follows:

H_0: *There is no relationship between the number of* ED *visits and the number of lab tests.*

H_a: *There is a relationship between the number of* ED *visits and the number of lab tests.*

To address our hypotheses, we must now determine a critical value of r to assess the likelihood of the relationship being because of chance. Although some computer programs give the actual probability or likelihood of the relationship with a p value, others do not. A p value is simply the probability of the test statistic calculated. Here, we present a table of critical r values, shown in **Table 3.7**, which gives the critical values of r at various sample sizes (n) at the alpha of .05. Alpha values are probability cutoffs to our decision rule, so in this case, we want to only consider likelihoods as significant when they occur at or less than 5% of the time. Another way to think about it is that the alpha is the converse or opposite of the confidence we have in our significance statement. So, if $p < .05$, we can be at least 95% confident that we can reject H_0. Given our example, we would use the critical value of r for $n = 14$ with degrees of freedom (df) = 12 (14 − 2), which is 0.532. If r (calculated) $\geq r$ (critical), we can be 95% confident that the association is not because of random chance. Note that analysis programs such as Excel will compute the correlation coefficient, r, but they do not provide the critical value of r or the probability associated with r. Here,

TABLE 3.7 Critical Values of *r*

n	*df*	*r*
5	3	0.878
6	4	0.811
7	5	0.754
8	6	0.707
9	7	0.666
10	8	0.632
11	9	0.602
12	10	0.576
13	11	0.553
14	12	0.532
15	13	0.514
16	14	0.497
17	15	0.482
18	16	0.468
19	17	0.456
20	18	0.444
22	20	0.423
24	22	0.404
26	24	0.388
28	26	0.374
30	28	0.361
40	38	0.312
50	48	0.279
60	58	0.254
80	78	0.222
100	98	0.196

Note: Correlation coefficient: $r = .855$; critical value of $r = .532$, $n = 14$.
df, degrees of freedom.

the calculated *r* value (0.979) is greater than the critical *r* value (0.532), so we can say that there is a statistically significant positive correlation between ED visits and lab tests. For each additional ED visit (1 unit), we would expect lab test volume to increase by 0.977 units. Video 3.4 shows how to calculate a correlation using the Excel analytic function.

t Tests

A second common analysis is to examine a continuously measured variable at two points in time or in two locations. For example, say we wish to compare the number of births at Port City

TABLE 3.8 Comparative Monthly Births for Port City Hospital Versus Other U.S. Hospitals Sample

	PORT CITY HOSPITAL	UNITED STATES SIMILAR-SIZED HOSPITALS
January	24	22
February	25	21
March	33	26
April	35	27
May	37	31
June	38	25
July	41	36
August	35	27
September	45	39
October	39	35
November	42	34
December	50	23
Mean	**37**	**29**

Hospital with other U.S. hospitals of comparable size. To do so, we collect data over 12 months, as shown in **Table 3.8**.

Examining the data, we see that that for all months, Port City Hospital facilitates more births than the average hospital of similar size in the United States and that the mean number of births over the period was 37 at Port City and 29 at other hospitals. Our question is whether the data we see here for 1 year represent the "true or authentic" relationship between Port City and other hospitals of comparable size. Because this is only a sample of data from 1 year, we must use statistics to assess this. First, however, we should state our hypotheses.

Step 1: State Hypotheses

H_0: *There is no difference between the mean number of births at Port City Hospital and other U.S. hospitals of comparable size.*

H_a: *There is a difference between the mean number of births at Port City Hospital and other U.S. hospitals of comparable size.*

Step 2: Determine the Appropriate Test Statistic

To test the difference between two means requires the use of a *t* test. *T* tests are used to compare means between two groups and can also be used to compare a mean value to some other hypothesized value. One may also use a *z* test if the sample size is >30. Here, we will use a *t* test. For group comparisons of means, the groups can be paired or different. A paired group analysis would be some group of individuals who is measured on some variable, for example, blood pressure, and then undergoes some intervention, for example, an exercise routine, and then blood pressure is remeasured. The groups can also be different, as is the case with our comparison of mean births at Port City Hospital with other hospitals. What cannot be compared are means for different variables, such as the mean average length of stay compared with the mean number of births. The means must be measured in similar units for comparison with a *t* test. One may also wish to see if a group mean is different from a static value. Say we know the mean blood pressure for all patients with prediabetes and wish to test our patient group against that value to see if it is truly "different." Here, we could use a t test as well.

Step 3: Create Our Decision Rule

If t (calculated) $\geq t$ (critical) we will reject H_0.

Step 4: Determine t (calculated)

All test statistics have formulas to calculate them out. We will not delve into these here. Most analytic software, including Excel, can calculate a number of tests, including t tests. What is important to note is that the different types of t tests (paired, assuming equal variances, and assuming unequal variances) revolve, as the names suggest, around variation of the data. For our purposes, we will assume that variances are unequal in cases other than paired data. In practice, this difference in variances would be analyzed with an F test, and some programs will provide output for both equal and unequal variances assumed. Because Excel does not do this, assume unequal variances. Rarely will the interpretation differ between the two, but it can. The t-test output for our data is shown in **Table 3.9**.

In **Table 3.9,** we are given a number of analytic outputs. The first is the mean of the data for both Port City Hospital and other similarly sized hospitals in the United States. We are also given the variance and the number of observations. The hypothesized mean difference is simply the null hypothesis restated. Examining the lower half of the table, we are given the t statistic, the probability of t for both one-sided and two-tailed tests, and the critical value of t that cuts off the upper or lower 2.5% of the distribution (one tailed) and the value of t that cuts off the upper and lower 2.5% of the distribution (two tailed). Thus, values of the t statistic that lie beyond the critical value are statistically significant (different) at the 95% level of confidence. Here, we would use a two-tailed p value because our hypothesis was not directional. That is, our null stated that the mean number of births was different but not in which direction (greater than or less than). Doing so would require a one-tailed test because we would only be interested in values at one end of the distribution. Here,

TABLE 3.9 t-Test Excel Output Comparing Mean Monthly Births at Port City Hospital to Those at Other U.S. Hospitals Sample

t TEST: TWO-SAMPLE ASSUMING UNEQUAL VARIANCES		
	Port City Hospital	**United States Similar-Sized Hospitals**
Mean	37	29
Variance	56	35.97
Observations	12	12
Hypothesized mean difference	0	
df	21	
t statistics	2.9499	
$P(T \leq t)$ one tail	0.0038	
t (critical) one tail	1.7207	
$P(T \leq t)$ two tail	0.0076	
t (critical) two tail	2.0796	

it does not matter, so we conduct and interpret the two-tailed test. Interpreting the t statistic, we see that t (calculated) = 2.95, t (critical, two tail) = 2.07, and $p(t)$ = 0.0007 which is <0.05. Video 3.5 examines the calculation of the t test using Excel.

Step 5: Make Conclusions

Recall our decision rule from Step 3, that if t (calculated) is ≥t (critical)—in this case, 2.95 ≥ 2.07— we reject H_0. This condition is met, so we would reject the null hypothesis. Otherwise stated, our hypotheses ask what the likelihood is of seeing a difference in observed means as large as the one we did (8 births) if in fact the real difference were zero (the null hypothesis). Examining our t (calculated) relative to the critical values tells us the likelihood is <5% of the time. Examining our p value tells us the exact likelihood, which is <0.7% of the time (0.0076). So, if we continue to collect samples of data, the means would likely only be the same in 0.76% of samples.

We may often be interested in analysis of two variables measured categorically through rates or proportions. Examples of these types of data include the following: What type of insurance does the patient have? What is their gender? Were they satisfied with their visit? Summarizing these involves creating counts and percentages. However, often we wish to compare how two groups of categories compare with one another. We do this using the chi-square statistic (X^2), which compares the observed differences in proportions with what would be expected if proportions were equal. For example, if we were to examine the satisfied/unsatisfied percentages of 40 men and 40 women on a satisfaction questionnaire, we would expect that if they were equal, 20 would say satisfied and 20 would not in each gender category (or 50% for each). When we observe actual data, however, we often see different results. The basic null and alternative hypotheses hold true here. The question we are asking is what is the chance of seeing a difference of the magnitude observed in the collected data if in fact there is no true difference (all proportions are equal) in the population. The chi-square statistic and its associated probability allow us to test these hypotheses. The simplest form of chi-square analysis is of two variables using a 2×2 contingency table, shown in **Table 3.10**.

Examine the data in **Table 3.11** that depict satisfaction responses from a survey at two campuses of a clinic group. The null hypothesis would state that there is, in truth, no actual difference between satisfied and unsatisfied respondents by campus location. The alternative would be that the difference observed is real. To calculate the chi-square, we use Equation 3.2:

TABLE 3.10   2 × 2 Contingency Table Layout

	GROUP 1	GROUP 2	TOTAL
Variable 1	a	b	$a+b$
Variable 2	c	d	$c+d$
Total	$a+c$	$b+d$	$a+b+c+d$

TABLE 3.11   Patient Satisfaction by Campus Location

	EAST CAMPUS	WEST CAMPUS	TOTAL
Satisfied	36	17	53
Not satisfied	30	35	65
Total	66	52	118

TABLE 3.12 Chi-Square Calculation of Table 3.11 Data

	OBSERVED (O)	EXPECTED (E)	O −	(O − E)²	$\frac{(O-E)^2}{E}$
	36	29.6	6.4	40.96	1.38
	17	23.4	−6.4	40.96	1.75
	30	36.4	−6.4	40.96	1.13
	35	28.6	6.4	40.96	1.43
Total	118	118	0	163.84	**5.69**

Equation 3.2

$$\chi^2 = \frac{\Sigma\,(\text{Observed} - \text{Expected})^2}{\text{Expected}}$$

where the expected count is:

$$\frac{(\text{Row Total} \times \text{Cplumn Total})}{n}$$

This formula yields the results in **Table 3.12** and the chi-square statistic of 5.69. Constructing the expected values will be further helpful when using Excel to calculate the chi-square statistic.

This generates a chi-square statistic that must then be examined relative to the distribution of chi-squares for the given *df*. *Df* are calculated by taking the number of rows minus one multiplied by the number of columns minus one. In this example, we have one *df*.

In practice, most computer programs and many applet-driven web pages provide the chi-square statistic and corresponding significance when examining two or more categorical variables. When examining any categorical variable with more than two response categories, such as satisfaction levels or agreement scales, the chi-square statistic has a slightly different interpretive meaning. The null hypothesis remains the same in this case. However, we now observe differences not just between two categories (one and two) but between multiple categories (two and three, one and three, three and four, two and four, etc.). The chi-square can only tell us if the differences overall between the categories is significantly different than what we would expect but does not test the differences between individual categories.

SUMMARY

This chapter has presented a tool kit of basic statistical techniques to help guide the health services manager with basic quantitative analysis. This was not meant to be an exhaustive statistical review but an applied, user-friendly introduction to statistics commonly used in making many healthcare-related decisions. The first step in any analysis is to determine whether one is examining one variable or data point or comparing more than one variable. When examining one variable at a time, we use descriptive statistics, and depending on whether the variable is continuous or categorical, different analyses are used.

Performing the appropriate type of analysis on the data at hand can often be confusing for many, which is why we have segmented analysis by the type of data being examined. Sound statistics and presentation skills afford the healthcare manager a clear and defensible way to both ask pertinent questions and construct evidence to answer those questions. The competent manager's job is to know which questions to ask and how to construct hypotheses and analyze data appropriately. By following the simple rules presented here, data can be categorized based on how they are measured (categorical or continuous), and from there, a defined set of analysis options can be applied to each type. It is further incumbent upon the analyst to present the data in a clear and understandable way but also to describe fully and cite the data used. These basic analyses will provide the foundation for many of the other managerial competencies described later in this book. It is also important to remember that all analyses rest within strategic considerations and questions. Knowing these is important prior to conducting analysis. Further, these methods utilize probability as the guardrails for making decisions; however, these too are just estimates. If you recall, they help us determine why we can be certain we are at least partially certain.

END-OF-CHAPTER RESOURCES

DISCUSSION QUESTIONS

1. Use the four basic guiding questions (Where are we now? Where do we want to go? How will we get there? Who will we know when we are there?) to plan a trip to Hawaii.
   a. How specific were you when answering?
   b. What questions came up or needed to be answered before answering the bigger questions?
   c. What types of measurement did you employ?
2. What is something in a health or healthcare setting that is described on a regular basis?
   a. Is it a continuously measured data element or categorical?
   b. What types of descriptive measurements would you employ for that variable?
   c. Pick another variable that represents the other measurement type (e.g., if you picked continuous, now pick a categorical variable). What types of descriptive measures would you now employ?
3. Describe a situation where you would be required to compare two variables or data measurements.
4. Describe something that would be useful to predict.
   a. What are the challenges with making those predictions? Be broad in your thinking.
   b. Are all of them surmountable?
   c. What happens to our prediction if we cannot account for all the unknowns?
5. Talk about the nature of having confidence and using hypotheses in your analysis. What are the benefits in doing so?
6. Develop an analysis from start to finish.
   a. Consider a question that could be of interest to answer.
   b. Define your hypotheses and consider what type of data you would need.
   c. Assuming you are able to collect a sample of that data, what statistical test would you need to conduct and what would be the criteria for rejecting your null hypotheses?

LEARNING ACTIVITIES

CourseConnect ▸

To access self-assessment questions and interactive, competency-based learning activities for this chapter, visit www.springerpub.com/courseconnect. See inside front cover and tear-out card for CourseConnect details.

REFERENCE

Morey, R. D., Hoekstra, R., Rouder, J. N., Lee, M. D., & Wagenmakers, E.-J. (2016). The fallacy of placing confidence in confidence intervals. *Psychonomic Bulletin & Review, 23*(1), 103–123. https://doi.org/10.3758/s13423-015-0947-8

CHAPTER 4

DATA DISPLAY

LEARNING OBJECTIVES

4.1. Select the most appropriate chart type for a given data set and communication goal.

4.2. Interpret data distribution patterns with histograms and box-and-whiskers charts.

4.3. Analyze the relationship between two continuous variables with scatterplots.

4.4. Construct line charts that illustrate changes in values over time.

4.5. Compare categorical variables with bar charts and column charts.

4.6. Examine composition with pie charts and donut charts.

4.7. Create pivot tables and pivot table charts to summarize and analyze data.

4.8. Apply design principles for visualizations to enhance clarity and effectiveness.

4.9. Recognize the advantages of dashboards for exploring and tracking dynamic data.

REAL-WORLD SCENARIO

As the director of maternal health at Metro General Hospital, Dr. Sophia Gonzalez has been closely monitoring the hospital's rates of cesarean section (C-section) deliveries. Recently, hospital administrators have raised concerns about an increase in C-section rates and rising costs associated with the procedures. They want to understand whether these trends are unique to their hospital or part of a broader pattern.

Dr. Gonzalez and her team have access to a rich data set containing detailed information on C-section patients at Metro General. The data set includes patient demographics, severity of illness, length of stay, payment types, and the total charges associated with each procedure. The hospital's leadership has tasked her with analyzing this data to uncover key insights. They need to know: What is the typical cost of C-sections at their hospital? Might there be some patients with unusually high costs who might be driving up the average? And might their patient population have unique characteristics (e.g., higher risk of mortality) that could be driving up costs? Dr. Gonazlez knows that she can use data visualizations to explore these questions and communicate her findings effectively to hospital leadership.

In the world of healthcare management, data is abundant, but its value lies in how effectively it can be translated into actionable insights. Data visualizations serve as a bridge between raw data and meaningful decision-making, offering healthcare managers the ability to identify trends, relationships, and outliers at a glance. Whether you are evaluating operational metrics, analyzing patient outcomes, or communicating findings to stakeholders, clear and well-designed visualizations are essential tools.

This chapter provides a practical guide to creating and interpreting data visualizations. We explore how to choose the right chart type based on the data you have and the story you want to tell. Starting with basic chart types such as histograms, box-and-whiskers charts, bar charts, and pie charts, we build a foundation for visualizing distributions, relationships, and comparisons. From there, we delve into design principles and ethical considerations that ensure your charts are both impactful and trustworthy. Finally, we end with a demonstration of dashboards, which allow managers to visualize, explore, and monitor complex, dynamic data.

INTRODUCTION TO THE C-SECTION DATA SET (DATA SET 4.1)

In this chapter, we work with a data set in the "C-Section Data" Excel workbook that accompanies this textbook (Data Set 4.1). The data has three parts, each in its own sheet that appears as a tab at the bottom of the Excel workbook. The first tab is "patient data," and it contains patient-level C-section data modeled after real data from a hospital in the New York City area in 2017. "Patient data" includes information on the patient's ethnicity, their length of stay (in days), and the type of admission (elective vs. emergency). There are also descriptions of the severity of illness and the risk of mortality, which range from minor to extreme. Finally, we have information on payment typology (i.e., insurance type); the total charges, which is the total cost for all the services that the patient received at the hospital; and the total cost, which shows the total payment that the hospital received for their services.

The second tab of the workbook is called "data summaries," and it shows different ways to group the patient-level data. For example, we can see the average length of stay for each of the mortality risk categories and the total number of patients for different races and ethnicities in this data set.

The third tab of the workbook has two sets of data. The first shows the annual average C-section rate (as a percentage of all births) for New York State between 2005 and 2022 (Centers for Disease Control and Prevention, 2022). The second set of data shows the annual average C-section rate (as a percentage of singleton births) for different races and ethnicities in New York state from 2003 to 2012 (New York State Department of Health, n.d.).

LEARNING OBJECTIVE 4.1: SELECT THE MOST APPROPRIATE CHART TYPE FOR A GIVEN DATA SET AND COMMUNICATION GOAL

Charts are indispensable tools for summarizing and communicating data. In this section, we focus on fundamental chart types that help visualize data distributions, relationships, and comparisons. From histograms and box-and-whiskers charts that uncover patterns in numerical data; to scatterplots that reveal relationships between continuous variables; to line charts that reveal trends through time; and bar, column, pie, and donut charts that clarify categorical data, these visualizations are versatile tools for healthcare managers. By mastering these basics, you can confidently interpret and present data in ways that inform evidence-based decision-making.

The first step in creating a chart is selecting a type that aligns your data with the message you want to communicate. The chart selection guide (**Figure 4.1**) in this chapter simplifies this process by outlining key chart types, the data they represent, and their primary purposes. By aligning your data format and communication goals to the right chart, you can create visualizations that deliver insights clearly and effectively. Let us explore each chart type, starting with the histogram.

FIGURE 4.1 Chart selection guide.

Data Type	Chart Purpose	Chart Type	
Numerical	Displaying data distributions	Histogram	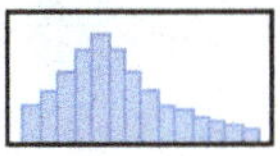
	Displaying quartiles, mean and median, and outliers	Box-and-whisker plot	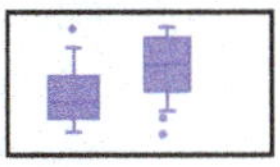
	Visualizing the relationship between two variables	Scatterplot	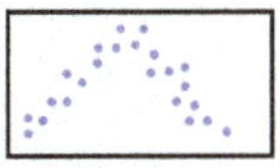
	Visualizing trends through time	Line chart	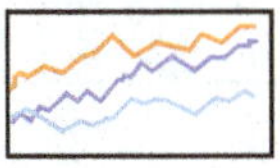
Categorical	Comparing a few categories	Column chart	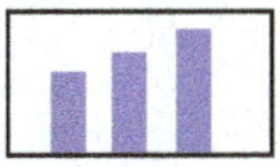
	Comparing many categories	Bar chart	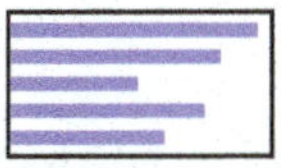
	Visualizing the contribution of parts to a whole	Pie chart	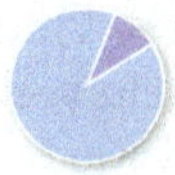
	Emphasizing the proportions of categories	Donut chart	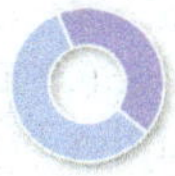

LEARNING OBJECTIVE 4.2: INTERPRET DATA DISTRIBUTION PATTERNS WITH HISTOGRAMS AND BOX-AND-WHISKERS CHARTS

 **VIDEOS FOR LEARNING OBJECTIVE 4.2**

- Video 4.1A How to Create a Histogram in Excel
- Video 4.1B How to Create a Histogram in Tableau
- Video 4.2A How to Create a Box-and-Whiskers Chart in Excel
- Video 4.2B How to Create a Box-and-Whiskers Chart in Tableau

A histogram takes a numerical variable and divides it into intervals of equal sizes. Then, it counts how many data points fall within each interval. For example, to create a histogram for the total charges in the "patient-level data" of our C-section data set (Data Set 4.1), we can divide that variable into bins of $10,000 (**Figure 4.2**). The histogram helps us see that there were

FIGURE 4.2 Histogram of total charges from the C-section data (Data Set 4.1).

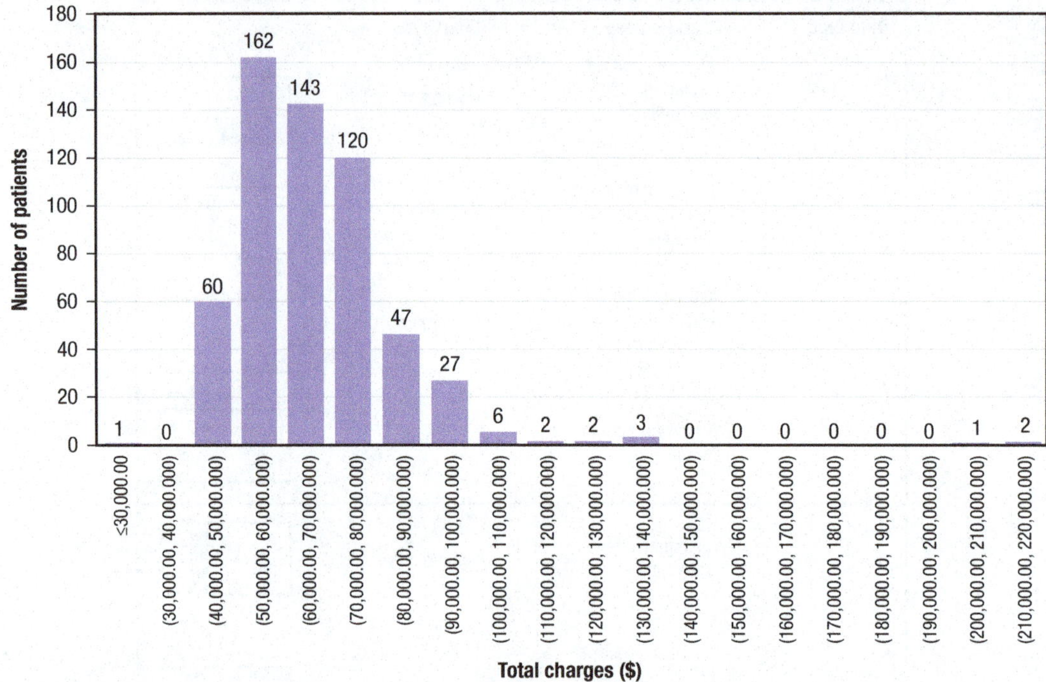

60 patients with total charges that were between $40,000 and $50,000, 162 patients with total charges that were between $50,000 and $60,000, and so on. Video 4.1A shows how to create this histogram in Excel. Video 4.1B shows how to create it in Tableau.

Histograms help you quickly grasp the distribution of the data—that is, they allow you to see its range and where your data points fall within that range. From the C-section histogram, we can see that the values for the total charges range from less than $30,000 up to $220,000. Most patients had total charges that fell between $40,000 and $100,000, with the majority having charges between $50,000 and $80,000. If someone asked you, "What is the typical total charge for a C-section at this hospital?" You could briefly glance at this histogram and answer, "Usually somewhere between $50,000 and $80,000."

The histogram also helps us see that the total charges variable also has a long "tail" at the right-hand side, meaning that there were a small number of patients who had total charges that were much higher than the typical patient. For example, one patient had a charge between $200,000 and $210,000, and two patients had a charge between $210,000 and $220,000. One drawback of histograms is that sometimes it can be hard to see the extreme values if the bars that represent them are very small. A better way to visualize these outliers in the data is to use a box-and-whiskers chart.

As its name suggests, the box-and-whiskers chart consists of a box with two "whiskers" extending from it. To create this chart, you first sort your data from least to greatest. Then, you find the median and the 1st and 3rd quartiles. These numbers will determine the position of the different components of the chart. Suppose your data consists of the following numbers:

1, 3, 4, 4, 5, 5 6, 7, 7, 9, 10, 10, 10

The median, or middle number, is 6. Next, we find the 1st quartile, which is going to be the midpoint between the lowest number (1) and the number before the median (5). In this case, the 1st quartile is between the numbers 3 and 4, so it takes the value of 3.5. Finally, we find the 3rd quartile, which is the midpoint between the number after the median (7) and the highest number (10). The 3rd quartile is between 9 and 10, so it takes the value of 9.5.

FIGURE 4.3 Box-and-whiskers chart of a sample data set.

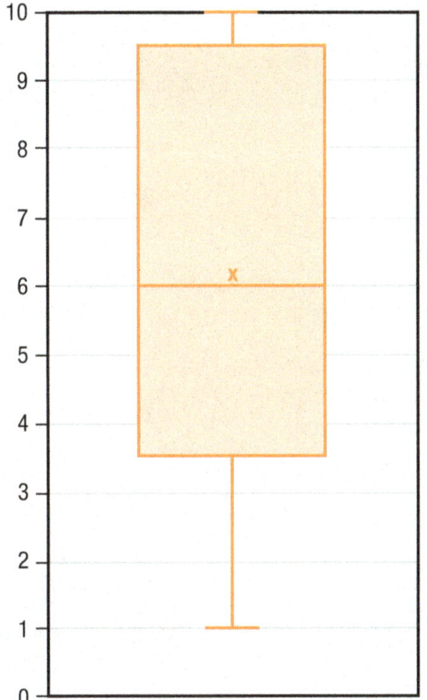

Figure 4.3 shows the box-and-whiskers chart that would result from these numbers. The lower bound of the box is at 3.5, which is the 1st quartile. The next horizontal line is the median (or 2nd quartile), at 6. There is an "x" just above the median. It represents the mean, which, for this data set, is 6.15. The upper bound of the box is at 9.5, which is the 3rd quartile. Finally, the whiskers extend down to the lowest number (1) and up to the highest number (10). The chart allows us to see that our data is skewed toward higher numbers because the box, which represents the middle 50% of our data, is not centered between 1 and 10. Instead, it is closer to 10, indicating a concentration of values near the upper bound.

Let us now examine a box-and-whiskers chart for the total charges in the C-section data (Data Set 4.1). In Figure 4.4, we can see that the lower whisker extends to the lowest value in the data set, which is $25,577.83. The lower bound of the box is at $55,033.96, the upper bound is at $74,914.92, and the upper whisker extends to $103,760.05. We see that there are additional data points beyond the upper whisker. These are the outliers in the data. Take a moment to compare this box-and-whiskers chart to the histogram we created with the same data in Figure 4.2. Video 4.2A shows how to create this chart in Excel; Video 4.2B shows how to create it in Tableau.

Data visualization applications may not always draw the whiskers in the same way. For example, Excel drew the upper whisker at the 95th percentile of our data. Other visualization applications may calculate the end of the upper whisker by adding the 3rd quartile plus 1.5 times the interquartile range (IQR). In this example, it would be:

$$\$74,914.92 + [1.5 \times (\$74,914.92 - \$55.033.96)] = \$104,736.40.$$

Likewise, the lower whisker may be at the 5th percentile of the data or at the 1st quartile minus 1.5 times the IQR. It is important to know which method is being applied so that the visualization can be interpreted correctly.

FIGURE 4.4 **Box-and-whiskers chart of total charges from the C-section data (Data Set 4.1).**

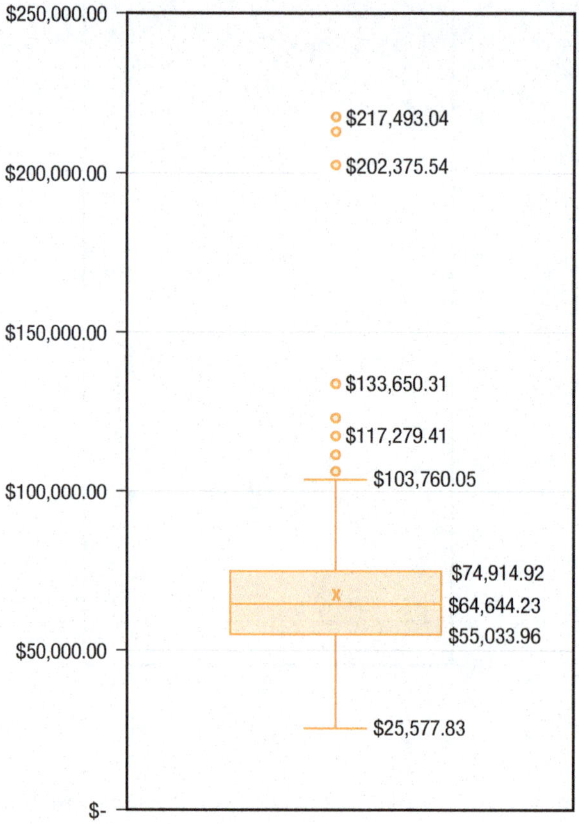

LEARNING OBJECTIVE 4.3: ANALYZE THE RELATIONSHIP BETWEEN TWO CONTINUOUS VARIABLES WITH SCATTERPLOTS

▶ VIDEOS FOR LEARNING OBJECTIVE 4.3

- Video 4.3A How to Create a Scatterplot Chart in Excel
- Video 4.3B How to Create a Scatterplot Chart in Tableau

Histograms and box-and-whiskers charts allow us to examine the distribution of a single, continuous variable. If we want to evaluate whether *two* continuous variables have a relationship with each other, we can use a scatterplot. Let us consider two continuous variables in our C-section data set (Data Set 4.1): total charges and total cost. Hospitals set standard dollar amounts for each of the services they provide. For any given patient, the amount in the total charges column reflects the grand total of these standardized costs. However, the hospital often receives a payment that is *less* than the total cost because payment rates are affected by the patient's insurance. The amount that the hospital actually receives for each patient is shown in the total cost column. Do you think it is likely that there is a relationship between total charges and total cost? Perhaps we can expect that a higher amount in the total charges column would also correspond to a higher amount in the total cost column. Is that true? A scatterplot can give us the answer.

To create the scatterplot, we use total charges on the horizontal axis (*x*-axis) and the total cost on the vertical axis (*y*-axis). Each dot on the scatterplot represents one row of data, which in this

FIGURE 4.5 **Scatterplot for total cost versus total charges from the C-section data (Data Set 4.1).**

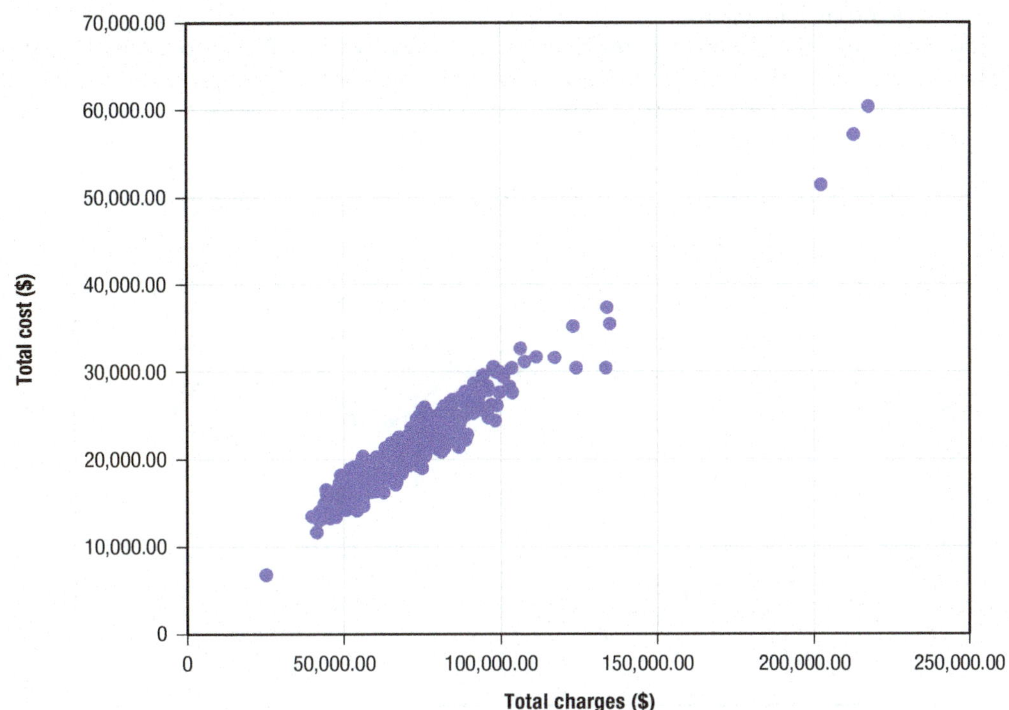

case, is one patient. Let us look at the very first row of the data set, in which the patient has total charges of $70,584.33 and total cost of $20,328.96. To place that person's dot on the scatterplot, we would first find the place along the horizontal axis where the total charges equals $70,584.33, and then we would travel up until the total cost equals $20,328.96. When we do this for every patient, we get a scatterplot like the one in **Figure 4.5**. Video 4.3A shows how to create this chart in Excel; Video 4.3B shows how to create it in Tableau.

There seems to be a relationship between total charges and total cost. As patients' total charges increase, the total cost increases as well. We can also see that most of the points tend to fall closely along an imaginary straight line drawn through the points. This suggests that there is a strong correlation between the two variables of total charges and total cost. The strength of this relationship could be quantified by calculating a correlation coefficient (see Chapter 3, "Statistical and Analytical Foundations"). If you wanted to create a model to predict a patient's total cost based on their total charges, you could use a simple linear regression (see Chapter 14, "Linear Regression Forecasting").

LEARNING OBJECTIVE 4.4: CONSTRUCT LINE CHARTS THAT ILLUSTRATE CHANGES IN VALUES OVER TIME

 ### VIDEOS FOR LEARNING OBJECTIVE 4.4

- Video 4.4A How to Create a Line Chart in Excel
- Video 4.4B How to Create a Line Chart in Tableau

Line charts are an excellent choice for visualizing how a numeric variable changes over time. The C-section Excel workbook (Data Set 4.1) has a sheet named "NY State Data." The first two columns of that sheet show the annual C-section rates as a percentage of all births from 2005 to 2022 in New York State. To create a line chart of this data, we place "year" in the *x*-axis and "C-section rate" in the *y*-axis (**Figure 4.6**). Video 4.4A shows how to create this chart in Excel; Video 4.4B shows how to create it in Tableau.

The chart shows that C-section rates increased steadily between 2005 and 2009 and then generally decreased, with some fluctuations. However, note that the *y*-axis ranges from 31 to 35.5. If we were to change the *y*-axis to start at zero, the changes in the data through time are not nearly as pronounced (**Figure 4.7**).

FIGURE 4.6 Line chart of C-section rates in New York State from 2005 to 2022.

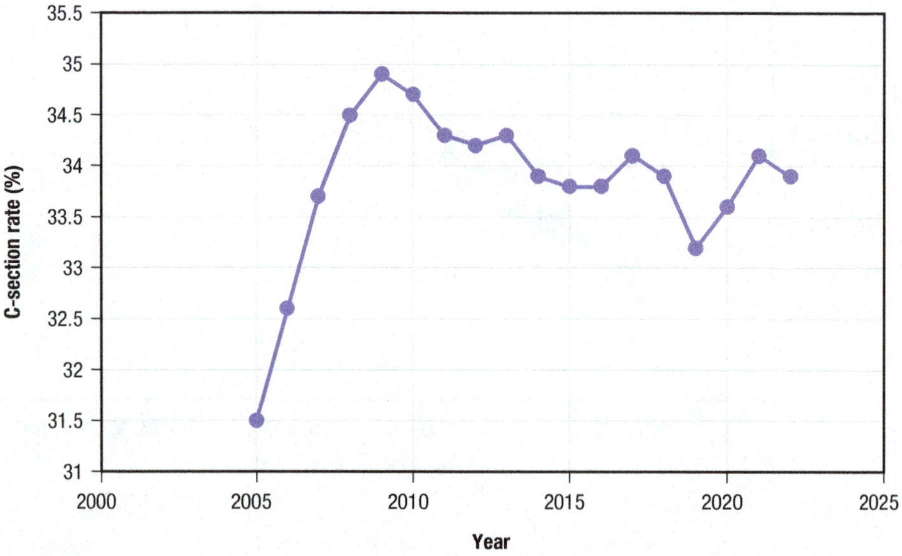

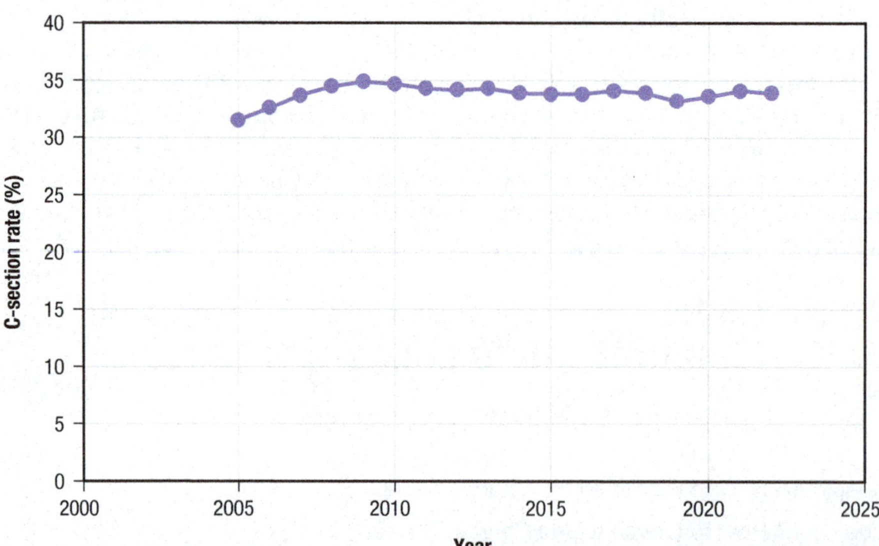

Source: Data from Centers for Disease Control and Prevention. (2022, February 25). *Cesarean delivery rate by state*. National Center for Health Statistics. https://www.cdc.gov/nchs/pressroom/sosmap/cesarean _births/cesareans.htm

FIGURE 4.7 Starting the *y*-axis at zero changes the appearance of the line chart.

Source: Data from Centers for Disease Control and Prevention. (2022, February 25). *Cesarean delivery rate by state*. National Center for Health Statistics. https://www.cdc.gov/nchs/pressroom/sosmap/cesarean _births/cesareans.htm

FIGURE 4.8 Line chart of C-section rates in New York State by race.

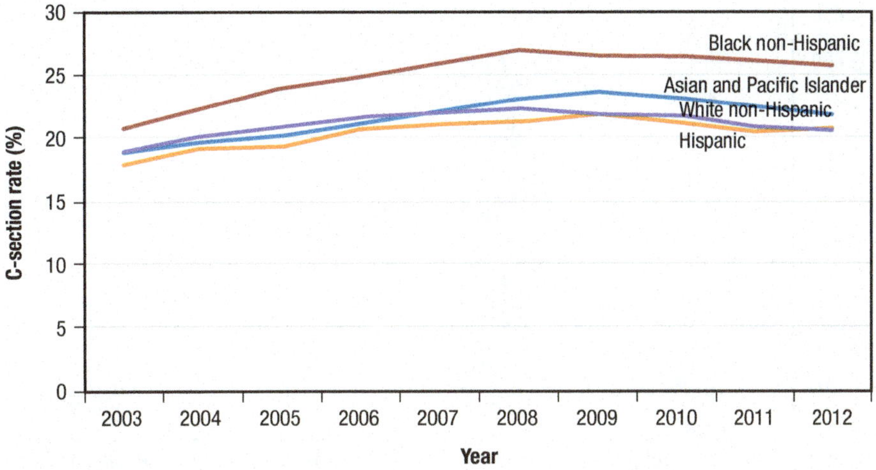

Source: Data from New York State Department of Health. (n.d.). *Primary cesarean delivery, 2003-2012.* https://www.health.ny.gov/statistics/vital_statistics/docs/primary_cesarean_delivery_2003-2012.pdf

When using line charts, the question of whether the *y*-axis should start at zero depends on the context and on the goal of the chart. If small differences in values are meaningful, or if you would like to determine whether there have been trends through a window of time, then it may be best *not* to start at zero because the differences or patterns may be diluted by the scale. However, if absolute values are important, then starting at zero ensures that the visual difference you see between points is proportional to their actual values. If you start the *y*-axis at anything other than zero, it is good practice to highlight this for your audience so that they are not inadvertently misled.

Line charts can also be used to visualize changes in the numeric values of multiple categories through time. The second set of columns in the "NY State data" Excel sheet shows the annual C-section rates of singleton births for four different races and ethnicities (Asian and Pacific Islander, Black non-Hispanic, Hispanic, and White non-Hispanic). A line chart created from this data (**Figure 4.8**) shows racial disparities in the rate of C-sections through time. Black non-Hispanics have had a consistently higher C-section rate than other groups. Asian and Pacific Islanders had similar rates to White non-Hispanics and Hispanics, but from 2008 onward, they diverged toward slightly higher rates. All groups seem to have had gradual increases in C-section rates that peaked around 2007 to 2009 and then declined very slightly.

LEARNING OBJECTIVE 4.5: COMPARE CATEGORICAL VARIABLES WITH BAR CHARTS AND COLUMN CHARTS

▶ VIDEOS FOR LEARNING OBJECTIVE 4.5

- Video 4.5A How to Create Column and Bar Charts in Excel
- Video 4.5B How to Create Column and Bar Charts in Tableau

The "data summaries" tab of the "C-section data" Excel file (Data Set 4.1) summarizes the patient-level C-section data by patient demographics, payment typology, risk of mortality, and type of admission. We use these data summaries to visualize relationships among different patient categories with bar charts and column charts. Let us use a column chart to visualize how many patients we had for each of the four payment typology categories: Blue Cross/Blue Shield, Medicaid, Medicare, and private health insurance (**Figure 4.9**).

FIGURE 4.9 Column chart of payment typology for C-section data (Data Set 4.1).

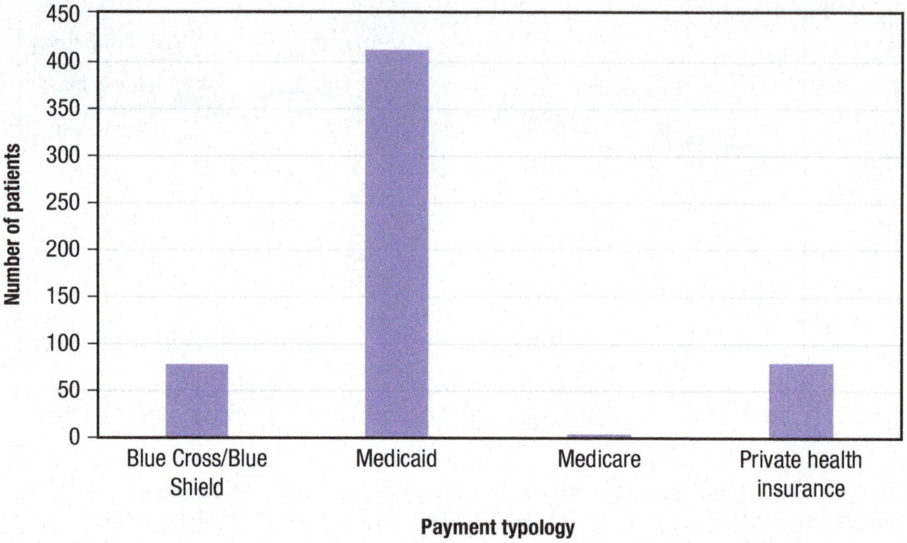

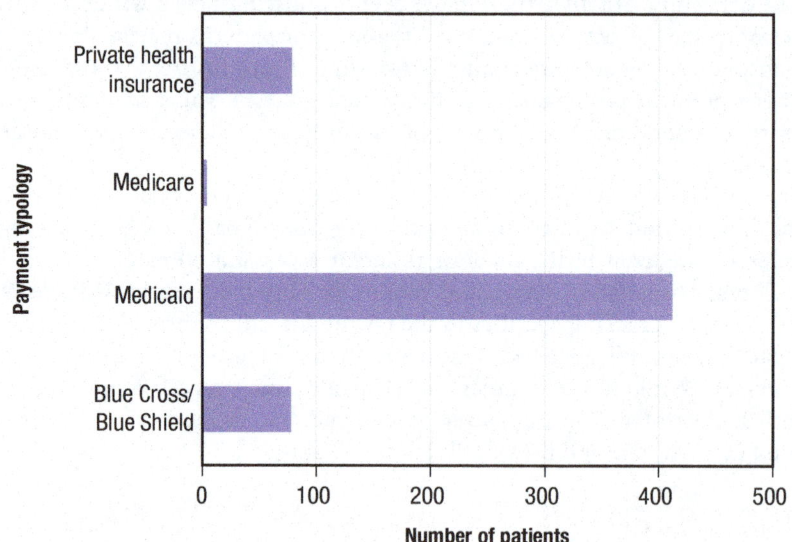

FIGURE 4.10 Bar chart of payment typology for C-section data (Data Set 4.1).

We can see immediately that most (>400) of the patients at this hospital used Medicaid to pay for their C-sections. A smaller number of patients used Blue Cross/Blue Shield or private health insurance, and a very small number of patients used Medicare.

Column charts use vertical bars to represent the data, while bar charts use horizontal bars (**Figure 4.10**). The decision to use one over the other usually comes down to personal preference, but there is one situation in which a bar chart has the advantage: if there are many categories to be displayed, a column chart can get crowded, and the labels may get truncated because there is usually a limited amount of horizontal space on a page. A bar chart, on the other hand, can keep expanding vertically to accommodate many more categories. Video 4.5A shows how to create column and bar charts in Excel; Video 4.5B shows how to create them in Tableau.

LEARNING OBJECTIVE 4.6: EXAMINE COMPOSITION WITH PIE CHARTS AND DONUT CHARTS

▶ VIDEOS FOR LEARNING OBJECTIVE 4.6

- Video 4.6A How to Create Pie and Donut Charts in Excel
- Video 4.6B How to Create Pie and Donut Charts in Tableau

Pie charts and donut charts are commonly used to visualize how different categories contribute to a whole. For example, let us examine how different categories of risk of mortality contribute to the overall number of C-section patients. This data can be found in the "data summaries" tab of the Excel file (Data Set 4.1). We can see four categories of risk of mortality (minor, moderate, major, and extreme), along with the number of patients in each category. A pie chart will divide a circle into slices, with each slice representing one of these four categories. The size of each slice in the pie will be proportional to the category's value as a percentage of the total. From the pie chart in **Figure 4.11**, we can see that the two categories with the highest number of patients are the minor and moderate risk of mortality. Accordingly, they have the two biggest slices of pie. Next is the major category, followed by extreme, which has such a small number of patients that its pie slice is just a sliver.

Pie charts are popular because they are visually appealing. They can be useful when you want to emphasize the relative contribution of each part to the whole. For example, if our goal is to highlight that the percentage of patients with extreme risk is very small, the pie chart can be an effective choice. As a rule of thumb, pie charts should only be used if there are fewer than five categories. Otherwise, the visualization can become cluttered, and as the number of categories increases, the size of the pie slices will decrease, which may make them harder to compare. This brings us to the main limitation of pie charts: the human brain is better at discerning differences in length than it is at discerning differences in angles or areas. If we had not labeled the pie chart

FIGURE 4.11 Pie chart showing the number of patients in each of the categories of mortality risk.

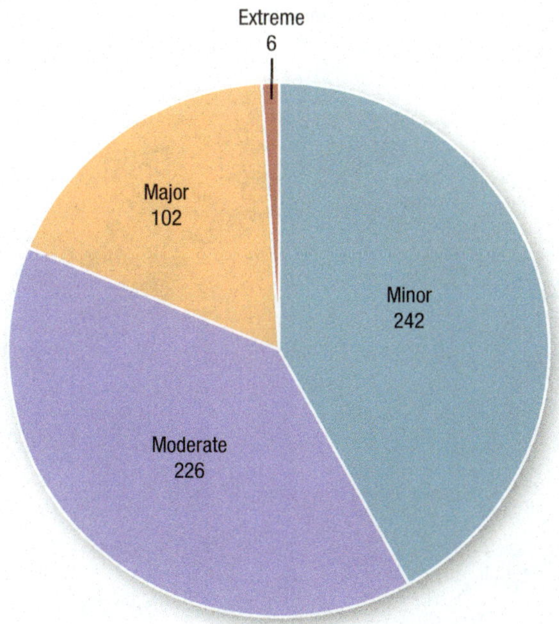

above with the number of patients in the minor or moderate categories, it probably would have been difficult for you to determine which one had more patients. However, if we represent the same data as a column chart (**Figure 4.12**), it is easier to see that the minor category had the most patients.

Donut charts are similar to pie charts, except that they have a hole in the center, like a donut. The advantage that a donut chart has over a pie chart is that it deemphasizes the role of the angles and areas and it draws more attention to the proportions instead. **Figure 4.13** shows the risk of

FIGURE 4.12 Bar chart showing the number of patients in each of the categories of mortality risk.

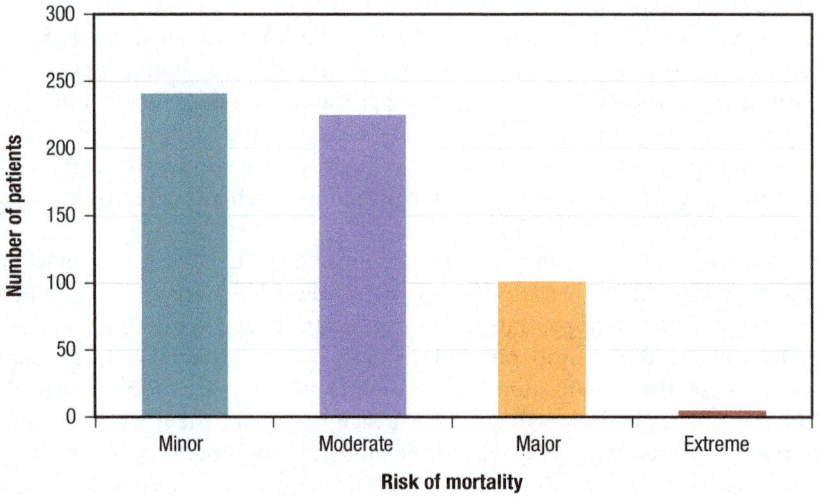

FIGURE 4.13 Donut chart showing the number of patients in each of the mortality risk categories.

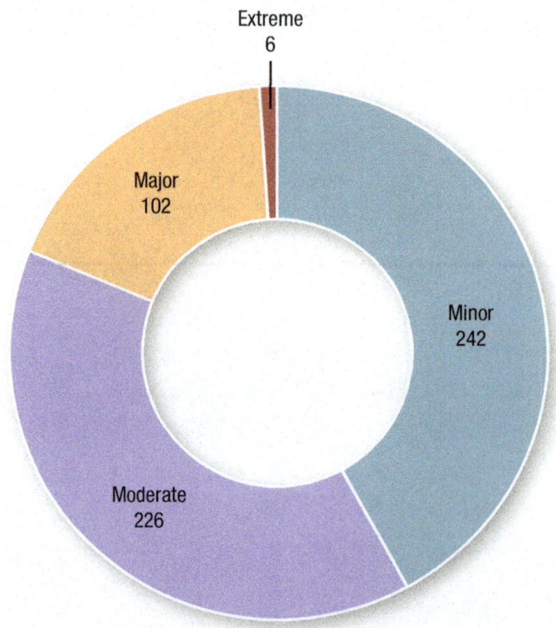

mortality data as a donut chart. Video 4.6A shows how to create pie and donut charts in Excel; Video 4.6B shows how to create them in Tableau.

Mastering the use of basic charts is a crucial step toward effective data visualization. Each chart type serves a specific purpose: histograms and box-and-whiskers charts illuminate the distribution of numerical data; scatterplots reveal relationships between continuous variables; line charts show trends through time; and bar, column, pie, and donut charts highlight comparisons and compositions in categorical data. These tools, when used thoughtfully, can transform complex data sets into clear, actionable insights. Understanding their strengths and limitations ensures that your visualizations communicate information accurately and effectively.

LEARNING OBJECTIVE 4.7: CREATE PIVOT TABLES AND PIVOT TABLE CHARTS TO SUMMARIZE AND ANALYZE DATA

 ### VIDEOS FOR LEARNING OBJECTIVE 4.7

- Video 4.7A How to Create a Pivot Table in Excel
- Video 4.7B How to Create a Pivot Table in Tableau

In some data visualization applications such as Excel, patient-level data cannot be used directly to create the column, bar, pie, and donut charts displayed in the previous section. Instead, the data first must be summarized or grouped by using pivot tables. Video 4.7A shows how to create a pivot table in Excel; Video 4.7B shows how to create their equivalent in Tableau. Once the variables of interest have been selected, pivot tables will provide different options for aggregating the values. For example, if we place the APR_Risk_Of_Mortality variable in the Rows section of the Pivot Table Fields and we place the Length_Of_Stay variable in the Values section, the data will be aggregated automatically by Sum. This means that, for each category of mortality (e.g., minor), Excel will find all the patients within that category and sum all their lengths of stay. If we change the aggregation type to Count, then Excel will count how many patients we have within each category. Selecting Average as the aggregation type will calculate the average length of stay within each category, and so on. Excel has additional aggregation types that can be used to summarize data in other ways.

LEARNING OBJECTIVE 4.8: APPLY DESIGN PRINCIPLES FOR VISUALIZATIONS TO ENHANCE CLARITY AND EFFECTIVENESS

Data visualizations are a powerful tool for communicating insights from data. Like any form of communication, it is important to tailor them to the audience and the context in which they will be received. When creating a chart, start by considering your audience's questions about the data. What are they trying to understand or decide? For example, healthcare administrators may need high-level summaries that provide actionable insights quickly, while clinical staff might need detailed, patient-level trends to inform day-to-day decision-making. Consider how much detail is appropriate for your audience. Too much detail can be overwhelming, but too little detail might leave critical knowledge gaps. By anticipating your audience's needs, you can ensure that your visualizations are relevant and effective.

When creating data visualizations, you will have many formatting options available. Should you include labels for each data point in a line chart? Do you need gridlines? What colors should you use for your bar charts? These questions go beyond the aesthetics of the charts—they directly influence the effectiveness of your visualizations. By following some simple design principles, you can increase the clarity of your charts and enhance their impact.

Avoiding Clutter

Charts use symbols to represent data. When we look at a chart, our brains must decode these symbols by considering their color, shape, position on the chart, and their relationships to one another. Every element in a chart requires cognitive effort to interpret. When a chart is cluttered, the audience must do more mental work to understand the message we are trying to convey. In some cases, the clutter may be so overwhelming that the viewer gives up on interpreting the chart altogether. If we eliminate unnecessary chart elements, we help our audience interpret the chart more quickly and with less effort. In **Figure 4.14**, notice how much more difficult it is to interpret a chart when there are unnecessary, distracting elements such as extra grid lines and labels for many data points. It also takes more mental work to use a separate legend to identify which line belongs to each group.

Focusing the Audience's Attention

Visualizations are often used to highlight significant trends, anomalies, or outliers within a data set. Through strategic design choices, we can focus our audience's attention to the aspects of the data that matter most. Look back at **Figure 4.8**, which shows the C-section rates for four different races and ethnicities through time. When all four groups have different colors with similar color intensity, then none of them stand out from the rest. If we want our audience to notice that the rate for Black non-Hispanics has been consistently higher than the rest, we can lower the color intensity for the other categories so that it becomes more prominent (**Figure 4.15**).

Another effective approach is to display the category of interest in bold black and color the other categories in the same shade of gray (**Figure 4.16**).

Data markers and labels can also be used to draw attention to important points. For example, if we wanted to highlight the highest C-section rate observed for Black non-Hispanic patients, we could add a label that shows the value and the year in which it was observed (**Figure 4.17**).

Using Colors Thoughtfully

Choosing colors thoughtfully can ensure that the visualization conveys its intended message effectively. One important factor to consider is the cultural significance of colors. For instance, in

FIGURE 4.14 Example of a cluttered chart.

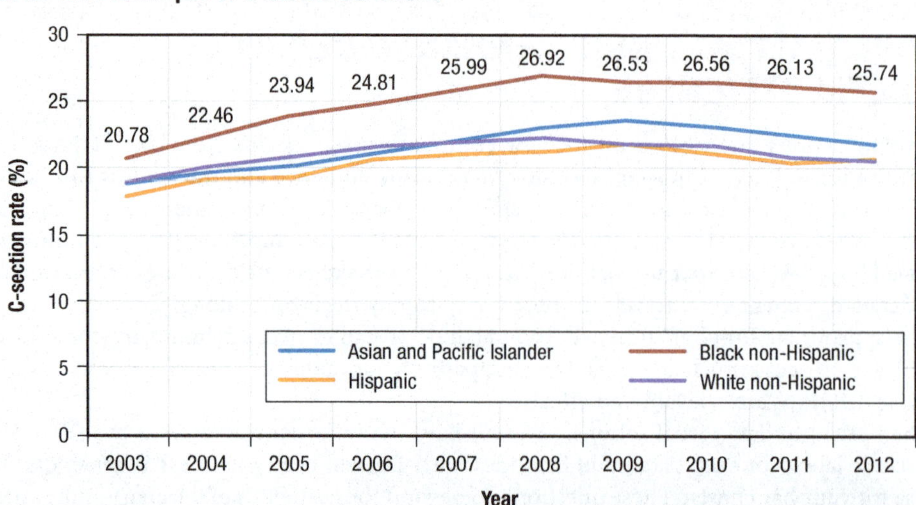

Source: Data from New York State Department of Health. (n.d.). *Primary cesarean delivery, 2003-2012.* https://www.health.ny.gov/statistics/vital_statistics/docs/primary_cesarean_delivery_2003-2012.pdf

FIGURE 4.15 Using color intensity to focus attention.

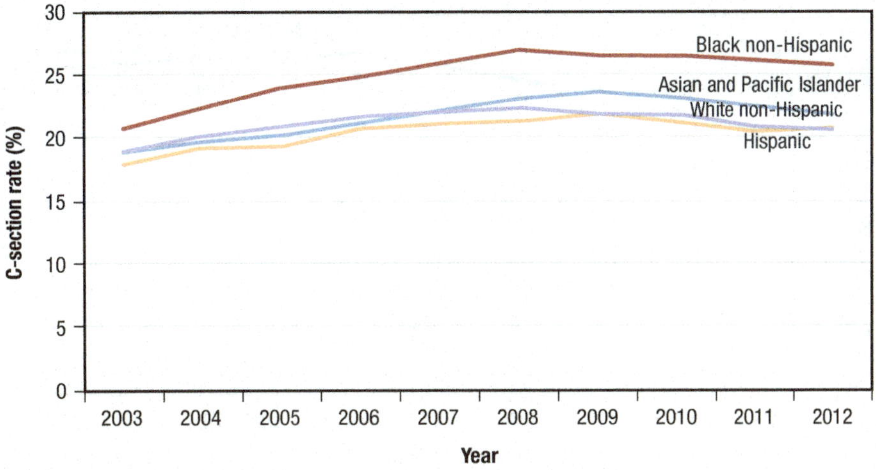

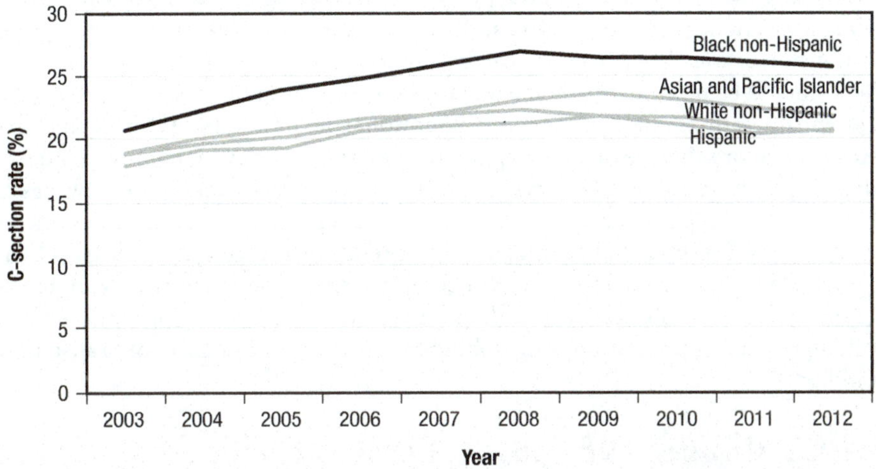

Source: Data from New York State Department of Health. (n.d.). *Primary cesarean delivery, 2003–2012.* https://www.health.ny.gov/statistics/vital_statistics/docs/primary_cesarean_delivery_2003-2012.pdf

FIGURE 4.16 Using gray and bold black to focus attention.

Source: Data from New York State Department of Health. (n.d.). *Primary cesarean delivery, 2003–2012.* https://www.health.ny.gov/statistics/vital_statistics/docs/primary_cesarean_delivery_2003-2012.pdf

North America, red often signals danger or urgency, while green suggests growth or success. In China, on the other hand, red is considered auspicious, and it is associated with luck, joy, and celebrations. Another important consideration is that not everyone perceives color in the same way. People with color blindness may have difficulty distinguishing certain colors, such as red from green or red from blue. To make visualizations more accessible, use colorblind-friendly color palettes and incorporate additional elements, such as labels or varying color saturation, to avoid relying solely on color hue to convey meaning.

Presenting Data Accurately and Ethically

In healthcare, where decisions based on visualizations can directly impact patient outcomes, presenting data accurately and ethically is a fundamental professional responsibility. Accuracy

FIGURE 4.17 Using a data label to highlight a data point of interest.

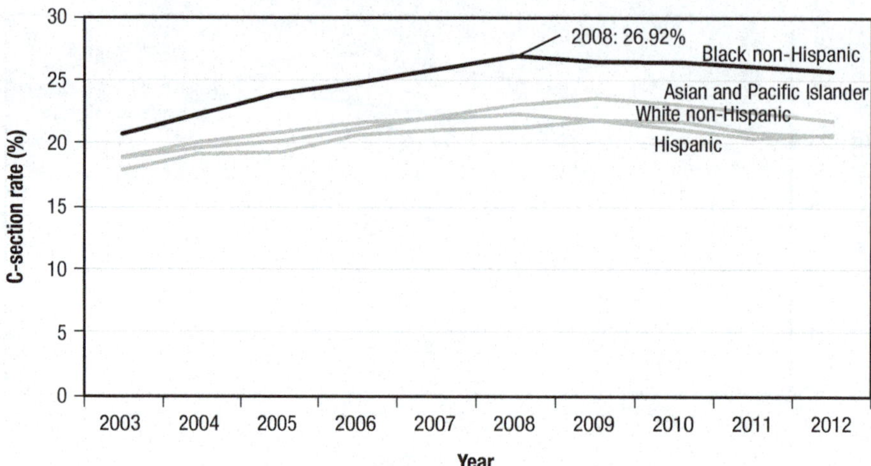

Source: Data from New York State Department of Health. (n.d.). *Primary cesarean delivery, 2003-2012.*
https://www.health.ny.gov/statistics/vital_statistics/docs/primary_cesarean_delivery_2003-2012.pdf

involves choosing the appropriate graph type for the data, using undistorted scales for the axes, and labeling axes and legends so that the audience is clear on the information being presented. Any data transformations (e.g., grouping categories or filtering data) and omissions (e.g., excluding outliers) should be prominently noted and explained to the audience.

Ethical considerations include avoiding intentional or unintentional bias that may arise from choices in color schemes, data grouping, or omission of relevant context. Understanding the audience's needs and potential interpretations is essential to anticipate how design decisions may shape perception and ensure that the visualization communicates its intended message accurately. It is essential to inform the audience of any limitations, caveats, or uncertainties associated with the data to provide a complete and honest representation of the information. Finally, verifying the accuracy of data sources and citing them appropriately reinforces the credibility of the visualization and upholds professional standards of transparency and accountability.

LEARNING OBJECTIVE 4.9: RECOGNIZE THE ADVANTAGES OF DASHBOARDS FOR EXPLORING AND TRACKING DYNAMIC DATA

Dashboards are a collection of charts, metrics, and data summaries that allow users to monitor data that are updated frequently. Dashboards can help healthcare managers monitor operations, track performance, and make data-informed decisions. An operational dashboard of patient flow might track patient admissions, transfers, and discharges in real time to assist in managing bed availability. An analytical dashboard of clinical quality can display historical data and uncover trends in metrics such as infection rates, patient outcomes, and compliance with clinical guidelines. A strategic dashboard might track high-level key performance indicators (KPIs) that are associated with an organization's long-term goals, such as overall hospital profitability or community health metrics.

Dashboards usually include a collection of visualizations such as charts and maps that are clearly organized to ensure a logical flow of information. They may also contain KPIs, displayed as prominent numbers, that highlight important metrics such as patients' average length of stay or patient satisfaction scores. Many dashboards allow for user interaction such as filtering data into subsets (e.g., displaying data for specific departments or patient demographics) or drilling down into different time scales (e.g., from yearly to monthly to daily summaries). Tableau Public maintains a collection of user-submitted dashboards that can be explored in a browser window. Healthcare-specific examples can be found at public.tableau.com/app/discover/healthcare.

A well-designed dashboard is tailored to the end user's needs. It delivers all the essential information while leaving out unnecessary details that could distract or overwhelm the user. It groups related metrics together and organizes them so that the most important information is found near the top left-hand corner, aligning with the natural reading pattern of viewers who scan from left to right and top to bottom. There is a consistent color scheme, typography, and layout across all visualizations. Any patient-level data is appropriately anonymized and secured. Finally, the dashboard provides transparency by clearly specifying assumptions and data limitations.

Dashboards offer a central location for visualizing complex, dynamic data. Their interactivity can allow users to explore data and uncover trends and anomalies that might otherwise go unnoticed. By displaying relevant key metrics, dashboards facilitate timely and data-informed decision-making, which can translate into improved operational efficiency and enhanced patient care.

SUMMARY

Data visualization is an essential tool for turning raw information into actionable insights. Effective visualizations depend on selecting the right chart type, aligning it with the structure of your data and the message you want to convey. Charts such as histograms, scatterplots, and bar charts each have unique strengths for exploring distributions, relationships, comparisons, and proportions. Understanding these strengths ensures that your visualizations are not only accurate but also impactful.

Clarity and design are equally critical. Well-designed charts avoid clutter, emphasize key points, and use colors thoughtfully to guide the audience's attention. Ethical considerations, such as accurate representation, transparency about data limitations, and accessibility, are fundamental to maintaining trust and ensuring that visualizations support sound decision-making.

Finally, dashboards bring these elements together by integrating multiple visualizations into a dynamic, user-friendly interface. They enable healthcare managers to monitor trends, uncover anomalies, and make data-driven decisions efficiently. By mastering these concepts, healthcare professionals can use visualizations to communicate effectively, inspire action, and drive improvements in a complex and data-rich environment.

END-OF-CHAPTER RESOURCES

DISCUSSION QUESTIONS

1. Suppose you are presenting data on patient wait times across different hospital departments. Would a histogram, a box-and-whiskers plot, or a bar chart be the most effective choice? Why? What insights might each chart reveal or obscure?

2. Consider the example of racial disparities in C-section rates. How might different visual representations either highlight or obscure disparities, and what responsibilities do healthcare managers have in presenting this information ethically?

3. Imagine you are designing a dashboard for a hospital emergency department. What KPIs would you include, and how would you structure the dashboard to maximize usability for healthcare professionals?

4. What are the trade-offs between simplicity and complexity in data visualizations? Simple charts may be easy to understand but might miss important nuances, while complex visualizations might provide detailed insights but could be overwhelming. How can healthcare managers strike the right balance to ensure effective communication?

LEARNING ACTIVITIES

CourseConnect ▶

To access self-assessment questions and interactive, competency-based learning activities for this chapter, visit www.springerpub.com/courseconnect. See inside front cover and tear-out card for CourseConnect details.

REFERENCES

Centers for Disease Control and Prevention. (2022, February 25). *Cesarean delivery rate by state*. National Center for Health Statistics. https://www.cdc.gov/nchs/pressroom/sosmap /cesarean_births/cesareans.htm

New York State Department of Health. (n.d.). *Primary cesarean delivery in New York State, 2003–2012*. www.health.ny.gov/statistics/vital_statistics/docs/primary_cesarean _delivery_2003-2012.pdf

INTERNAL EFFICIENCY

QUALITY AND PROCESS IMPROVEMENT

REAL-WORLD SCENARIO

A multispecialty group practice is striving to serve its patients promptly. It has defined a late patient as one who is brought into a medical examination room more than 5 minutes after the scheduled appointment. Patients who wait in the waiting room more than 5 minutes after the scheduled time of their appointment are late patients. The practice has collected the following data over a 10-day period (**Table 5.1**).

It should be noted that this multispecialty group practice gives approximately the same number of available appointments each day. Based on this, does the clinic need to redesign its patient care systems to better serve its patients? Is there a problem? What might be the best approach to addressing it?

LEARNING OBJECTIVE 5.1: DEFINE QUALITY AND ITS CHARACTERISTICS IN HEALTHCARE

Quality is a general term that was first introduced in the manufacturing and production sectors and then extended to service sectors such as healthcare and hospitality. As such, initial definitions of quality were limited to characteristics of physical and tangible products. In general, these definitions included characteristics that are either *must have* or *good to have*. *Must-have* characteristics relate to the core functionality of the product such as performance, reliability, and conformance. *Good-to-have* characteristics include extra features, durability, serviceability, and overall look of the product.

Consider x-ray machines as an example of a physical product. Performance, as a must-have characteristic, relates to the core functionality of the x-ray machine, which is to take x-ray images accurately. Reliability, as another must-have characteristic, refers to consistency in performance over time. A reliable x-ray machine should produce accurate and consistent x-ray images any time that is needed. Conformance, as another must-have characteristic, refers to the alignment of the product with established standards and requirements. For instance, a cabinet x-ray system must have a permanent floor as one of the requirements. In addition to these characteristics, users (i.e., clinics) will be interested in more durable x-ray machines that are also easy to service for repairs and maintenance, equipped with additional alarming and safety features, and look stylish.

It is worth mentioning that these quality characteristics contribute differently to the overall quality of physical products. Depending on the core function and requirements of a physical product, some of these quality characteristics might be less or more important. For instance,

TABLE 5.1 Number of Patients Who Waited (Data: Clinic Records for June)

DAY	NUMBER OF PATIENTS WHO WAITED
1	12
2	16
3	26
4	4
5	8
6	17
7	13
8	16
9	22
10	18
Mean	15.2
Standard deviation	6.4
Median	16

reliability (i.e., the probability a product works correctly) of 99.90% is completely acceptable for a pregnancy test kit, but it is not sufficient for products that work under highly sensitive environments such as nuclear power plants or airplanes. With 99.90% reliability, there will be one missed landing every day in an airport with 1,000 daily flights.

Applied to service, quality characteristics slightly differ from that of physical products. Products are physical and tangible items that are produced or transformed through a production process. Service, on the other hand, refers to experiences that are delivered through a service system such as call centers, hospitals, education systems like universities, cleaning services, and hospitality and tourism. Consider a typical physical therapy session as a service. What characteristics would make the physical therapy session a quality experience for patients? Could we use the same quality characteristics of physical products (i.e., performance, reliability, conformance, features, durability, serviceability, and overall looks) to assess the quality of service? The answer is yes, but not all of them. When it comes to service, durability and serviceability become irrelevant. Overall looks could refer to cleanliness of the environment and equipment; reliability and performance could refer to preparedness of trainers; and remaining characteristics could refer to more specific aspects of the service such as empathy, openness, responsiveness, assurance, and so forth.

Healthcare is also a service with more specific characteristics for quality. These characteristics are mainly tailored around patients and their experiences (i.e., patient-centered care). One of the popular quality frameworks in healthcare is called Triple Aim that was introduced by the Institute for Healthcare Improvement. As the name suggests, the framework focuses on three major areas for quality, which are patients, population as a whole, and cost. Under this framework, healthcare organizations should strive to improve both patient care and population health with minimum costs.

The Triple Aim can guide the strategic planning of healthcare organizations as it focuses on broad yet important goals. It is important to understand the relationship between these goals. It is easy to think that investing in any effort to improve patient care or population health can directly increase the cost. Hence, these goals might seem contradictory at first. However, the term *cost* refers to long-term and overall cost that both the healthcare system and society as a whole bear. For instance, investing and utilizing the full potential of electronic health record (EHR) systems within hospitals can improve patient handoffs; physician efficiencies; discharge planning; and patient outcomes such as length of stay, readmission, and misdiagnosis. Any improvement in these outcomes can improve the hospital's ranking and reimbursement rates from the Centers for Medicare & Medicaid Services (CMS). Another important relationship lies between patient care (i.e., delivered through inpatient and ambulatory settings) and population health. Health systems and health organizations have been actively involved in community-based efforts that support the health and well-being of populations and communities. These involvements include fundraising, sports events, educational workshops, and supporting affordable housing, among others.

The Triple Aim provides strategic and high-level goals for quality improvement in healthcare. These goals could be broken down into more specific aims or areas. In 2001, the Institute of Medicine (IOM) identified six aims or areas, known as **S**afety, **T**imeliness, **E**ffectiveness, **E**fficiency, **E**quity, and **P**atient centeredness (STEEEP), that hospitals need to focus on for quality improvement. Each of these aims include various initiatives and sub-aims that might require hospital-wide collaborations. For instance, safety as one of the aims refers to delivering care that is *safe*. Under this aim, hospitals are encouraged and incentivized to reduce the number of safety violations such as patient falls, patient burns, hospital-acquired infections, medication errors, misdiagnosis, pressure ulcers, patient misidentifications, unsafe blood transfusion, and unsafe surgical procedures.

Timeliness refers to hospitals' ability to provide the needed care as soon as it is recognized. This aim is also connected to many operations management topics such as resource planning and supply chain management, staffing, inventory management, scheduling and triaging patients, forecasting demands and needs, risk managements, and budgeting.

The next two aims, effectiveness and efficiency, were introduced in Chapter 1, "Using Quantitative and Analytic Methods for Managing Healthcare Services." Effectiveness focuses on achieving desired care outcomes, usually related to treating patients, making effectiveness one of the most important aims. Effectiveness is also related to and is dependent on prior aims (i.e., timeliness and safety). Effectiveness is also the driving force for evidence-based medicine, which seeks to use current data and evidence to improve healthcare decisions. Efficiency focuses on better utilizing resources to achieve the best outcome. Efficiency directly improves costs (i.e., one of the Triple Aims) because it helps to achieve the same outcome with less resources. Examples include increasing the utilization of healthcare equipment such as beds and operating rooms, reducing no-show appointments in ambulatory settings, and optimizing staffing. Equitable care refers to giving the same quality of care to patients, irrespective of gender, race, economic strata, and other factors. Like previous aims, equity also depends on many other sub-aims such as improving access, organization's culture, improving care coordination between teams, involving community members in the care delivery process, and expanding telehealth. Lastly, patient-centered care refers to treating patients with respect and empathy and involving them in decision-making processes such as treatment options and privacy concerns.

LEARNING OBJECTIVE 5.2: EXPLAIN KAIZEN METHODOLOGY AND ITS DIFFERENT PHASES

Depending on the scope and characteristics of quality improvement initiatives, one or some of the existing methodologies for performing the improvements may apply. The term *methodology* refers to a collection of tools or steps to achieve a broad goal. Kaizen, as a methodology, is a four-step process to achieve better efficiency and effectiveness across the organization.

Kaizen is a Japanese term for continuous improvement and the Kaizen methodology was first introduced by Toyota Motor Corporation in order to improve its production systems. The term *continuous* refers to the idea that quality improvement initiatives should be viewed as a continuous effort through cycles, in which organizations should always find room for improvement. Kaizen is a well-adopted methodology in healthcare as it focuses on both processes and people (i.e., culture). Under Kaizen, continuous improvement cycle includes four phases—**Plan**, **Do**, **Check**, and **Act** (also known as PDCA)—as shown on **Figure 5.1**.

FIGURE 5.1 Kaizen phases for quality improvement cycles.

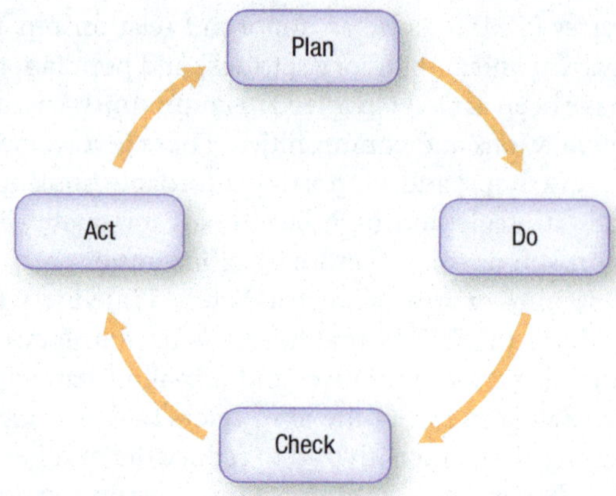

- **Plan:** In this phase, current state is investigated to identify problems and potential solutions.
- **Do:** This phase refers to a pilot implementation where selected solutions are tested in a controlled, small-scale environment.
- **Check:** Performance of the selected solutions is evaluated against expected outcomes.
- **Act:** In this phase, the final solution is implemented in full scale.

Example: Timeliness in care is one of the key quality characteristics in healthcare. Suppose your goal is to reduce the patient wait time in an ED using Kaizen methodology. You would take the following steps under each phase of the PDCA cycle:

- *Plan:* Investigate the current state by measuring current patient wait time, potential solutions to reduce the wait time (e.g., improving the triage process), and setting a goal (e.g., reducing the patient wait time by 10% over the next quarter).
- *Do:* Prepare the ED for the new change or solution (e.g., training, awareness, buy-in from the leadership), and pilot test the solutions.
- *Check:* Monitor the situation and waiting time metrics before and after the pilot test. Also, address the unanticipated issues during the pilot period.
- *Act:* If the final solution passes the check phase, roll out the solution in full scale, and continue to monitor the waiting time. Document the process and identify new solutions for the next cycle of PDCA (e.g., offering online check-in).

LEARNING OBJECTIVE 5.3: APPLY SIX SIGMA METHODOLOGY FOR QUALITY AND PROCESS IMPROVEMENT

Six Sigma is another popular methodology in quality improvement that aims to reduce defects and errors by reducing variation in processes. Six Sigma is a powerful methodology in healthcare. Any quality improvement initiative that aims to reduce some sort of errors can benefit from Six Sigma methodology. For example, Six Sigma can help reduce the number of misdiagnosis, billing and insurance errors, patient falls, and misidentification errors, as well as achieve broader goals such as improving patient satisfaction, reducing patient wait time, and enhancing hospital operations.

In Six Sigma, a process is considered acceptable (i.e., quality is assured) if its sample measurements fall within a predefined acceptable limit or specification. These specifications are reported around the mean with some multipliers of sigma (i.e., standard deviation). Hence, Six Sigma refers to a specification with six standard deviations on each side of the mean. The idea is to reduce variation in the process such that the samples gather nearer the mean so that we can increase the number of acceptable samples and decrease the number of defective or unacceptable samples. The goal in Six Sigma is to keep reducing variations such that we achieve 3.4 defects per million opportunities (DPMO) which translates to 99.99966% accuracy. If the process specification becomes narrower—say four sigma instead—then the number of defects will increase because more samples will fall outside the specification limit, leading to a more lenient quality specification.

Beyond a statistical definition, Six Sigma also refers to a collection of tools and steps to improve the quality measures of interest. Similar to Kaizen, Six Sigma quality improvement projects are broken down into a number of phases that repeat as a cycle until the desired quality is achieved. For improving *existing* processes, we use a **Define, Measure, Analyze, Improve, and Control (DMAIC)** cycle definition. For improving *new* processes, we use DMADV cycle which stands for **Define, Measure, Analyze, Design, and Verify**. We discuss each of these phases in detail and include relevant tools and techniques that you can use.

Define

Defining the problem is the first step in Six Sigma. In this phase, we define the problem, goals, processes, and stakeholders and customer needs. In defining the problem, the quality issue or improvement opportunity is clearly defined in a way that it aligns with the organization's overall strategy. If there is more than one improvement opportunity, we can use an impact-effort matrix to choose the one with highest impact and lowest effort (i.e., quick wins) as shown in **Figure 5.2**.

Next is to define the goals and objectives for the quality improvement project. These goals should be **S**pecific, **M**easurable, **A**chievable, **R**elevant, and **T**ime-bound (SMART). An example of a SMART goal is to reduce the average wait time for patients in an ED by 10% over the next 6 months.

Next is to define processes through different mapping and visualization techniques. This step will ensure all process details are well understood by team members and that everyone sees processes as they are. Among these tools, mind mapping is a good starting point that allows one to visualize different themes or categories and their relationship with each other. There is no strict rule on how to create these maps. They are simply a visual representation of a *busy mind* with interconnecting variables and their relationships. Activity mapping is another mapping tool that is used for tracking the alignment between the organization's value proposition and its activities to deliver these values. For example, if fast and affordable service is in the clinic's value proposition, these activities would be the center of the activity map and any activities that facilitate this value will be connected to it.

FIGURE 5.2 Impact-effort matrix to prioritize quality improvement projects.

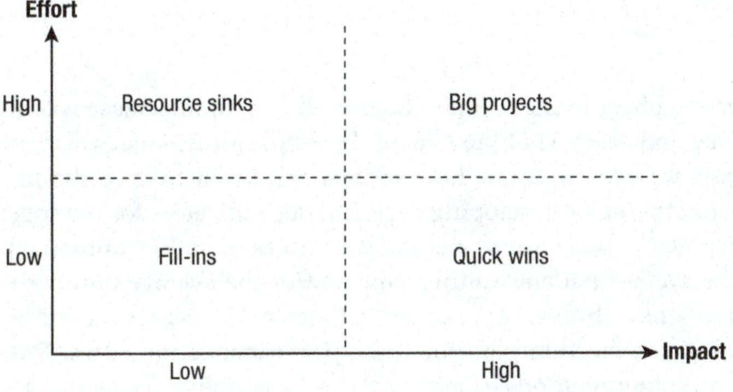

FIGURE 5.3 **CTQ diagram for patient hospitalizations.**

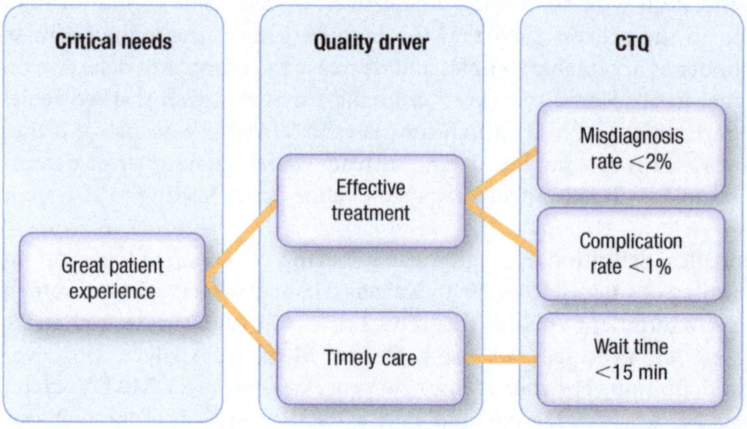

CTQ, critical to quality.

Service blueprinting is another mapping tool that separates processes into different layers based on their visibility and interactions with customers. It is used to design service prototypes and to convert high-touch customer points into low-touch customer points to understand how customers see and experience the service. Creating service blueprints is a time-intensive work that requires capturing complex details of the service in different levels such as frontstage, backstage, and support layers that exist behind the service scene.

Another popular mapping tool is flowcharts. Flowcharts are more structured mapping tools that are used to visualize process flows in a sequential manner. The flow could be a movement of physical items or individuals across the system or a sequence of intangible processes such as information sharing, decision-making and logics behind them, or data sharing. In creating flowcharts, we use different shapes to indicate different processes or actions. For example, arrows are used to show the flow direction, and diamonds are used to show decision points, while rectangles are used to show a task or process. Flowcharts are explained in detail in Chapter 18, "Project Management."

The next step in the *define* phase is to identify key stakeholders and their requirements. Depending on the scope of the project, these stakeholders can include customers, employees, management, suppliers, distributors, third-party entities, and investors. Among these, customers play a key role when it comes to healthcare services. As such, understanding their needs and expectations becomes a must. Critical to quality (CTQ) is a visualization tool that translates customers' high-level critical needs into a set of specific quality performance measures that are easy to understand, measure, and monitor. **Figure 5.3** represents an example of simplified CTQ for patient hospitalizations.

Measure

Measure is the second phase in Six Sigma. The overall goal in this phase is to measure and quantify the current state and baseline of the system. In simple terms, once we identify a quality issue in the define phase, we want to know how serious this problem is in the measure phase. This phase starts with identifying or developing performance indicators for the specified quality issue. For instance, if the CTQ quality issue is long patient wait times in an ED, potential performance indicators could be the average patient waiting time and/or the average number of patients waiting in the ED during different shifts or days of week. Once performance measures are identified, we need to identify a data collection plan for these performance measures. Data collection plans include different sampling methods, sample sizes, and sampling frequencies. Once the data are collected, we then need to check for data quality to ensure repeatability and reproducibility of the experiment. This phase involves advanced statistical analysis such as precision and bias measurements that are beyond the scope of this book. The next step is to analyze the current behavior of the process measures using descriptive statistics and visualization techniques. In the case of average wait time as the performance measure, simple histograms can provide information on skewness of the wait time distribution, potential outliers, the range values, and measures of central tendency. Lastly, we calculate baseline performance such as DPMO and its associated sigma level and process capability measures.

Analyze

The overall goal of this phase is to understand the quality problem from a systems perspective and identify its possible causes or root causes. It involves both statistical analysis such as hypothesis testing and correlation analysis (Chapter 3, "Statistical and Analytical Foundations") and management tools such as brainstorming, affinity diagrams, the five whys technique, fishbone or cause-and-effect diagrams, tree diagrams, failure mode and effects analysis (FMEA), Pareto charts, and scatterplots. A brief review of each of these tools is provided in the following section.

Brainstorming and Affinity Diagrams

Brainstorming is useful to gather a lot of ideas in a short period of time. Brainstorming is usually a team effort with a moderator that writes any and all ideas on a board or using sticky notes. Once all ideas are all listed, they can be moved around until different themes are formed around subsets of ideas. Ideas are then listed under each theme which results in an affinity diagram.

The Five Whys Technique

Five whys is a root cause analysis tool to find root causes or a critical root cause of a quality issue. In this technique, one starts with a problem and keeps asking "why" for five times or iterations (as a rule of thumb) until the root cause issue is found. It is important to stay on the same problem throughout the sequence of "whys." While brainstorming expands the issue horizontally, the five whys technique attempts to stretch the issue vertically. Further, the five whys technique is a retrospective technique. It is used after a problem is observed. FMEA, on the other hand, is a prospective technique that is used to prevent problems before they take place.

Example: Patients in an ED who are admitted to the hospital but stay in the ED while waiting for a hospital bed for a period of time. This waiting period is called ED boarding time, and patients who experience this wait time are called ED boarders. Accumulation of ED boarders can fill up the ED beds, which can result in delayed ED admission or ED diversion. Therefore, it is crucial to keep ED boarding time short. Long ED boarding time is a well-known and persisting quality issue in most hospitals because it is a complex issue that stretches throughout the entire care continuum. In this case, using the five whys technique could help to identify the root cause of the issue. **Figure 5.4** shows the five whys application for this problem.

Fishbone or Cause-and-Effect Diagram

When there is more than one root cause, we use fishbone or cause-and-effect diagrams to visualize the causes and their relationships. The diagram looks like a fish skeleton, with multiple major bones that each indicates a group of causes and the main problem depicted as the fish head. Causes are usually grouped into the following categories: *personnel, environment, materials, methods, measurement, and machines/equipment.* **Figure 5.5** represents a fishbone diagram for the long ED boarding time problem.

Tree Diagrams

A tree diagram is similar to a fishbone diagram in that it is used for breaking down a problem into subproblems in order to have a more detailed picture of the issue. Tree diagrams are also called hierarchy diagrams, given their hierarchical structure. The main quality problem sits at

FIGURE 5.4 Application of the five whys technique for long ED boarding time issue.

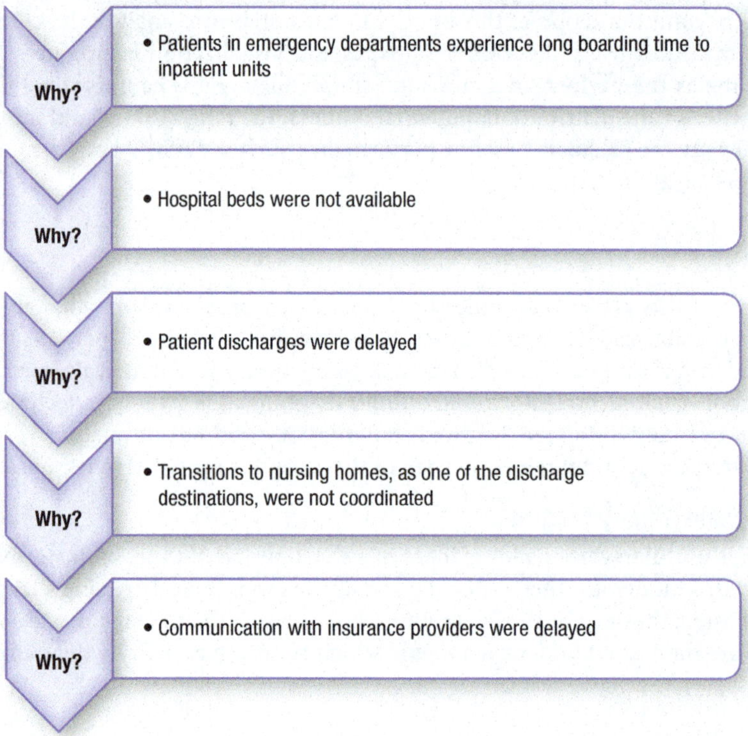

FIGURE 5.5 An example of a fishbone diagram for long ED boarding time issue.

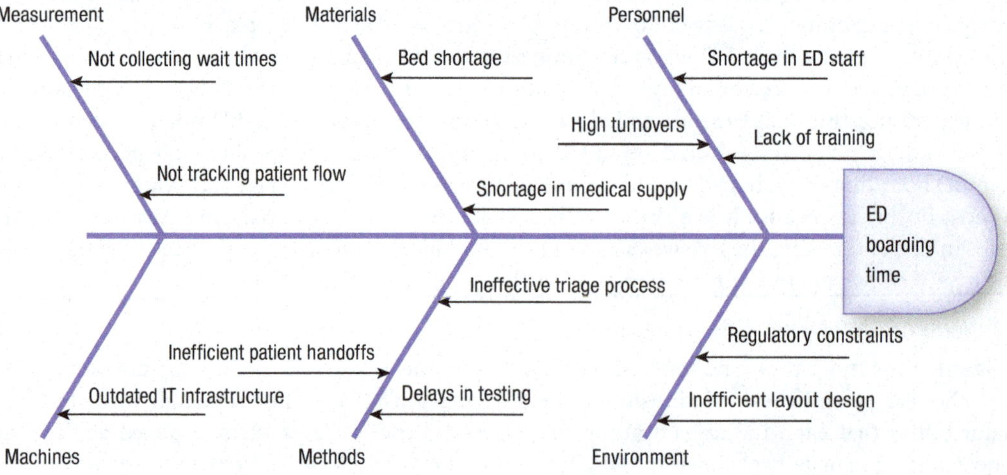

the top node of the tree (i.e., parent node), then categories that contribute to this problem are listed under the parent node. The tree expands with more detail added in each level, either from top to bottom or left to right. **Figure 5.6** represents an example of tree diagram for long ED boarding time issue.

FIGURE 5.6 Example of tree diagram for long ED boarding time issue.

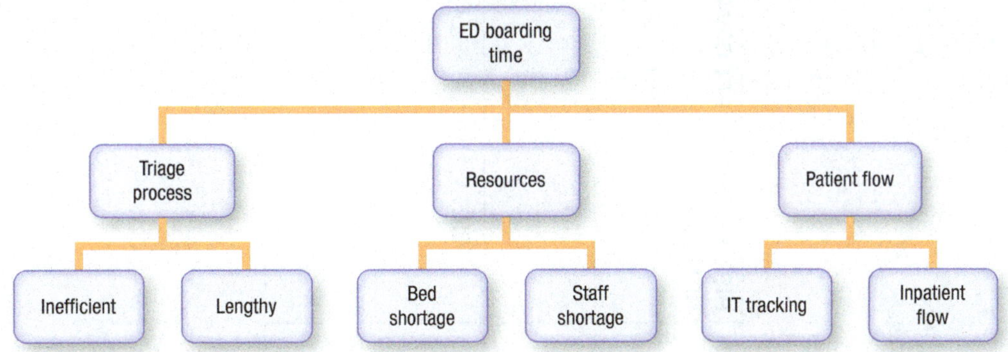

IT, information technology.

Failure Mode and Effects Analysis

FMEA is different from previous tools. Instead of looking backward, FMEA looks forward to assessing potential failure points in the process. FMEA is reported as a table. Each row represents a step in the process and columns represent numerical scores (between 0 and 10) for occurrence, severity, and detection of error in these steps. Their product becomes the risk priority number (RPN). Scores for each step should be determined in relation to other steps. For example, if a failure mode leads to a high-risk event, its severity score should be the highest among the steps. Hence, relative values are more important than the actual scores. The last column provides recommendations for the highest RPN. Some FMEA tables include recommendations for each step, regardless of their RPN. **Table 5.2** shows an example of FMEA for patients visiting an ED.

Pareto Charts

A Pareto chart is a vertical histogram that lists the most common problems or problem causes in descending order from the leftmost margin of the chart. Pareto charts are based upon the belief that, in general, "80% of the problem derives from 20% of the factors." The purpose is to focus on the major problems or the major causes of the problem (**Figure 5.7**). Like all histograms, these charts are efficient approaches to visually present relative frequencies of events. They are easy to read as long as the number of bars is kept to a minimum and labels are used to present the scale, the title, and the legend for each individual bar.

Scatterplots

Scatterplots are used to illustrate the relationship between two variables or process characteristics. These were first introduced in Chapter 3, "Statistical and Analytical Foundations," relative to correlation. At best, such plots can suggest associative properties, as is the case with correlation analysis. However, such plots provide no basis to conclude a causal relationship. Any scatterplot should report the correlation coefficient between the two variables with associated critical value or p value. By providing a picture, they are very efficient at calling attention to the relationship between variables. Consider the following example of a scatterplot (**Figure 5.8**). This chart indicates the graphical relationship between the total number of visits and the *total number of patients who waited* over a 20-day period. For more details on scatterplots, please review Chapter 3, "Statistical and Analytical Foundations."

Improve

After identifying critical root causes of the quality issue, we need to list potential solutions to address the root cause issue and select the best solution. In the improve phase, we consider

TABLE 5.2 Example of FMEA for Patients Visiting an ED

STEPS OF THE PROCESS	FAILURE MODE	FAILURE EFFECTS	SEVERITY	FAILURE CAUSES	OCCURRENCE	CURRENT CONTROLS	DETECTION	RISK PRIORITY NUMBER	RECOMMENDATIONS
Triage	Incorrect assessment	Patient harm	8	Lack of training	8	Automated algorithms	9	576	Better training the triage staff
Bed assignment	Lack of beds	Long ED wait time	8	Bed shortage	6	Monitoring bed availability	7	336	
Diagnosis	Delays in lab work and testing	Delayed diagnosis	9	Poor layout design	4	Early initiation	7	252	
Boarding	Delayed boarding	ED crowding	7	Poor discharge planning	8	Monitoring hospital beds	6	336	

FMEA, failure mode and effects analysis.

FIGURE 5.7 **Example of a Pareto chart.**

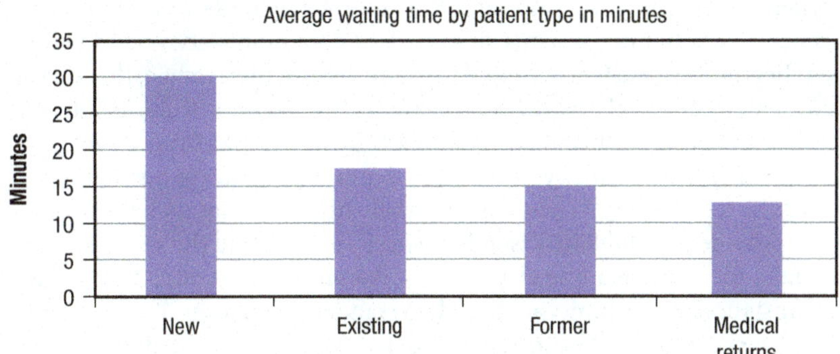

FIGURE 5.8 **Example of a scatterplot.**

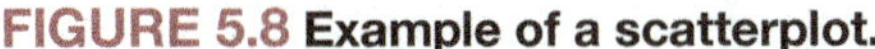

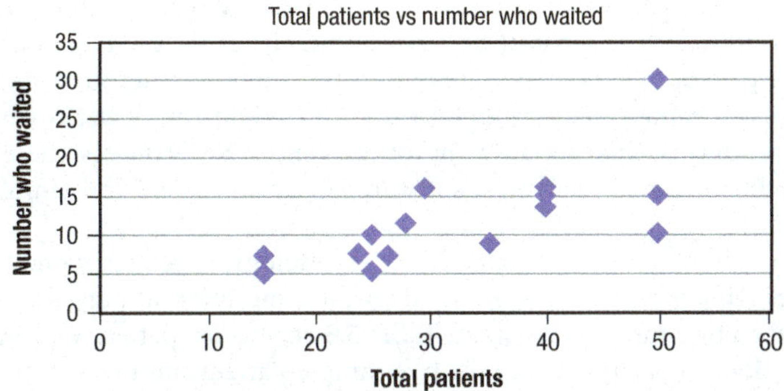

feasible solutions for the root cause and conduct optimization or cost-benefit analysis to select the best solution. We then pilot test the solution at small scale, and then implement it at full scale. Feasible solutions are identified using brainstorming or other techniques mentioned in the *analyze* phase. To compare these solutions based on cost measures, we can use various cost-benefit analyses. If performance measures are not cost related (e.g., average patient wait time), we can use simulation or optimization methods. Chapter 8, "Simulation Modeling," and Chapter 9, "Discrete-Event Simulation and Its Applications," provide details on how to develop and analyze simulation models for complex systems.

Control

The primary goal of this phase is to make sure that the implemented solutions are being integrated into the system. This requires monitoring over time and documentation of the process. To monitor the process over time, we use run charts and statistical process control charts. These are both considered time series as they show the variation of the performance measures over time. In both charts, the horizontal axis is a time element (e.g., hour, day, week, month, and quarter) and the vertical axis is the performance measure of interest (e.g., average wait time, average number of patients left without being seen, and average patient satisfaction rate).

Run charts are used to illustrate patterns of data collected over time. They are intended to indicate patterns. Run charts can be used to monitor a system over time and plot occurrence against the average or desired average or desired level of service to monitor performance. They are also used to identify when a system is not in compliance with a desired outcome or process indicator.

Over the long term, the run chart provides a data image of the system in operation. Such a chart can indicate when the system is functioning within acceptable limits and when the overall average changes. In general, functioning systems should yield data points above and below the average. When a system begins to consistently yield data points above the average, this may mean that the average is shifting up. Conversely, when the system begins to demonstrate a pattern of data points consistently below the average, this may mean that the average is shifting down.

Run charts are used to monitor systems. They report the status of a system as well as trends that have or may be developing. When desired levels of service are added (in place of the average), run charts provide the ability to visually inspect and evaluate the system. Statistical process control charts take the approach one step further. A control chart adds to the data plot control limits. In some instances, these limits are based on standard deviation. When standard deviations are used, a line that represents 1.96 and 1.96 standard deviations is added to the chart. Deviations beyond this line represent, by definition, abnormal events.

Unlike run charts, there are various types of control charts that are used for different types of variables. For instance, X-bar chart is used if the performance measure is the average of a continuous variable (X indicates a continuous variable, and bar in statistical term means average). An R chart is used if the performance measure is the range of a continuous variable. A P chart is used for proportions such as satisfaction rates, and C charts are used for count variables such as the number of patient falls per day. The reason for differentiating these charts is related to their control limits. Specific equations that are used for calculating lower control limits (LCLs) and upper control limits (UCLs) are different for each chart. Nevertheless, these limits are rarely calculated manually. Advanced statistical software like Minitab or Excel templates are used to calculate these limits.

Example: Suppose we have used Six Sigma methodology to reduce patient wait time at an outpatient clinic. *Patient wait time* is defined as the time interval between patient check-in and until being seen by a medical assistant. **Table 5.3** represents patient wait time in this clinic over a 15-day period. In each day, we take five sample patients and record their waiting time in minutes.

Since patient wait time is a continuous variable, we are interested in constructing an X-bar chart and an R chart to monitor the impact of Six Sigma efforts on the wait time.

X-Bar Chart

To construct the X-bar chart, we need to plot daily average wait times with three curves on the chart: the center line, the LCL, and the UCL. The center line is average of the averages. We indicate each datapoint with X_{ij} where i refers to a day and j refers to a sample number. For instance, X_{35} is the wait time for sample patient 5 on day 3, which in this example is 22.55 minutes.

We use $\bar{X}_i$ to indicate the average of the wait times on day i. For instance, $\bar{X}_1 = 11.24$. Similarly, we use $\bar{\bar{X}}$ to indicate the average of all $\bar{X}_i$. In our example, $\bar{\bar{X}} = 11.60$ denotes the center line for the X-bar chart.

For LCL and UCL in X-bar charts, we use the following formulas:

$$LCL = \bar{\bar{X}} - A_2\bar{R}$$
$$UCL = \bar{\bar{X}} + A_2\bar{R}$$

where $\bar{R}$ is the average of daily ranges, $\bar{R} = 16.52$, and A_2 is a constant number that is determined based on the sample size ($n = 5$ in our example). **Table 5.4** provides control chart constants for different charts. In our example, sample size is 5, so we will use 0.577 as A_2 constant. **Table 5.4** also includes constants d_2, D_3, D_4, B_3, and B_4. These constants are used for other control charts, as we see later.

$$LCL = \bar{\bar{X}} - A_2\bar{R} = 11.6 - 0.577 \times 16.52 = 2.07$$
$$UCL = \bar{\bar{X}} - A_2\bar{R} = 11.6 + 0.577 \times 16.52 = 21.13$$

TABLE 5.3 Patient Wait Time (Minutes) at an Outpatient Clinic

DAY	SAMPLE 1	SAMPLE 2	SAMPLE 3	SAMPLE 4	SAMPLE 5
1	7.69	7.43	22.7	12.07	6.3
2	12.79	20.26	24.9	7.3	10.64
3	24.12	14.74	6.83	3.4	22.55
4	6.27	9.77	11.7	19.03	19.41
5	21.09	4.47	11.3	3.51	3.09
6	23.06	2.04	3.83	10.93	21.96
7	5.71	2.58	18.44	11.09	16.73
8	11.95	1.84	5.05	4.24	5.96
9	0.43	10.78	4.32	18.42	4.95
10	3.24	23.99	18.58	6.97	14.64
11	15.15	6.78	0.75	0.55	22.93
12	8.4	0.73	13.06	18	23.94
13	3.38	16.15	21.28	17.54	13.93
14	14.58	16.92	17.2	12.7	18.14
15	6.03	5.74	13.07	12.23	5.74

We can now construct the X-bar chart as shown in **Figure 5.9**. It is important to interpret the control chart in detail and highlight the key trends, the natural variations due to sample difference, and abnormal variations due to some external factors (such as extreme weather, holiday and staff shortage effects, etc.). In this example, we do not see extreme abnormalities or obvious trends. We have three points near the average, seven points above the average, and five points below the average. The overall trend is downward during the first 8 days, followed by an upward trend until day 14, then downward again. Perhaps extending the analysis to a longer time period could help to reach a more robust conclusion.

R Chart

Similar to X-bar chart, we need a center line and control limits to construct the R chart. We use $\bar{R} = 16.52$ as the center line and the following formulas to calculate the control limits. Constant D_3 and D_4 are also used from **Table 5.4**.

$$LCL = D_3 \times \bar{R} = 0$$
$$UCL = D_4 \times \bar{R} = 2.11 \times 16.52 = 34.86$$

Figure 5.10 shows the R chart for the clinic. Based on the R chart, we can see that the range shows an oscillating pattern with a wider range over time. This is a concerning sign that needs to be monitored more closely over a longer period.

LEARNING OBJECTIVE 5.4: APPLY LEAN METHODOLOGY FOR QUALITY AND PROCESS IMPROVEMENT

Lean is another quality and process improvement methodology that focuses on eliminating waste from the system. In this definition, *waste* refers to any non–value-added processes or resource from the customers' perspective. TIMWOODS is the acronym for common types of waste in

TABLE 5.4 Control Chart Constants

Sample Size	A_2	A_3	d_2	D_3	D_4	B_3	B_4
2	1.88	2.659	1.128	0	3.267	0	3.267
3	1.023	1.954	1.693	0	2.574	0	2.568
4	0.729	1.628	2.059	0	2.282	0	2.266
5	0.577	1.427	2.326	0	2.114	0	2.089
6	0.483	1.287	2.534	0	2.004	0.03	1.97
7	0.419	1.182	2.704	0.076	1.924	0.118	1.882
8	0.373	1.099	2.847	0.136	1.864	0.185	1.815
9	0.337	1.032	2.97	0.184	1.816	0.239	1.761
10	0.308	0.975	3.078	0.223	1.777	0.284	1.716
11	0.285	0.927	3.173	0.256	1.744	0.321	1.679
12	0.266	0.886	3.258	0.283	1.717	0.354	1.646
13	0.249	0.85	3.336	0.307	1.693	0.382	1.618
14	0.235	0.817	3.407	0.328	1.672	0.406	1.594
15	0.223	0.789	3.472	0.347	1.653	0.428	1.572
16	0.212	0.763	3.532	0.363	1.637	0.448	1.552
17	0.203	0.739	3.588	0.378	1.622	0.466	1.534
18	0.194	0.718	3.64	0.391	1.608	0.482	1.518
19	0.187	0.698	3.689	0.403	1.597	0.497	1.503
20	0.18	0.68	3.735	0.415	1.585	0.51	1.49
21	0.173	0.663	3.778	0.425	1.575	0.523	1.477
22	0.167	0.647	3.819	0.434	1.566	0.534	1.466
23	0.162	0.633	3.858	0.443	1.557	0.545	1.455
24	0.157	0.619	3.895	0.451	1.548	0.555	1.445
25	0.153	0.606	3.931	0.459	1.541	0.565	1.435

FIGURE 5.9 *X*-bar chart for the patient wait time example.

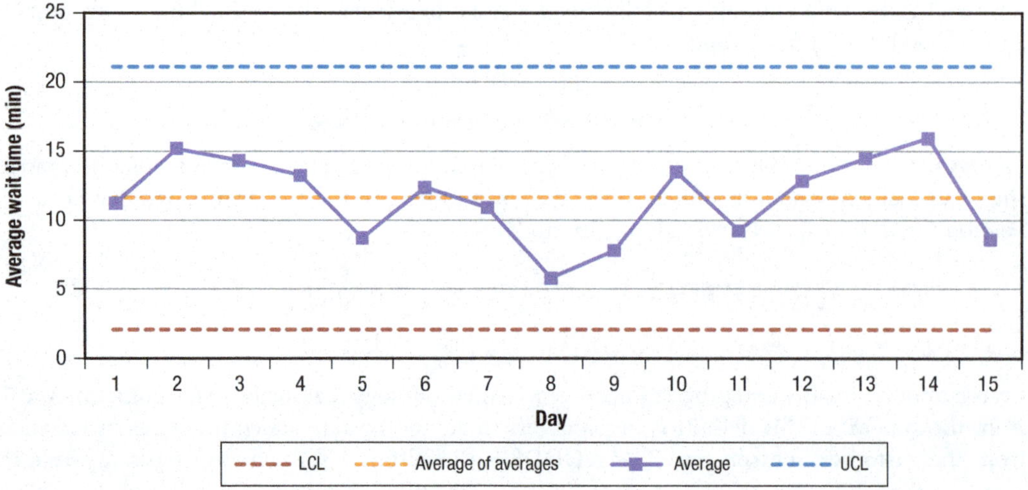

LCL, lower control limit; UCL, upper control limit.

FIGURE 5.10 *R* **chart for the outpatient clinic example.**

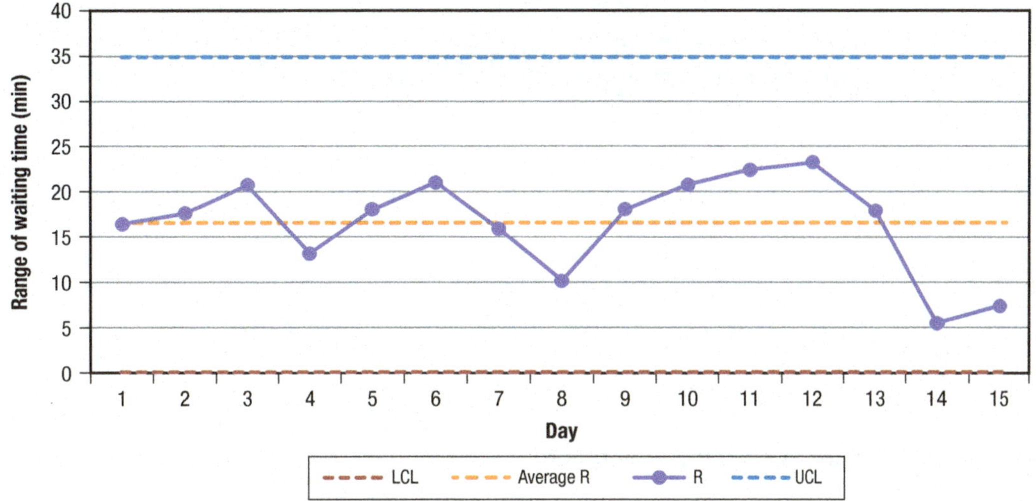

LCL, lower control limit; UCL, upper control limit.

production and service systems and stands for **T**ransportation, **I**nventory, **M**otion, **W**aiting, **O**verproduction, **O**verprocessing, **D**efects, and **S**kills.

Transportation

Transportation refers to unnecessary movements of materials and equipment. Examples in healthcare include the movement of beds, ventilators, and other equipment across the hospital that could be minimized. Spaghetti diagrams and the 5S method are common techniques to identify and reduce unnecessary transportations. To create a spaghetti diagram, we follow the movement of items or people within a facility and visualize their paths with different colors. Each color represents an item or a person or type of an item or a person. Repeating these steps results in spaghetti-like paths that can highlight frequently travelled paths and destinations. The 5S includes five steps that each starts with S: Sort, Set in order, Shine, Standardize, and Sustain. Sort refers to sorting items and prioritizing tasks. Set in order refers to positioning items, tools, equipment, and resources in the most efficient place. Shine refers to keeping the work environment clean and organized. Standardize refers to making previous phases standard procedures. Sustain refers to sustaining the previous phases over time.

Inventory

Inventory is a vital and necessary part of any healthcare system. Without sufficient blood and medication inventories, hospitals run the risk of shortage. Besides reducing the shortage risk, inventory has several other functions such as facilitating production and service systems, taking advantage of quantity discount and seasonality patterns, and protection against price fluctuations. However, inventory as a waste refers to unnecessary inventory that leads to unnecessary inventory holding costs (e.g., rent, insurance, and utility) and blocked capital that could have been invested elsewhere (i.e., opportunity costs). Chapter 12, "Foundations of Forecasting," provides various inventory management models to optimize the cost and risk trade-offs.

In Lean thinking, inventory is minimized using the *just-in-time* technique that was developed by Toyota. The idea is to produce goods or provide services only when they are needed. A system that runs *just in time* is called a pull system. Basically, a pull system waits for the customer (i.e., demand) to arrive. The demand then signals the system backward, all the way to raw inventory,

FIGURE 5.11 Pull system representation.

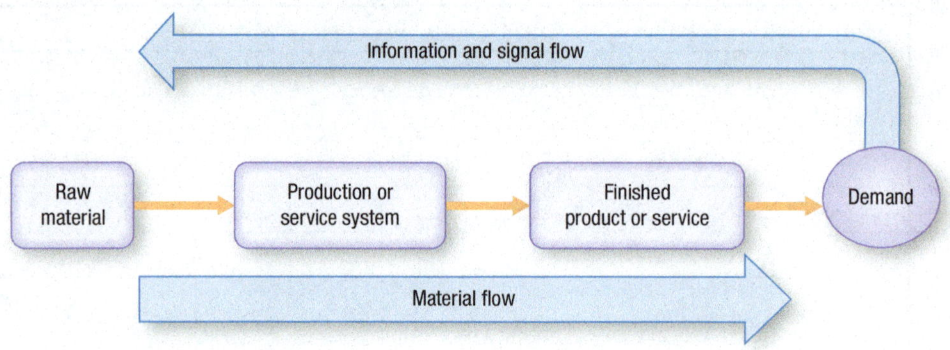

FIGURE 5.12 Push system representation.

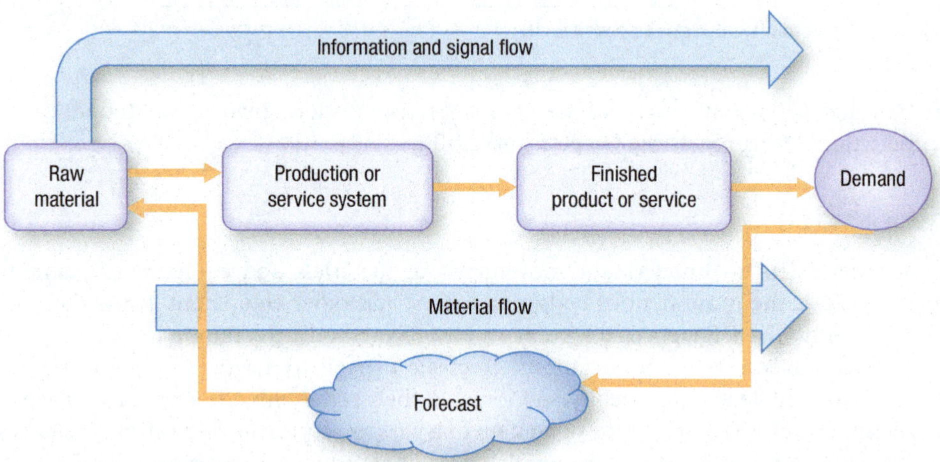

to start producing the good or providing the service. If there is no customer in the system, the system will remain idle with no inventory (either raw material or finished goods) being held. **Figure 5.11** represents a pull system and flow directions for both material and information (note that they are in opposite directions). The signaling is usually done using Kanban (a Japanese term for visual cards) or electronic methods.

The opposite of a pull system is called a push system, where goods are produced (or services provided) constantly and are being pushed into the market. Hence, push systems require an inventory of raw materials to run constantly and then to hold finished products until they are demanded. **Figure 5.12** shows a push system with material and information flow directions. Unlike a pull system that uses real-time signal of demand arrivals, push systems utilize historical demand patterns for forecasting future demands in order to plan the production or service system.

Motion

Motion refers to inefficiencies in the movement of people. These could include unnecessary micromovements such as bending and turning to pick up medical tools and equipment or walking longer distances such as the movement of nurses, providers, and patients between hospital units. Time and motion study is a well-known technique in industrial engineering that is used to identify unnecessary micromotions in a system. Another Lean tool for minimizing unnecessary motions is the 5S technique.

To minimize travel distance and motions in the system, layout redesign algorithms such as Automated Layout Design Program (ALDEP), Computerized Relationship Layout Planning (CORELAP), and Computerized Relative Allocation of Facilities Technique (CRAFT) are used. Details of these algorithms fall beyond the scope of this book, but interested readers may find online resources for more details.

Waiting

Waiting is one of the most common wastes in healthcare. Waiting is a non–value-added activity that negatively impacts patient experience and care quality. Waiting could include short periods that patients experience after entering the system (e.g., waiting for a nurse or physician, for lab results, or for a bed) or longer periods before they enter the system (e.g., waiting for the appointment or surgery day to come). Waiting is the effect of mismatched supply and demand. To minimize waiting, various simulation, scheduling, and queueing models are used. These models are discussed in Chapter 8, "Simulation Modeling;" Chapter 9, "Discrete-Event Simulation and Its Applications;" and Chapter 11, "Inventory and Supply Chain Management."

Overproduction

Overproduction is producing or providing products or services unnecessarily. Overproduction in healthcare is a common issue. Examples include prescribing unnecessary medications, keeping patients in hospital beds beyond their needs, and providing higher levels of care than needed (e.g., ICU instead of general wards). Determining the right level of care and what constitutes "unnecessary" in healthcare is challenging, which might require inputs from clinicians and experts in the field.

Overprocessing

Overprocessing includes extra unnecessary steps in a process (e.g., collecting unnecessary patient data on the electronic health record, overtesting for diagnosis purposes, including multiple approval levels for routine processes, printing electronic forms for signature and approval and converting them to an electronic version again, or unnecessarily complicated scheduling procedures).

Defects

Defects and errors are also common waste types in healthcare. Examples include safety errors such as patient falls, burns, misdiagnosis, and medication errors. To prevent system errors and defects from happening, the Poka-Yoke (the Japanese term for mistake proofing) concept from Lean is used. Daily examples of Poka-Yoke are dishwashers and microwaves that will not start until the door is shut. Similar examples exist in healthcare equipment with CT scan and x-ray machines. Jidoka, or "intelligent automation," is another Lean concept that refers to a system's ability to detect errors and shut down the system automatically before it trickles down the system. A Jidoka example is modern printing machines that automatically stop if papers get jammed. Another Lean concept for minimizing errors is Andon (Japanese term for light). Andon refers to any alarm or signal to indicate potential errors in the system. These signals could be either visual, audible, or both. Examples include code announcements in hospitals, smoke detectors, and crosswalk lights.

Skills

Skills refer to underutilized talents, knowledge, experiences, and skills in the system. Improving employee engagement, listening to their needs and ideas, and supporting their careers can help to minimize the skills waste.

SUMMARY

We have provided a summary of quality characteristics and their relative importance for healthcare managers. We have also provided two popular methodologies for quality improvement projects: Kaizen and Six Sigma. Both run as cyclic efforts to improve quality; however, their phases and tools differ significantly. Each phase of Six Sigma has its own objectives and tools that can guide healthcare managers throughout projects. We have introduced statistical process control or simply control charts for monitoring processes over time. Although we have used them in the control phase of Six Sigma, their applications cover beyond the Six Sigma methodology. Lastly, we have covered Lean methodology and tools to identify and reduce waste in systems.

END OF CHAPTER RESOURCES

DISCUSSION QUESTIONS

1. Describe the differences between Kaizen and Six Sigma methodologies.
2. Discuss how quality and process improvement in healthcare impacts other areas including finance, patient satisfaction, and health outcomes.
3. Explain the steps of Six Sigma methodology through a healthcare example.
4. What waste types are more common in healthcare?

LEARNING ACTIVITIES

CourseConnect >

To access self-assessment questions and interactive, competency-based learning activities for this chapter, visit www.springerpub.com/courseconnect. See inside front cover and tear-out card for CourseConnect details.

CHAPTER 6

DECISION ANALYSIS

LEARNING OBJECTIVES

6.1. Use decision trees as a method to examine decision alternatives.
6.2. Calculate expected payoff and select a decision based upon maximum payoff.
6.3. Develop and solve decision trees for sequential decisions.

REAL-WORLD SCENARIO

Amherst Clinic is one of 10 clinics in the Hancock Medical System. Recently, the clinic has been realizing higher than average visit volumes. The director of the clinic has examined this using statistical control charting and found evidence to suggest that some fundamental change had occurred. Upon further investigation, it was found that the population in the clinic's service area had increased by 5%, largely because of the relocation of a large employer, Bayside Systems, to the neighboring town of Gardner, which the Amherst Clinic serves. In talking to management from Bayside, they conveyed that further growth was likely, as they had plans to relocate two additional divisions to the Gardner facility. This would add an additional 400 employees. They could not, however, provide a definite assurance of this or a timeline for the addition. At the clinic, wait times have increased, appointment times have been extended to the future, and the staff has begun to hear rumblings of patient dissatisfaction. The director must decide on a course of action for the clinic, examining all possible options.

Managerial life is full of decisions. Managers must decide, given available resources, how best to meet their organization's mission. Often, managers must adjust organizational goals and objectives based upon changes in internal capacity or the external environment. They often investigate ways to enhance the efficiency and effectiveness of their organization, which often requires making decisions involving the reallocation of resources that in turn affect the work and process flow within the organization. And most important, they have to make decisions in a systematic way that relies on informed assessments and not purely on gut reactions and incomplete or false information.

This chapter examines the art and science of decision analysis. Although it is a process influenced by many qualitative factors, such as organizational culture, precedents, and the values of the managers, it is also a process in which quantitative analytic frameworks can be effectively applied.

LEARNING OBJECTIVE 6.1: USE DECISION TREES AS A METHOD TO EXAMINE DECISION ALTERNATIVES

Most decisions are made under conditions of uncertainty. It is rare that one knows with full certainty the consequences of their decisions. Some decisions are simple, having only two or limited potential outcomes, but others are complex, having any number of potential outcomes. The outcomes associated with decision outcomes are further governed by unknown probabilities that those outcomes can or will occur. At times, the decision-maker will have some insight into these probabilities, such as the chance of rain from a weather forecast. Other times, decisions must be made in an environment of complete uncertainty.

Finally, all decisions carry implications. A decision might mean that a fewer or greater number of resources are used in the future. It might mean extending the types of services currently being offered or offering them at a new location or that certain diseases get more attention or resources depending on prevalence or predictive impact. In health management, many outcomes are assessed in terms of some monetary cost or person time or cost. What is the value of adding 10 more appointment slots to a clinic? What is the cost? And thus, what is the net revenue? Here, these are termed payoffs, and they can be either negative or positive. It is important to note, however, that in practice, not all payoffs are monetary. In the medical professions, these can also be expressed as years of life gained or quality-adjusted life years (QALYs), to name a few.

When thinking about decisions, it is useful to also think about what is in the control of the decision-maker and what is not. There are three parts to any decision, only two of which are under the control of the decision-maker. They are as follows:

1. Stating the *alternatives* from which a decision can be made. These are the decision options, and they are under the control of the decision-maker. Examples are whether to hire more staff or not or to invest in equipment or not. Listing these should also be realistic and exhaustive.

2. Conceptualizing the state of the world that *could* occur *in the future*. These are unknowns at the time the decision is made. These are not under the control of the decision-maker. Examples are whether or not visit volume increases or a new technology is developed. These also have some *probability* of potentially occurring that can be estimated but is not truly known.

3. Determining the potential payoffs of the decision in whatever terms is meaningful (cost, quality improvement, etc.). These are then combined with the potential states of the world that may or may not occur and their probability of occurring. Estimating these costs are within the control/consideration of the decision-maker and should be assessed in the most complete manner possible.

Managers are expected to consider alternatives before making a decision. Most alternatives are different strategies intended to realize a similar outcome or payoff that matches the strategic objective of the organization. In other instances, managers consider very different alternatives given their assessment of the payoffs and outcomes associated with each alternative, for example, to carry an umbrella on a given day. Intuitively, each person makes this decision using reasoned judgment. We listen to the weather reports and then think about how far we must walk. We also might think about what we are wearing that day and where we are headed (e.g., home or work). In this simple case, the decision alternatives are to carry an umbrella or not. The future states of the world will be that it either rains or it does not. Because states of the world are unknown, regardless of which alternative we choose, there is a chance that any of the states of the world could actually occur. When using decision analysis, we must list all the alternatives for each potential future state of the world. We then determine the payoff for each interaction of alternative and state of the world.

For this example, let us say the payoffs are the cost of an umbrella, should we carry one (lose it or break it), and the cost of ruined work clothes (should we get rained upon). There are obviously others, but we will use these for simplicity. There are always as many possible payoffs as the product of the number of alternatives times the number of states of the world. In this case, for example, there are two alternatives and two states of the world for a total of four payoffs. This is shown in **Table 6.1**.

This example demonstrates the basic decision analytic approach covered in this chapter—the explicit identification of decision alternatives, states of the world, and comparison of outcomes and payoffs. Missing from this simple analysis, however, is an assessment of the likelihood of rain.

TABLE 6.1 Decision to Carry an Umbrella

ALTERNATIVE	STATE OF THE WORLD	PAYOFF
Carry an umbrella	It rains	Lose umbrella: −$1
	It does not rain	Lose umbrella: −$1
Do not carry an umbrella	It rains	Ruin clothes: −$150
	It does not rain	No loss: $0

FIGURE 6.1 Decision tree for carrying an umbrella.

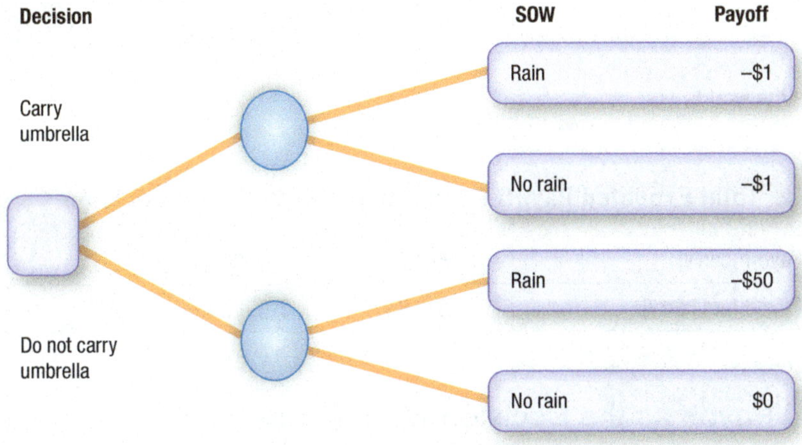

SOW, state of the world.

It is rarely the case that we have no information on the day's weather. Decision analysis allows us to assign each state of the world a probability of occurrence to better assess the payoffs. It is a formal process very similar to the intuitive processes we use every time we hear of the chance of showers. The difference, however, is that the explicit approach has the power to assist health services managers identify alternatives and select among the alternatives.

One way of looking at the chronology and payoffs of a decision is to construct a decision tree. A decision tree looks like a tree with branches for each decision alternative and each state of the world. A square is used for a choice node and a circle is used for the states of the world nodes. The decision tree for the previous example is shown in **Figure 6.1**. Note that this tree shows the decision being made first and the weather condition occurring second. When you choose to carry the umbrella, you are choosing under conditions of uncertainty; you do not know for certain whether it will rain or not. If it is raining when you leave the house, you are choosing under conditions of certainty; you know the payoff, so you choose correctly every time. On a day when it is not raining as you leave the house, you do not know the state of the world later that day so you cannot be certain of choosing correctly. In this instance, you would no doubt consult a weather forecast for assistance. In our example, let us suppose that there is an 80% chance of rain. You will notice that in our decision tree diagram, this probability is added after each state of the world in **Figure 6.2**. From this information, we can calculate our total expected payoffs for each decision.

FIGURE 6.2 Decision tree for carrying and umbrella with probabilities and payoffs.

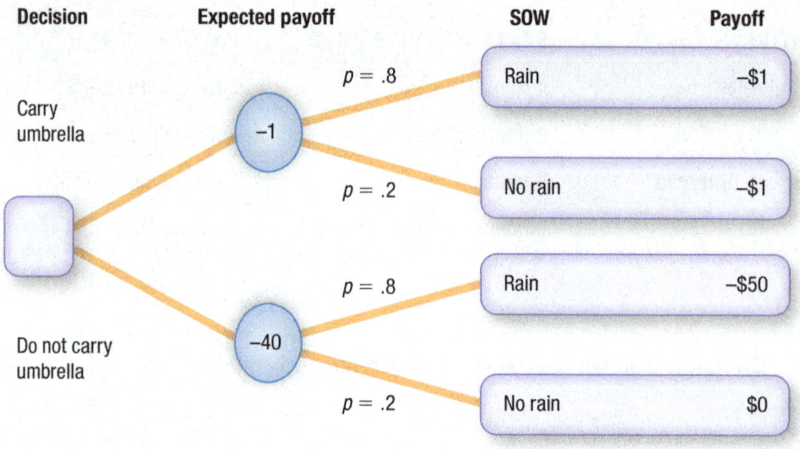

SOW, state of the world.

TABLE 6.2 Total Expected Payoff Calculations for Umbrella Decision

Expected Payoff [carry]	$= (.8 \times \$1) + (.2 \times \$1) = \$1$
Expected Payoff [not carry]	$= (.8 \times \$50) + (.2 \times \$0) = \$40$

Expected Payoff as the Decision-Making Criterion

From statistics, recall the idea of the expected value of some outcome, x. Here, x is our payoff. The formula of the expected value of x, $E(X)$ is Equation 6.1:

Equation 6.1: Expected Payoff Formula

$E(X) =$ [probability of $(X_1) \times$ payoff (X_1)] + [probability of $(X_2) \times$ payoff (X_2)] + [probability of $(X_3) \times$ payoff (X_3)] + . . . [probability of $(X_n) \times$ payoff (X_n)] where the Xs are the possible outcomes.

Each decision alternative has an expected payoff. When the expected payoffs have been calculated, you would then choose the alternative whose expected payoff is "best" by whatever definition of best you assign. With monetary outcomes, this is often the expected value that is greatest or highest or where the cost is lowest. In the example of carrying the umbrella, we examine the expected cost or financial consequences for each alternative. **Table 6.2** shows the expected payoffs for this example. We stated our probability of rain at 80%. Knowing that the probabilities of states of the world must add to one, if there is an 80% chance of rain, then there is a 20% chance it will not rain. This is also illustrated in the decision tree in **Figure 6.2**. Note that the expected payoffs are written inside the state of the world nodes. If we carry the umbrella, there is a chance of leaving it somewhere, but that cost is low (loss of $1) compared with not carrying the umbrella and ruining our clothes ($40). We should choose, under these probabilities of rain, to carry an umbrella as the expected cost to us is lowest.

Break-Even Analysis

Using the preceding example, one question that may come to mind would be, "How low does the probability of rain have to be before we leave our umbrella at home?" In essence, we are asking at what probabilities for future states of the world we are *indifferent* to our decision choices. This is a break-even question. Expressed as a break-even question, with the payoffs we have estimated, what probability value will give an expected payoff if we do not carry an umbrella equal to the expected payoff if we do?

In this case, we would set the expected payoff of not carrying an umbrella be equal to $-\$1$, which is the value of the expected payoff for carrying an umbrella. We can state this algebraically:

$$-\$1 = (p \times \$50) + [(1 - p) \times 0]$$

Here, p represents the probability of rain. Remembering that all probabilities add to 1, we use p to represent the probability of rain and $1- p$ to represent the remaining probability of no rain.

Solving this equation, we find

$$-1 = p \times -50$$

and thus

$$p = \frac{1}{50}$$

$$.02 \text{ or } 20\%$$

Given the parameters used in this example, when the chance of rain equals 2%, we are indifferent as to whether we carry an umbrella or not. If the chance of rain is <2%, we choose not to carry our umbrella.

Again, it is important to realize that our payoff amounts for losing an umbrella or the value of our clothes are often estimates. At times, we may need to alter those estimates and reassess our analysis. If, for example, we estimate the value of our clothes to be equal to $20 rather than $50 when our clothes got wet, then the break-even probability for carrying an umbrella changes to:

$$-1 = p \times -20$$

and thus

$$p = \frac{1}{20}$$

$$.05 \text{ or } 50\%$$

Changing the value of our expected loss from ruined clothes from $50 to $20 changes the break-even point for our decision alternatives—in such an example, the probability of rain must be 5% or less for us not to carry an umbrella.

LEARNING OBJECTIVE 6.2: CALCULATE EXPECTED PAYOFF AND SELECT A DECISION BASED UPON MAXIMUM PAYOFF

▶ VIDEOS FOR LEARNING OBJECTIVE 6.2

- Video 6.1 Building a Decision Analysis Table

Health services managers make decisions under conditions of uncertainty all the time. In some instances, uncertainty may be relatively low. For example, purchasing a new imaging device to meet existing volume demands more efficiently involves a low level of uncertainty. Conversely, purchasing a new imaging device to meet an unknown demand, or to compete with another similar service provider, might represent a situation characterized by a high level of uncertainty. Consider the examples in the next section.

Expanding Ambulatory Services: Renovate Existing Space or Build New Space

An ambulatory care clinic administrator is trying to decide how to expand to accommodate increased future demand. The manager could plan a new space costing $1,700,000 that would allow 100 patients per day to be served or a minor renovation costing $700,000 that would allow 50 patients a day to be served. The final alternative is to do nothing, thus keeping the status quo by not renovating. This continues the existing capacity of accommodating the current 35 patients per day but no more. Presently, the clinic earns an average of $175 per patient served. Assume that the clinic is open 300 days per year and that management wants to cover the costs of the renovation from first-year earnings.

To begin quantitatively analyzing our decision options, we first go back to the three decision steps listed previously. The first step is to state the alternatives. These are to do nothing, undergo a minor renovation, or undergo a major renovation. The second step is to determine the future states of the world. These are the unknowns in our decision. Here, they are the estimates of future demand. Because our decisions limit future capacity, we will use these limits as estimates of future demand. Thus, let us describe the potential for 35 patients per day, 50 patients per day, or 100 patients per day to be served, defined by current capacity, capacity given a minor renovation, and capacity given a major renovation.

There are three alternatives and three possible states of the world. This means that there are nine possible outcomes. These are listed in **Table 6.3**. The third step is to determine the payoffs for each of the potential outcomes.

Earnings are based upon patients served; therefore, part of the payoff involves earnings. For each state of the world of future demand, there are different *potential maximum patients* who can be seen. Each of these brings in an average revenue of $175. This amount is then multiplied by the 300 days the clinic is open yearly to calculate the total revenue per year. The maximum revenue generated in each state of the world can be seen in **Table 6.4**.

In addition to revenue, however, clinic renovations cost money that must be charged against these earnings. Remember that doing nothing carries no renovation expense, whereas minor and major renovations cost $700,000 and $1,700,000, respectively. **Table 6.5** lists both the revenues and costs and payoff for each decision alternative.

It is important to remember that the potential demand is uncertain. The clinic does not know for certain whether the demand will continue to be 35, 50, and 100 patients per day or something in between. It is quite possible that if a major new building renovation is undertaken, only

TABLE 6.3 Clinic Expansion—Expected Outcomes From Service Expansion

DECISION ALTERNATIVES	FUTURE STATE OF THE WORLD DEMAND CAPACITIES (PATIENTS SERVED)	OUTCOME
Do nothing/no expansion	35 patients per day	Demand can be met
Do nothing/no expansion	50 patients per day	Demand is not met
Do nothing/no expansion	100 patients per day	Demand is not met
Minor expansion/existing space	35 patients per day	Demand can be met
Minor expansion/existing space	50 patients per day	Demand can be met
Minor expansion/existing space	100 patients per day	Demand is not met
Major expansion/new space	35 patients per day	Demand can be met
Major expansion/new space	50 patients per day	Demand can be met
Major expansion/new space	100 patients per day	Demand can be met

TABLE 6.4 Clinic Expansion—Potential Monetary Payoffs by Future States of the World

FUTURE DEMAND (PATIENTS SERVED)	AVERAGE PAYMENT PER PATIENT	DAYS OPEN	TOTAL YEARLY REVENUE
35	$175	300	$1,837,500
50	$175	300	$2,625,000
100	$175	300	$5,250,000

TABLE 6.5 Clinic Expansion—Revenues, Expenses, and Payoffs by Decision Alternatives

DECISION ALTERNATIVE	FUTURE DEMAND (PATIENTS ABLE TO BE SERVED)	TOTAL YEARLY REVENUE	RENOVATION EXPENSE	PAYOFF
Do nothing/no expansion	35	$1,837,500	$–	$1,837,500
Do nothing/no expansion	35	$1,837,500	$–	$1,837,500
Do nothing/no expansion	35	$1,837,500	$–	$1,837,500
Minor expansion/ existing space	35	$1,837,500	$700,000	$1,137,500
Minor expansion/ existing space	50	$2,625,000	$700,000	$1,925,000
Minor expansion/ existing space	50	$2,625,000	$700,000	$1,925,000
Major expansion/ new space	35	$1,837,500	$1,700,000	$137,500
Major expansion/ new space	50	$2,625,000	$1,700,000	$925,000
Major expansion/ new space	100	$5,250,000	$1,700,000	$3,550,000

35 patients per day show up or are booked. At this point in this example, one management approach would be to use expert opinion or mathematical forecasting to predict the future demand and base the subsequent analysis upon the "certainty" associated with the forecast. Such insight may help determine how probable future demand might be and could assist in choosing an alternative. It should also be noted that future demand may be influenced by marketing the new space, so other elements of demand forecasting would be employed at this point to best estimate these volumes.

If, however, we are making a decision in complete uncertainty about the future, one approach is to assume that all states of the world are equally likely to occur. In this example, doing so would mean that the probability of current demand (35 patients per day) would be 0.3333, moderate demand (50 patients per day) would be 0.3333, and high demand (100 patients per day) would be 0.3333, thus setting them equal.

Remember that states of the world are future unknown events. They are beyond the power of the decision-maker to know. However, there may be data or other information that can assist in altering our probabilities of a future event, such as the case with the decision to carry an umbrella earlier in the chapter. In that instance, a weather forecast could have provided valuable information about setting the probabilities of rain. When the future is truly unknown, setting probabilities equal is a good starting rationale. Once probabilities for each state of the world have been determined, the expected total payoff (ETP) for each can be determined. Remember again that each state of the world in this example has three potential outcomes (see **Tables 6.3** and **6.5**). Only one of these will occur. Thus, for each state of the world, all probabilities must add up to 1 (or 100%). To calculate the ETP for each state of the world, we simply multiply each outcome's payoff by its probability of occurrence and sum them up.

Using equal probabilities our ETP for each decision payoff we find:

1. Expected payoff [no renovation] =

$$\left(\frac{1}{3} \times \$1,837,500 \right) + \left(\frac{1}{3} \times \$1,837,500 \right) + \left(\frac{1}{3} \times \$1,837,500 \right) = \$1,837,500$$

2. Expected payoff [minor renovation] =

$$\left(\frac{1}{3} \times \$1,137,500 \right) + \left(\frac{1}{3} \times \$1,925,000 \right) + \left(\frac{1}{3} \times \$1,925,000 \right) = \$1,665,125$$

3. Expected payoff [major renovation] =

$$\left(\frac{1}{3} \times \$137,500 \right) + \left(\frac{1}{3} \times \$925,000 \right) + \left(\frac{1}{3} \times \$3,550,000 \right) = \$1,557,625$$

Table 6.6 shows this in table form.

In this case, the clinic management would choose the higher of the ETPs, or the decision associated with $1,665,125—to conduct a minor expansion. What is important to note, however, is how close the expected future payoff (EFP) values are for decision alternatives. One might wonder, as we did in the umbrella example, what probability would cause us to make a different decision. Because we are dealing with three and not two decisions, we cannot calculate a break-even set of probabilities per se. What we can do is alter our probabilities slightly to assess the changes in our EFP and thus our choice.

Perhaps the clinic management anticipates they would conduct marketing in the community concurrent with construction to increase demand. Let us say that they think there is a 10% chance that demand will remain at 35 per day and there is a 50% chance that demand will increase to 50 per day. This means they are implicitly assigning the probabilities of 0.1 to low future demand and 0.5 to moderate future demand, leaving 0.4 left over for high future demand or a 40% chance.

1. Expected payoff [no renovation] =

    $(0.10 \times \$1,837,500) + (0.50 \times \$1,837,500) + (0.40 \times \$1,837,500) = \$1,837,500$

2. Expected payoff [minor renovation] =

    $(0.10 \times \$1,137,500) + (0.50 \times \$1,925,500) + (0.40 \times \$1,925,500) = \$1,665,125$

3. Expected payoff [major renovation] =

    $(0.10 \times \$137,500) + (0.50 \times \$925,500) + (0.40 \times \$3,550,000) = \$1,557,625$

In this case, the clinic management would change their decision to choose a minor renovation strategy because the expected payoff is the greatest. Notice that this is true even though the probability of high demand is less than that of moderate demand. Thus, with all conditions before the decision being equal, decision analysis tells the manager to choose a minor renovation. What is nice in this example is that once a simple decision analysis table is built in Excel, changing the future scenarios by probability becomes easy. We demonstrate this in a step-by-step tutorial in Video 6.1, "Building a Decision Analysis Table."

TABLE 6.6 Clinic Expansion—Revenues, Expenses, and Payoffs by Decision Alternative Equal Probabilities

DECISION ALTERNATIVE	FUTURE DEMAND (PATIENTS ABLE TO BE SERVED)	TOTAL YEARLY REVENUE	RENOVATION EXPENSE	PAYOFF	PAYOFF BY DECISION ALTERNATIVE $p = .33$
Do nothing/no expansion	35	$1,837,500	$–	$1,837,500	
Do nothing/no expansion	35	$1,837,500	$–	$1,837,500	
Do nothing/no expansion	35	$1,837,500	$–	$1,837,500	$1,837,500.00
Minor expansion/ existing space	35	$1,837,500	$700,000	$1,137,500	
Minor expansion/ existing space	50	$2,625,000	$700,000	$1,925,000	
Minor expansion/ existing space	50	$2,625,000	$700,000	$1,925,000	$1,665,125.00
Major expansion/ new space	35	$1,837,500	$1,700,000	$137,500	
Major expansion/ new space	50	$2,625,000	$1,700,000	$925,000	
Major expansion/ new space	100	$5,250,000	$1,700,000	$3,550,000	$1,557,625.00

LEARNING OBJECTIVE 6.3: DEVELOP AND SOLVE DECISION TREES FOR SEQUENTIAL DECISIONS

Similar to one-time decision-making problems, decision trees can be used for formulating and solving sequential decisions. In real life, often each decision leads to new future states, where each new future state can have implications on subsequent decisions. Suppose the manager of a small clinic is considering whether to invest in a new telehealth system. The system could either be successful, leading to increased patient engagement and revenue, or it could fail, resulting in financial losses. The manager has two options:

Option 1. Do not invest in the telehealth system: In this case, the clinic continues to perform with current situations, with no change in profit.

Option 2. Invest in the telehealth system: The cost of investing in the telehealth system is $20,000, which will be subtracted from the profit if the system is successful or added to the loss if it fails.

Based on the data from similarly sized clinics, we estimate that the probability of the telehealth system being successful is 70% and the probability of it failing is 30%. If the telehealth system is successful, it will increase the clinic's annual profit by $30,000.

If it fails, the manager has another decision to make: to do nothing (with no additional impact on annual profit) or add new services that could potentially benefit from the established telehealth system such as routine checkups with patients in remote areas. The cost of adding new services is $10,000. If there is a strong demand for the new services (probability of 50%), it will generate an additional $22,000 profit per year. Otherwise, it will not affect the annual profit.

In this example, we can see how one decision leads to potentially another decision in future. The most important step in sequential decisions is to formulate the problem correctly as a decision tree. Once the tree is drawn, we use the same concept of maximizing expected payoff to solve the tree. Note that we start from the end of the tree and solve backward. **Figure 6.3** shows the decision tree with probabilities and payoffs for the telehealth implementation problem.

To solve the tree, we start from the end of the tree and move backwards. For chance nodes (circles), we calculate expected values, and for decision nodes (rectangles), we choose the best decision, in this case, maximum profit. Note that negative numbers indicate cost and positive numbers denote revenue.

For node 3, the expected payoff is $11,000. We can write this number on top of node 3 to make it easier to track. The next node is a decision node; thus, we should make a decision (highlight one of the arrows). For the "Yes" branch, the expected payoff is $1,000. For the "Not" branch, the expected payoff is $0. So, we chose the "Yes" branch. In other words, in the future, if we end up deciding between whether to add new services or not, we should in fact add new services. The expected payoff for this decision is $1,000. Again, we can write this number on top of the decision node.

For node (1), the expected payoff is $0.7 \times 30,000 + 0.3 \times 1,000 = \$21,300$.
For node (2), the expected payoff is $0.

The last node is a decision node "Implement Telehealth." Thus, we should choose either "Yes" or "No" options. For the "Yes" option, the expected payoff is $21,300 - 20,000 = \$1,300$. For the

FIGURE 6.3 Decision tree for telehealth system with probabilities and payoffs.

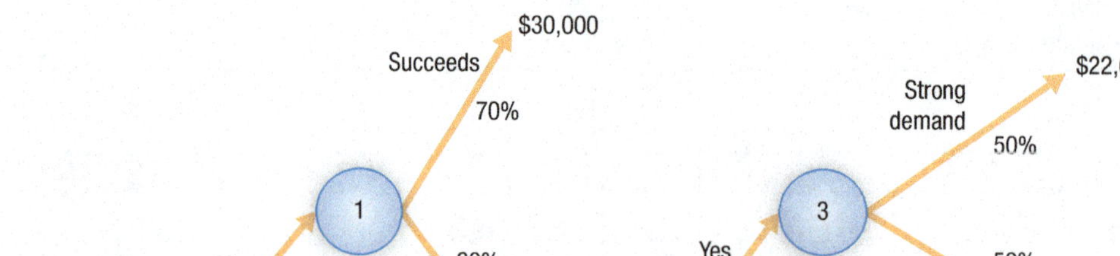

"No" option, the expected payoff is $0. Thus, we chose the option "Yes." The overall expected payoff of this decision is only $1,300. The actual payoff will be different from this number (why?).

SUMMARY

Decision analysis provides a quantitative method for choosing among options in the face of uncertainty. It allows us to specify alternatives and estimate payoffs of decisions based on our assessment of their likelihood of occurrence. It further allows the healthcare manager to assess how different probabilities of future states of the world affect decision-making. Decision analysis has three core component parts: the alternatives, the anticipated or forecasted state of the world that will occur after the decision is made, and the payoffs assigned to each. It is important to note, however, that in healthcare management decision-making, expected payoff is not always the only criterion we use for assessing choices. It is important to consider patients' quality of life and other values important to the community because it is not just the decision but the consequences of that decision that are ultimately most important.

END-OF-CHAPTER RESOURCES

DISCUSSION QUESTIONS

1. Think about each of the components of calculated highest expected value. What ultimately drives your decision? How subject to change are these decisions and why?

2. What might be the ramifications of a decision-maker not being robust or complete enough in their assessment of the potential alternative decisions?

3. What might be the ramifications of a decision-maker not being robust or complete enough in their assessment of the potential future states of the world?

4. How might one employ decision trees when attempting to predict new influenza strains that could strike the United States? What if the infectiousness of the strain is unknown?

LEARNING ACTIVITIES

CourseConnect >

To access self-assessment questions and interactive, competency-based learning activities for this chapter, visit www.springerpub.com/courseconnect. See inside front cover and tear-out card for CourseConnect details.

MATCHING DEMAND AND SUPPLY

CHAPTER 7

CAPACITY ANALYSIS

LEARNING OBJECTIVES

7.1. Describe the capacity of a medical care service system.
7.2. Describe the relationship between costs and capacity.
7.3. Estimate the production capability of a service system.

REAL-WORLD SCENARIO

The Fairborn Clinic (FC) is located in a large industrial park adjacent to a major midwestern city. It provides nonemergency care for work-related injuries covered by the state's workers' compensation program and many types of physical examinations. Physicals are paid for by employers. FC's primary market is the corporations and factories in or near its location in the industrial park. FC is owned and operated by Meadowood Occupational Health, Inc., a regional corporation with multiple sites in a six-state regional market. FC provides on-site treatment for work-related injuries and many types of physical examinations. Its services include laboratory testing and radiographic imaging. Generally, two types of services are provided. Both involve the direct actions of a receptionist/billing clerk, a registered nurse who is also able to take simple x-rays, and a physician. No emergency care is provided. Visits include work-related injuries paid for by workers' compensation rules and regulations and employer-paid physicals.

LEARNING OBJECTIVE 7.1: DESCRIBE THE CAPACITY OF A MEDICAL CARE SERVICE SYSTEM

The capacity of any service system is finite. Capacity is defined by the resources devoted to providing the service and how those resources are managed. For example, in a commercial passenger airplane, capacity is defined by the number of seats. Commercial airlines have learned that reservation systems, in contrast to open, first-come, first-served seat selection systems, lead to higher level of utilization of this capacity and less customer chaos and uncertainty. Reserved seating also has become an industry standard. Most important is that higher levels of utilization of capacity (e.g., full flights) typically enhance profitability.

Capacity analysis identifies the production capability and constraints of a given service system or function. Doing so, in conjunction with associated costs and revenues, allows managers to determine the efficient mix of resources—given constraints—to provide service at peak operational capacity as well as ways in which resources can be managed to accomplish specific operational goals. Capacity analysis prioritizes service efficiency. "Efficiency" is the ratio measure of system output, such as the number of patients served and system inputs (e.g., staff hours available to provide services). Efficiency can be enhanced if output can be increased for the same level of inputs. It can also be increased if the level of output is held constant and input resources are reduced. Examples of input resources include worker hours, supplies, equipment, and facilities. Examples of outputs are measures used to describe specific systems, including patient days, ambulatory care visits, meals served, and number of surgeries. Determining the maximum capacity of a medical service system and the resources needed to establish a specific level of capacity are the primary competencies associated with capacity analysis.

Managers monitor service systems to ensure that system capacity is close to the actual demand for service. If capacity is significantly above actual demand, then some resources may need to be subtracted to increase the efficiency of the system. If capacity is below the actual or forecasted demand, then resources may need to be added to ensure that an adequate service capacity exists to provide an effective as well as efficient service. In either case, to achieve reasonable levels of efficiency, the manager needs to know when, where, how to act, and what resources need to be added or subtracted to enhance operational profitability.

Service systems used to provide medical care are complex. Typically, they include multistep processes, with each step governed by specific procedures and protocols, and may potentially involve many service stations or servers. For example, admit-treat-discharge is a simplified process map for any inpatient or outpatient medical process. Each of these steps or phases in this multistep process also involves multiple steps. Each phase also requires the coordinated actions of many individuals and service stations in the hospital, some of which deal directly with the patient and others that respond to patient-oriented actions and needs.

Patients come to a hospital or clinic for medical treatment and expect the needed treatment to be provided. Typically, medical treatment is a multistep process potentially involving multiple servers or service stations including imaging and laboratory testing. As this process evolves, the treatment plan may change as the medical care team clarifies both the diagnosis and treatment options and plans.

As stated, providing medical care services is a complex process involving many steps and the coordinated actions of many servers or services. This complexity is reflected in the system used to classify and report what has been done after admit and before discharge. Note that the American Medical Association (AMA)'s formal system used to classify specific medical services uses 11,000 individual Current Procedural Terminology (CPT) codes to classify medical services. This suggests the potential complexity and difficulty associated with precisely forecasting the demand for medical services. The mission and market of each medical care organization also influences its treatment capabilities.

Medical Care Service Systems

Two general service protocols are used by medical care services: on demand and appointment. On-demand systems allow patients to present themselves for service anytime during the time period (i.e., hours of operation) established by the service to treat patients. There are two types of on-demand patient: emergency and urgent care. Appointment systems are also used to address the needs of urgent as well as routine care (e.g., physical examination) patients.

Given the earlier scenario at FC, it is important to acknowledge the influence of mission on service demand. For example, someone seeking prenatal care would not use the FC. FC physicals are provided to address the needs of specific workers, employers, and occupations (e.g., police, fire, and airline pilots). Annual physical exams are traditionally scheduled as service appointments. This occupational clinic, as described, also provides urgent, but not emergency, care for injured workers. Demand for urgent care services is stochastic, meaning it is variable and difficult to predict. Faced with this type of situation, any medical care service system must reserve capacity for unanticipated demand. As an aside, if an emergency patient arrives at this clinic, staff immediately request ambulance services to transport the patient to a local hospital or medical center.

Service units such as patient days, ambulatory care visits, and lab tests provided are based on demand and reflect the productivity of the servers as well as by their technologies and other resources used to produce a service unit. Recognizing that determining the capacity of a system or subsystem is as much an art as a science, it is sometimes appropriate to analyze service time periods when patient wait time exceeded planned parameters, meaning that planned capacity has been exceeded. This also recognizes the difficulty associated with a priori estimates of operational capacity of a specific medical service system. For example, in the cited scenario, the mix of planned service demands addressed with appointments (e.g., physicals) and stochastic service demands (worker injuries) may justify these types of special study to assess planned and actual capacity. As stated, it is important to recognize that the actual capacity of any medical service system is influenced by the type and mix of service demands and that the capacity of any service system is finite.

LEARNING OBJECTIVE 7.2: DESCRIBE THE RELATIONSHIP BETWEEN COSTS AND CAPACITY

Costs can be described by type such as the cost of personnel, utilities, supplies, equipment, and facilities. Costs also are described by their behavior. Some costs are "variable," meaning that their total cost is influenced by service volume. For example, the monthly total cost of postage is a variable expense; it reflects the number of bills mailed per month, which reflects service volume. Typically, healthcare organizations are dominated by fixed costs—costs that do not change as the volume of service changes. For example, salaries and benefit expenses are fixed costs. The majority of expenses associated with physical structures (e.g., heat, light, and insurance) are fixed costs. Other fixed costs typically involve expenses associated with equipment, debt, and taxes.

Cost analysis and the general field of financial management indicate that certain costs also behave differently in terms of service volume. As stated, a fixed cost does not change based upon the volume of service provided. Conversely, a unit of "variable" cost is added when an additional unit of service is provided. For example, supply costs are typically linked to the volume of services provided. Similarly, a variable cost is avoided when a unit of service is not provided. Variable costs are service specific, reflecting the specific diagnosis and treat protocol. Total variable costs also change as the volume of service changes.

The total operational cost (TC) of a service system is equal to the sum of fixed costs (FC) plus the variable costs (VC) associated with the volume of service (VO; in units) as stated in Equation 7.1:

Equation 7.1: Total Cost Formula

$$TC = FC + (VC \times VO)$$

This relationship has special relevance in healthcare organizations. Although variable costs do exist, many of the costs associated with providing health and medical care service are fixed costs. Other service-oriented organizations such as schools, colleges, airlines, hospitals, and long-term care facilities share the same challenge. When the concept of fixed costs and variable costs are added to the relationship between volume and revenue production, the classical "break even" or cost–volume–profit relationship emerges. **Figure 7.1** illustrates this relationship. It is important that the features and characteristics of this relationship are appreciated in this context. Note that:

- At the break-even point in volume, total costs equal total revenue. Both financial profit and loss are zero.
- The contribution margin (CM) equals the revenue or price per service unit minus the variable cost per service unit.
- Below the break-even point in volume, the CM is contributed to paying for the fixed costs.
- Above the break-even point, the CM is contributed to profits—excess revenue left after all costs (fixed and variable) have been paid.

Given these relationships, a manager has choices. To prosper financially, fixed-cost intensive systems require volume. In contrast, variable costs are managed by ensuring that a unit of variable cost is at the lowest possible level. For example, medical supplies are typically a variable cost. The challenge of efficiency and effectiveness requires that the manager ensures that the organization

FIGURE 7.1 The cost-volume-profit relationship.

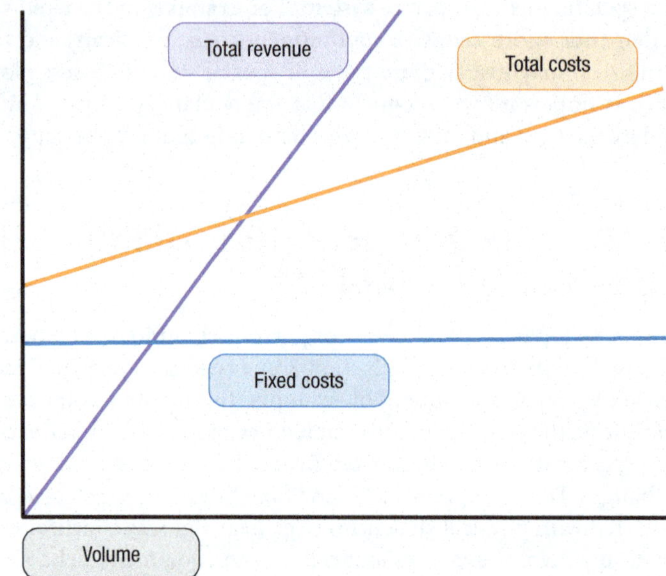

uses technically competent supplies (i.e., quality) and secures these supplies at the lowest cost possible.

Managing fixed costs is different. Fixed costs require that the actual or forecasted volume of services correspond to the capacity created by the fixed costs. To accomplish this, managers have the option of changing a fixed cost into a variable cost by redefining certain practices. For example, changing personnel expenses from a fixed salary to a per-patient fee paid to each employee changes a fixed cost to a variable cost. In healthcare, however, most professionals are compensated based upon a guaranteed salary or an hourly rate guaranteed for 37.5 or 40 hours per week. Because many fixed costs found in healthcare organizations lie in personnel, lowering staffing levels and changing the staffing mix are options that usually attract managerial interest when fixed costs need to be reduced. Note that lowering fixed costs typically lowers the financial break-even point.

Another option is to change a fixed cost into a semifixed cost. A semifixed cost changes in increments of volume. It is under this option that the manager becomes especially interested in the capacity associated with specific levels of resources. When combined, these last two choices present an interesting approach. Staffing could be held at one (i.e., basic) level when the volume is or is expected to be between X and Y units of service and increased to a higher staffing level (i.e., enhanced) when volume exceeds or is expected to exceed a specific amount. This type of approach, for example, changes salary costs from a fixed to a semifixed cost. The cost of personnel increases or decreases only when the volume exceeds the threshold established, such as Y units of service. This last option establishes a different break-even point in volume depending upon the fixed or semifixed costs used to create the needed capacity.

Numerous mathematical models and utilization methodologies have been used to forecast service demand. Each has its strengths and limitations. In the final analysis, a manager must make a decision based on imperfect information in order to plan and operationalize the service capacity to meet the anticipated demand for service. Generally, past utilization may be a reliable predictor of future utilization. Equally relevant is that "service times" typically vary by service rendered, meaning that an ideal forecast must include volume of service by type of service.

In general, the challenge of fixed costs must be met with increased volume. Actions must be taken so that capacity and service volumes are reasonably close and that when volumes change, to the degree possible, capacity is lowered. Balancing service capacity with service demand is the ongoing challenges faced by the manager.

LEARNING OBJECTIVE 7.3: ESTIMATE THE PRODUCTION CAPABILITY OF A SERVICE SYSTEM

The capacity of any medical care organization is defined by its human and physical resources. For example, if a community hospital has 100 staffed beds, then its annual operational capacity is 36,500 inpatient days. Its actual number of inpatient days is based on admissions and the length of stay of each admitted patient. Length of stay also reflects medical protocols and how patients respond to their medical care.

The capacity of the FC is defined as a finite number of physicals and a finite number of ambulatory care services. As described, one service is provided by appointment (i.e., physicals) and the other service (i.e., walk-in occupational urgent care) is provided on demand during its operating hours. As described, the FC uses the same service team (i.e., receptionist, registered nurse, and physician) to service all patients. As such, this clinic faces an interesting paradox. For each physical it provides, FC precludes—to some degree—providing ambulatory urgent care during the same time period.

All service systems have inherent inefficiencies. Anytime actual usage is less than the production frontier, inefficiency is present. Maximum system utilization is referred to as the system's "production frontier," the highest level of possible utilization. Consider the concept of a production frontier. Any one medical service system typically provides many types of services. For example, a walk-in patient at the FC may want a comprehensive physical examination or need attention for a simple laceration. One service could require 60 minutes of staff time, while the other could require 10 minutes. Since every medical service has its own specific resource profile in terms of the amount of staff time and supplies, capacity analysis must consider the mix of services likely to be provided when estimating a system's capacity. Since the capacity of all service systems is finite, all service systems are limited by their maximum service capacity. This is also known as its "production frontier." As resources are increased, more service units are possible. For example, as the size of an airplane assigned to a specific flight increases, the number of service units that can be generated increases. If the 250-seat airplane is substituted for the 100-seat airplane on a specific flight, capacity shifts from 100 passengers to 250 passengers. As notes, a change in capacity changes the production frontier. The production frontier establishes a quantitative measure of the upper limit of production also known as the system's capacity.

Airlines measure their output based upon "passenger miles." Each mile one passenger flies is one passenger mile. If an airplane flew 100 passengers over 400 miles, this would generate 40,000 passenger miles. If an airplane flew 250 passengers over 400 miles, the output of the flight would be 250 passengers times 400 miles, or 100,000 passenger miles. Knowing the production frontier associated with specific levels of resources (e.g., a 100- vs. 250-seat airplane) establishes the upper limit of output. Hospitals and medical centers use "patient days" as a primary measure of inpatient utilization. In this case, the number of "inpatient beds" is analogous with airline seats. For example, the annual capacity of a 100-bed hospital is 36,500 inpatient days. Inpatient utilization is measured by patient admissions and the length of stay in the hospital. Knowing the upper limit of service output provides the ability to compare actual service output with potential upper limit service capacity. This provides the ability to assess and manage the relationship between input resources and output. For example, if this 100-bed hospital over the last year reported 23,725 patient days, then inpatient utilization (of capacity) would be estimated at

$$65\% = \left(\frac{23,725}{36,500} \right) \times 100.$$

"Visits" are typically used to describe utilization in outpatient systems. Similarly, "procedures" are used to describe the utilization of ancillary services such as laboratory and imaging services. Measures of system utilization include the following:

- Patient days describe the number of days a patient was served by hospital inpatient patient services.

- Resident care days are used to express the service output of a nursing home.

- Visits are used to express the output of ambulatory care services and home health agencies.

- Ancillary and related services are described by the number and type of procedures or processes performed such as scans, laboratory tests, assessments, and treatments.

Measures of utilization also are the metrics used to estimate service system capacity and related service production rates such as the number of procedures per minute, hour, day, week, or year. The number of procedures possible (e.g., production frontier) is the system's capacity. The number of procedures done is the system's output.

The process of designing and analyzing service systems can be accomplished using a multistep process:

1. Identify the system or subsystem in question and identify the general process (e.g., admit) and the microsteps associated with the process. Typically, general system flowcharting is used to accomplish this step.

2. Determine who (e.g., occupation) is responsible for each microstep.

3. Estimate the system's current capability. This estimate should include historical data as well as current estimates.

4. Compare the system's current capacity with its utilization.

5. Change the resource mix of the service system, as necessary, to enhance the system's efficiency.

The critical step in this process is the determination of a service system's capacity. The time it takes staff to do a specific procedure or task can be measured. Repeated measures can be taken to enhance reliable and valid estimates. Industrial engineering provides numerous approaches to measure the capacity of systems. Most involve observing a service system and timing different steps or stages.

Measuring and estimating the capacity of service systems should focus on the components of the service system. In some instances, categories of activities must be used. For example, a typical radiology department in a hospital can do in excess of 200 different imaging procedures. The time and resources it takes to do each type of procedure can be estimated. Grouping specific procedures into resource-based categories can facilitate analysis. Once categorized, the resources needed for each step in the production process can also be estimated. In most instances, interviewing the professional staff to determine their perspectives is essential. Service system capacity also can be estimated using peak volumes. Although using past levels of performance to estimate capacity may not be as precise as capacity based upon formal study, it does provide the manager with a usable surrogate to estimate capacity.

SUMMARY

As presented, capacity analysis estimates the production frontier associated with multistep production processes. It is used to develop strategies to increase or reduce resources so that service output is a reasoned investment on the part of a medical service provider. The primary challenge, however, remains estimating the demand for service and the need to adjust resources based on demand. While some quantitative models can describe the economically optimal mix of services that could be provided by a medical service system, this information is of limited value. The primary management issue is matching the demand for service and the provision of service. Medical care service systems are driven by demand that require sufficient capacity to respond as needed.

Unlike many service sectors, capacity can also influence demand, which in healthcare can lead to capacity-induced demand. Estimating the cyclical nature of demand, the systems' response, and the systems' capabilities are the key components to effective capacity analysis.

END-OF-CHAPTER RESOURCES

DISCUSSION QUESTIONS

1. Capacity is defined by the resources devoted to providing service and the demand/need for service is stochastic. As such, capacity may need to be flexible rather than fixed. Agree or disagree with this statement and discuss the management implications of your position.

2. From the perspective of "capacity," which type of costs (fixed or variable) are more significant and why?

3. For ambulatory care service systems, identify and discuss the advantages and disadvantages of "appointment-based" versus "walk-in" medical service systems. Does this system characteristic have implications on decisions involving capacity? Explain your answer.

4. All service systems have inherent inefficiencies. One example of an inefficiency is "idle time," which is time not devoted to providing a service. For example, consider a hospital cafeteria as a service system. Discuss why some planned idle time may be appropriate for health and medical care services and approaches that could be used to minimize idle time when it is a system inefficiency.

LEARNING ACTIVITIES

CourseConnect ▶

To access self-assessment questions and interactive, competency-based learning activities for this chapter, visit www.springerpub.com/courseconnect. See inside front cover and tear-out card for CourseConnect details.

SIMULATION MODELING

REAL-WORLD SCENARIO

Rivercare Health System serves a diverse community of approximately 80,000 residents. Amidst a recent worldwide health emergency, the system encountered formidable obstacles as it attempted to efficiently distribute vital resources and handle a swift surge of patients. Rivercare saw a dramatic spike in admissions as the outbreak worsened, putting a heavy burden on the hospital's intensive care units, EDs, and ventilator capacity. The management of medical equipment, staff, and bed occupancy became even more complex due to the unpredictable nature of disease transmission and changing patient care needs.

Rivercare's leadership used different simulation modeling as a crucial decision-making tool to enhance its response strategy. In order to replicate patient arrival rates, disease progression scenarios, and resource utilization patterns, they created dynamic models using simulation methodology. Through these simulations, the team was able to assess a variety of tactics, including redistributing resources, optimizing staffing schedules, and increasing intensive care unit capacity under various infection rate scenarios. Rivercare was able to predict resource shortages, find possible bottlenecks, and improve operational plans in a risk-free setting by virtually testing interventions.

Rivercare realized the long-term benefits of simulation-based emergency planning after gaining new insights. In order to improve readiness, expedite decision-making, and guarantee adaptable, data-driven responses to quickly changing healthcare demands, the leadership team is currently investing in cutting-edge simulation technology. This strategy seeks to improve adaptability, optimize effectiveness, and uphold superior patient care even in the face of adversity.

This chapter reviews simulation framework and its components. It provides insights on when and how to use simulation modeling as a primary decision-making tool that is used in health services administration.

LEARNING OBJECTIVE 8.1: DESCRIBE THE SIMULATION FRAMEWORK

Simulation is an abstract representation of a usually complex process or system in order to better understand its outcomes. Thus, the goal of simulation is always to estimate some measure of outcomes. Simulation is useful when the process or system has some uncertain parameters or

FIGURE 8.1 Simulation framework.

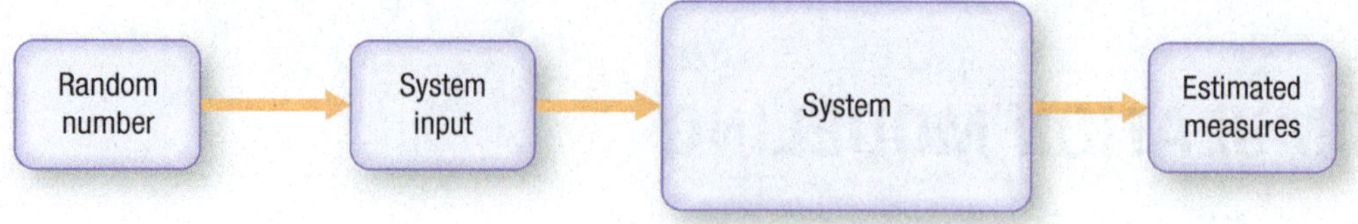

complexity that makes it difficult to mathematically derive the outcomes. For example, simulation could be used to understand the spread of a virus within a community. In this example, the community is a complex system with different age groups that interact in various and uncertain forms. The outcome of interest could be the number of infected people within a certain time period.

Sometimes, simulation is used to verify theory. For example, we can use probability theory to calculate the probability of having an even number when rolling a die. This probability is

$$probability\ (dice\ comes\ 2\ or\ dice\ comes\ 4\ or\ dice\ comes\ 6) = \frac{1}{6} + \frac{1}{6} + \frac{1}{6} = \frac{1}{2}.$$

Alternatively, we can simulate this process and estimate the probability. To do so, we roll a die repeatedly for a large number of replications (for instance, 10,000 times) and count the number of times that the die comes up as 2 or 4 or 6. The estimated probability is then the total number of times that the die came up as 2 or 4 or 6, divided by the total number of rolls. As the total number of rolls increases, the estimated probability gets closer and closer to the actual probability of .5. This is generally true, meaning, if you increase the number of replications in the simulation, the estimations become more accurate.

Whether we use simulation to model a complex system or to verify a known outcome, the overall simulation framework is the same. **Figure 8.1** shows the overall simulation framework. Any simulation starts with a series of numbers that are generated randomly. These random numbers are then converted into the distribution of the system input so that the system can take them and generate outcomes for estimating the measures of interest.

Example: ED crowding is a common issue for hospitals and health systems. One way to alleviate this issue is to proactively manage the ED capacity by estimating patient length of stay (LOS) in the ED using simulation. Components of the simulation framework for this example are as follows:

- **Random number:** Randomly generated numbers that will be converted into the distribution of system inputs.
- **System input:** Patient characteristics such as age, severity of illness, sex, and so forth that are given as probability distributions. Through some mathematical processes, random numbers are converted into system inputs in a way that they follow the same distributions.
- **System:** The ED and its detailed operations such as number of beds, nurses and doctors, care pathways, labs, and durations.
- **Estimated measures:** It could be any outcome measure of interest such as percentage of ED patients with LOS of >2 days.

In this example, simulation is a preferred method for analyzing the LOS because the ED is a complex system with various uncertain parameters. Simulation also allows for testing what-if scenarios in order to study the impact of changes on outcomes without implementing them in reality. For instance, one can increase the number of ED beds or expedite the admission process and observe their impact on LOS over a long period of time, say within the next 2 years.

Now that we have a general understanding of the simulation framework, let us take a closer look at each component in the following sections.

LEARNING OBJECTIVE 8.2: APPLY BASIC RANDOM NUMBER GENERATORS

Random numbers are the starting and essential point of any simulation model. Unreliable random numbers that feed into a simulation model will result in unreliable simulation outputs. In simple terms, we call a sequence of numbers random if they lack any pattern or predictability. Generating true random numbers requires physical experiments such as spinning a wheel, rolling a die, radioactive decay, or electronic noise. However, these experiments are slow and computationally expensive. Therefore, we use pseudorandom number generators. These generators are mathematical recursive equations that start with a fixed number (i.e., seed) and generate a pseudorandom number in each iteration. For a given seed, the sequence of generated random numbers remains the same (i.e., reproducible). The goal of these algorithms is to generate a sequence of random numbers that are uniformly distributed. For one random number at a time, the uniform distribution will be a one-dimensional distribution (random dots on a line segment). For two random numbers at a time, the uniform distribution will be a two-dimensional distribution (random dots on a rectangle). In three dimensions, the uniform distribution will be random dots within a box. In the next section, we will use these uniformly distributed random numbers and convert them into specific distributions of system inputs (e.g., generating patient ages based on a normal distribution).

There are several algorithms to generate pseudorandom numbers including mid-square method, linear congruential generator, multiple recursive generators, and Mersenne Twister.

Mid-Square Method

Mid-square method is one of the initial and simpler methods of generating pseudorandom numbers. We start with a four-digit, positive integer number as a seed. We then square the number and take the four digits in the middle (add zeros to the left if needed) as the next random number and repeat the process. This method is simple and easy to understand, but it can quickly fall into repeating cycles and result in degenerate sequences. This is a general problem for all algorithms. In a way, each pseudorandom number generator can be viewed as a giant wheel. We start somewhere on the wheel (i.e., seed) and travel over the perimeter of the wheel in every iteration. Eventually, we cover the entire perimeter of the wheel. At that point, we start repeating the sequence of random numbers that are degenerate and not random anymore. The number of iterations that it takes for an algorithm to start repeating itself is called *period*. The mid-square method usually has a small period and is prone to repeat itself quickly.

Example: Use mid-square method to generate three random numbers.

Step 1. We start with a four-digit, positive integer number as a seed. $X_0 = 1234$

Step 2. We square X_0 and add zeros to the left in order to get an eight-digit number. Then, pick the middle four-digits and add decimals which will be the new random number that is uniformly distributed between (0,1). $X_0^2 = 1522756$. Thus, the new eight-digit number is 01522756 and $X_0 = 05227$.

Step 3. $X_1^2 = 27321529$ and $X_2 = 0.3215$.

Step 4. $X_2^2 = 10336225$ and $X_3 = 0.3362$.

The following are the three random numbers using mid-square method: $X_1 = 0.5227$, $X_2 = 0.3215$, and $X_3 = 0.3362$.

Linear Congruential Generator

The linear congruential generator (LCG) is another simple and easy to understand algorithm to generate pseudorandom numbers. The LCG uses the following formula and starts with a seed number (X_0) and three constant numbers: a, c, and m.

$$X_{n+1} = (a \times X_n + c) \bmod m$$

where mod is a function to calculate the remainder of $(a \times X_n + c)$ divided by m.

The LCG also has a period which depends on parameters a, c, and m. Finding the best parameters in order to increase the period is not trivial and takes extensive experimentation.

Example: Use LCG to generate three random numbers.

Step 1. We initialize the algorithm parameters and the seed.

$$a = 5, c = 2, m = 4, X_0 = 7$$

Step 2. Using the formula, we calculate the first random number.

$$X_1 = (a \times X_0 + c) \bmod m = (5 \times 7 + 2) \bmod 4 = 37 \bmod 4 = 1$$

Step 3. We repeat step 2 until we have the desired number of random numbers.

$$X_2 = (a \times X_1 + c) \bmod m = (5 \times 1 + 2) \bmod 4 = 3$$
$$X_3 = (a \times X_2 + c) \bmod m = (5 \times 3 + 2) \bmod 4 = 1$$

The three random numbers are 1, 3, and 1. We can see that the next numbers will start to repeat, indicating the improper values of selected parameters.

Multiple Recursive Generators

Multiple recursive generators (MRGs) extend the LCG by incorporating multiple past values rather than just one, which helps to increase the period and statistical properties of the generator. MRG uses the following formula that incorporates past k values. When $k = 1$, the MRG is the same as the LCG with c = 0.

$$X_n = (a_1 X_{n-1} + a_2 X_{n-2} + \ldots + a_k X_{n-k}) \bmod m$$

In order to run the MRG, we need initial values of multipliers and their corresponding seeds.

MRGs are widely used in scientific simulations, statistical sampling problems, cryptography, and other applications that require high-quality randomness. Variants of MRGs such as MRG32k3a are widely used in modern random number libraries.

Mersenne Twister

The Mersenne Twister is one of the popular pseudorandom number generators due to its fast performance, long period, and high-quality randomness. The *RAND* function in Excel software uses the Mersenne Twister to generate pseudorandom numbers. The Mersenne Twister is a complex algorithm that uses a state vector of 624 numbers (32-bit integers) to generate pseudorandom numbers. The period of the Mersenne Twister is $2^{19937} - 1$, indicating its ability to generate a large set of high-quality pseudorandom numbers.

Suppose we have a pseudorandom number generator that generates uniformly distributed random variates. To convert these uniform random variates into other specific distributions (e.g., normal distribution), we use different transformation methods. Depending on the desired probability distribution, these methods could be simple or complex mathematical functions. Some of the popular methods include inverse transform method, composition method, Box–Muller method, and rejection sampling method. Much of the simulation theory focuses on these methods. Although details of these methods fall beyond the scope of this book, we need to recognize the importance of this step within the overall simulation framework. In practice, most commercial simulation software has built-in features to generate random samples from any probability distribution without the need to understand its underlying details.

LEARNING OBJECTIVE 8.3: EXPLAIN THE SYSTEM COMPONENT OF THE SIMULATION FRAMEWORK

A system is a collection of components that work together to achieve a unified goal. Despite this simple definition, systems can differ in many ways. Systems could be simple or complex, actual or abstract, deterministic or stochastic, static or dynamic, and discrete or continuous. These features determine which type of simulation model to be used.

Mathematical Solution

Simple and deterministic systems or problems can be analyzed mathematically, without needing to simulate. Consider an M/M/1 queue (single server, with exponential interarrival times and service distributions). We can precisely estimate the expected wait time in the queue with a mathematical expression.

Monte Carlo Simulation

For analyzing complex systems that are static (i.e., do not evolve over time), we can use Monte Carlo simulation. It is useful for both deterministic and stochastic systems or problems.

Example: Calculate the area of the following irregular shape, shown in **Figure 8.2**. This is an example of a static, deterministic, and complex problem. We can use Monte Carlo simulation to solve this problem.

We can draw a rectangle with known width (*w*) and length (*l*) and cover the given shape as shown in **Figure 8.3**. Then, cover the entire area of the rectangle with small balls (each ball representing a random coordinate).

The estimated area of the given shape can be calculated as the proportion of balls that fall within the shape to the total number of balls, multiplied by the area of the rectangle.

$$\textit{area of the shape} = \textit{area of the rectangle} \times \frac{\textit{number of balls within the shape}}{\textit{total number of balls}}$$

Example: Let us consider a stochastic process that involves uncertainty in outcomes. Suppose we are interested in estimating the likelihood of getting exactly three heads if we flip a fair coin five times. Since this is a fairly simple process, we can use either probability theory or Monte Carlo

FIGURE 8.2 Irregular shape.

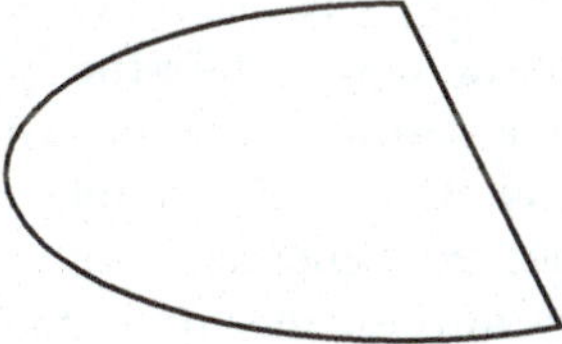

FIGURE 8.3 Irregular shape covered with a rectangle.

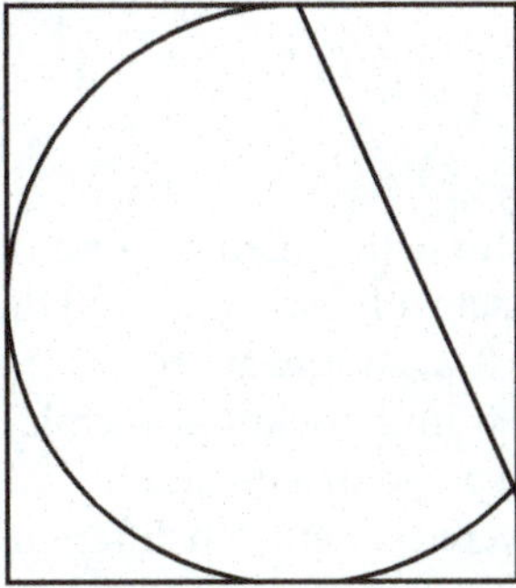

simulation to estimate the given probability. We can use binomial probability formula to calculate the given probability:

$$p(3\ H\ in\ 5) = \binom{5}{3} \times \frac{1}{2}^{3} \times \frac{1}{2}^{2} = 0.3125$$

Alternatively, we can use Excel to run a Monte Carlo simulation of this problem. We can use the RAND function to generate five random numbers between (0, 1) at a time. If the random number is <0.5, we consider it as a head; otherwise, it is a tail. We repeat this experiment 10,000 times and count the number of times that we observe exactly three heads. The estimated probability will be the proportion of times that we observe exactly three heads. If we repeat the simulation for large enough times (i.e., replication), the estimated probability should be close to 0.3125.

Discrete-Event Simulation

If a system changes at specific points in time, we can use discrete-event simulation (DES) to model the system and understand its behavior. Examples include queueing systems (where the queue size changes only when a patient arrives or leaves) that are present in various industries such as healthcare, manufacturing, transportation, airlines, and retail. Due to its popularity and extensive applications, there are many DES software (e.g., Arena, Simio, AnyLogic, and FlexSim) that are easy to learn and use. Nevertheless, building a DES requires extensive amounts of data, effort, and details.

Given the popularity of DES in healthcare, we introduce its components, terminologies, and examples in detail throughout Chapter 9, "Discrete-Event Simulation and Its Applications."

System Dynamics

If a system changes over time in a continuous manner, we can use system dynamics to model the system. Details and building block of system dynamics are different from DES. While DES is useful for modeling processes, system dynamics is useful for modeling big-picture dynamics involving accumulations and feedback loops (e.g., economics, ecosystem behavior, and policy impacts). Examples of system dynamics include modeling population growth or resource depletion over time.

Main building blocks of system dynamics include stocks (levels) that accumulate or deplete over time (e.g., population level, inventory level), flows (rates) in which stocks change (e.g., birth rate, demand rate), and feedback loops within the system that are either positive (reinforcing) or negative (balancing). In a reinforcing loop, a change in one direction leads to further changes that amplify the initial effect. For example, money in a savings account earns interest, which increases the balance and generates even more interest over time. In contrast, balancing loops oppose change by introducing forces that act in the opposite direction to restore stability.

System dynamics is a powerful modeling technique in healthcare for evaluating the system-wide effects of various policies and understanding the feedback loops within the system. Similar to DES, there are numerous software that are used for building system dynamics models such as Vensim and AnyLogic.

Agent-Based Modeling

Agent-based modeling (ABM) is a simulation method for modeling dynamic systems where entities (agents) within the system interact with each other and the system. Unlike DES where entities do not interact with each other, in ABM, entities are agents that can behave differently in different conditions. The ABM is widely used in modeling epidemic and social behaviors. For example, the ABM can be used to model the spread of a disease in which people with different conditions (e.g., susceptible, infected, and recovered) interact in different ways. For instance, each interaction between an infected and susceptible person may transmit the disease. Similar to DES and system dynamics, ABM is also widely used in different applications and industries and being supported in commercial software such as AnyLogic and NetLogo.

Hybrid Systems

Sometimes, a system consists of several subsystems that all need to be integrated within the simulation model. When the subsystems differ in type (e.g., one subsystem changes continuously and one subsystem changes at specific points in time), we may end up using different simulation models simultaneously (e.g., system dynamics with DES). In this case, the aggregated model is referred to as a hybrid model. For example, consider a health system network as the main system. Patient flow in its hospitals and clinics could be modeled as DES models. The dynamics of its overarching policies could be modeled as a system dynamics model, and the interaction between the clinics and hospitals could be modeled as an ABM. Due to the increasing popularity of hybrid models in practice, some commercial software, such as AnyLogic, supports all three simulation models and provides a platform to build hybrid models within the same software.

LEARNING OBJECTIVE 8.4: ASSESS THE ESTIMATED MEASURES AS ONE OF THE COMPONENTS OF THE SIMULATION FRAMEWORK

The main goal of any simulation model is to estimate some parameters. For example, we might be interested in average ED boarding time in the next 10 years or average number of ED admissions per day if we increase the number of beds by 10%. Often, the actual and true value of these parameters are unknown or difficult to calculate. Without knowing the true values, how are we going to verify if simulation estimates are in fact accurate and reliable?

One way to verify the estimates is to first build a base simulation model. In the base model, we do not include any intervention (e.g., increasing the number of beds by 10%). We then compare the base simulation outputs with actual data. For example, we can run the base ED simulation and collect its reported statistics such as average ED boarding time, average number of ED admissions per day, and ED throughput. We can then compare these statistics with real data using appropriate hypotheses tests. If they are not significantly different, simulation should be close to reality. Otherwise, the simulation details need to be adjusted. Once the base simulation model is verified, we can then run the model for a longer time period (e.g., 10 years) for predictions or test different intervention impacts (e.g., increasing beds, hiring more nurses). Each of these models are called scenarios.

Apart from basic comparison and post hoc analyses, advanced statistics and simulation theory provide insights on how to rigorously verify simulation outputs, reduce its variance, build confidence intervals around the parameter estimates, understand the convergence of the simulation estimates, and determine the required simulation time to reach a steady state. These are advanced topics that fall beyond the scope of this book. The following sections outline some of the important simulation verification concepts.

Warm-Up Period

Typically, simulation models need to run for some time, known as warm-up period, until the system reaches its steady state. Consider simulating ED operations. At the beginning of the simulation, the ED beds are empty. As the simulation evolves, patients begin to arrive, and the system begins to look like an actual busy ED. During the warm-up period, no statistics are being collected. One way to determine the warm-up period is to plot the system performance over time and see when the plot begins to stabilize. **Figure 8.4** shows the warm-up and data collection periods for a performance measure. For example, we can plot the ED occupancy over time. The plot

FIGURE 8.4 Warm-up and data collection periods of a performance measure.

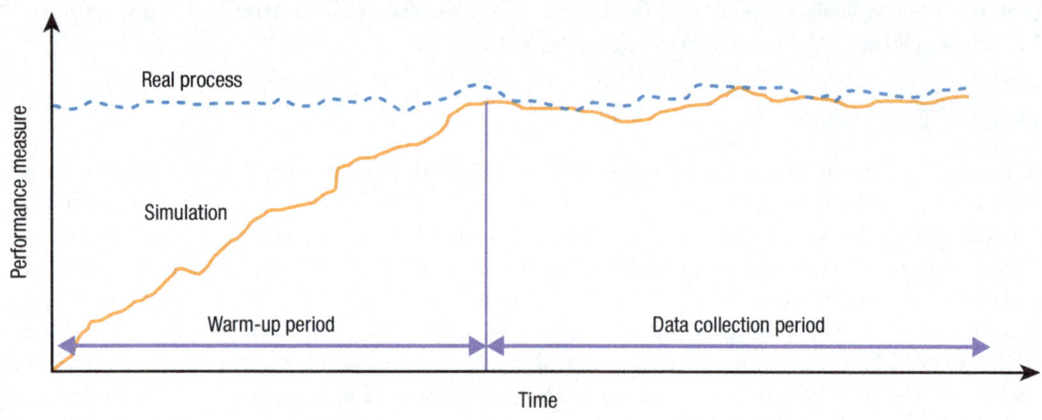

should increase steadily, reach a certain level (e.g., 80%), and then continue to fluctuate around that level.

To achieve reliable estimations, we should always allow simulation models to warm up for some period of time. Most modern simulation software allows you to specify the warm-up period.

Replication

We know from statistics that larger sample size results in more accurate (i.e., smaller standard error) estimates of mean. Similar analogy applies to simulation. To minimize the estimation error of a simulation, we can simply increase the number of simulations, which is known as replications. Note that this method will only reduce the natural variability due to randomness and not going to address modeling discrepancies or external variability.

A simulation model with 100 replications provides more accurate estimations than the same simulation model with only 10 replications. Almost all modern simulation software allows users to specify the replication number. At the end of the simulation, estimated measures are reported as averages of these replications.

Sensitivity and Robustness Analysis

Sensitivity analysis is a necessary step in both simulation verification (before running the simulation) and post hoc analysis (after running the simulation and collecting the estimated measures). In sensitivity analysis, we change simulation or system parameters one at a time and observe the impacts on simulation outputs. Sometimes, small changes in input parameters can result in significant changes on simulation outputs. If simulation outputs are less sensitive to its inputs, then the results are considered to be robust. Sometimes, sensitivity is due to the nature of the system, and sometimes it is due to poor modeling. Either way, sensitivity and robustness analysis help to identify sensitive parameters and inputs.

SUMMARY

In this chapter, we explored the foundational concepts of simulation modeling and its essential components. The framework for simulations consists of key elements, including random number generators, system inputs, the system itself as the primary model, and the estimated performance measures derived from system outputs. Random number generators play a crucial role in introducing variability and stochastic behavior, which are critical for modeling real-world uncertainty. System inputs, such as probability distributions and initial conditions, drive the simulation and influence the outcomes, while the system model represents the process or system being studied, whether physical, abstract, or hybrid. Estimated measures based on outputs, such as performance metrics, efficiency, and cost-effectiveness, help evaluate and interpret the results of the simulation.

We also discussed when simulation is an appropriate and effective tool for analysis. Simulation is particularly useful when analytical solutions are infeasible due to the complexity of the system or when randomness and variability must be considered. Understanding different types of simulations (e.g., Monte Carlo, discrete-event, system dynamics, and agent-based modeling) allows us to choose the most suitable approach for a given system. We examined scenarios in which each type is preferable and how to tailor simulation strategies to match specific system characteristics and objectives.

Lastly, we reviewed the critical steps necessary to ensure the reliability and robustness of simulation outputs. These steps include proper model formulation, verification to confirm the model operates as intended, and validation to ensure it accurately represents the system. Techniques such as sensitivity analysis, scenario testing, and the use of appropriate warm-up period and replications were highlighted as essential practices for improving the credibility of simulation results.

Ultimately, this chapter provided a comprehensive framework for designing, executing, and interpreting simulations to support decision-making and problem-solving across various domains.

END-OF-CHAPTER RESOURCES

DISCUSSION QUESTIONS

1. Discuss how simulation contributes to understanding and predicting the behavior of complex systems.

2. Why is sensitivity analysis important in model validation, and how does it improve decision-making?

3. What are the key differences between agent-based simulation, discrete-event simulation, and hybrid modeling?

4. Why is it essential to consider warm-up periods and replications when assessing the reliability of simulation results?

5. How do random number generators impact the accuracy of simulation experiments?

LEARNING ACTIVITIES

CourseConnect ›

To access self-assessment questions and interactive, competency-based learning activities for this chapter, visit www.springerpub.com/courseconnect. See inside front cover and tear-out card for CourseConnect details.

CHAPTER 9

DISCRETE-EVENT SIMULATION AND ITS APPLICATIONS

LEARNING OBJECTIVES

9.1. List the building blocks of discrete-event simulation.

9.2. Explain when to use discrete-event simulation.

9.3. Create simple discrete-event simulation model.

9.4. Name simulation software for complex discrete-event simulation models.

9.5. Identify the applications and potential of discrete-event simulation in healthcare management.

REAL-WORLD SCENARIO

A recent public health emergency presented major operational challenges for Central Valley Medical Center, which serves a community of about 120,000 people. The hospital's ED, surgical units, and inpatient bed availability were all under extreme strain as a result of a sharp increase in patient admissions. Managing patient flow and guaranteeing prompt care delivery became more challenging due to irregular patient arrival patterns, differing lengths of stay, and complex resource allocation issues.

In order to address these issues, the hospital administration used discrete-event simulation (DES) to model important procedures and improve patient flow control.

LEARNING OBJECTIVE 9.1: LIST THE BUILDING BLOCKS OF DISCRETE-EVENT SIMULATION

DES is a powerful tool to model complex and stochastic systems that change at different points in time. In DES, the state of the system changes in discrete times rather than a continuous time. State refers to a variable or set of variables that contain just enough information to describe the system at any given time. The state is usually defined together with events. Events are occurrences that change the state. For example, suppose we are simulating a laboratory testing center that processes samples for diagnostic testing. In this type of system, state and events could be defined as follows:

- **State:** Number of samples in the queue, number of samples being processed, number of lab technicians currently working. We represent each state variable with a mathematical variable.
- **Events:** Sample arrivals, sample completions

Note that with each new event, the state is updated. For example, with a new sample arrival, the number of samples in the queue increases by one unit. Similarly, with any sample completion, both the number of samples being processed and the number of lab technicians currently working decrease by one unit.

TABLE 9.1 Definition of Discrete-Event Simulation Components

TERM	DEFINITION
State	Variable or set of variables that contain just enough information to describe the system at any given time
Event	Occurrences that change the state
Entity	Virtual objects of interest in the system
Attribute	Characteristics that describe entities
Resource	Entities compete for resources
Clock	Virtual clock that keeps track of the simulation time
Simulation period	User-specified time period for the simulation to run

In order for events to occur, the simulation should have entities and resources. Entities are virtual objects of interest in the system. They are generated and fed into the system according to a specified probability distribution. For example, walk-in patients to an outpatient clinic could be an entity type. With a certain interarrival probability distribution (i.e., determined by historical data), these entities are fed into the model. Entities may have differentiating characteristics (e.g., age, severity of illness). These characteristics are called attributes.

Once entities are generated, they compete for resources, which are often limited in scope. Resources can be hospital beds, nursing staff, medical equipment, or any type of service that are limited in quantity. When there are more entities needing the same resource, there will be a queue that forms to allocate that resource. Lastly, DES needs a clock or time tracker to reorder events to run over time. Simulation time or duration is specified by the user. For example, we can build a DES of a hospital and run the model for 6 months. The actual running time of the model in computer software processing time might only be a few seconds or minutes (depending on the model complexity). Users can also speed up the simulation. When the full simulation duration is reached, the simulation stops. In this case, the stopping criteria is called the simulation period. **Table 9.1** summarizes the definitions of discrete-event simulation components.

Example: Consider toll gates in highways that we drive through every day. Sometimes, there will be a long queue of cars behind the gates. We can simulate these toll gates using a DES in order to optimize the traffic flow. In simulating a toll gate system with a DES, identify the state, events, entities, resources, queues, and attributes. Explain how DES can be useful to improve the system.

When simulating a toll gate system, we can estimate average wait time for cars, average queue length, and average number of cars that pass through the gates. To improve the system, we can define scenarios (based on expert opinions, literature review, or other methods) and test their impacts on performance measures. Scenarios could include increasing the number of gates (scenario 1) or speeding up the processing time at the gates (scenario 2). We can create different solutions, compare them with each other, and conduct cost-effectiveness analyses among the scenarios. Speeding up the processing time may be a more cost-effective scenario in a short term, but increasing the number of gates might be a more cost-effective scenario in the long term. Our inputs in this case are as follows:

- **State:** Number of cars in each gate (note that the total number of gates does not change over time, so it is not a state variable)
- **Events:** Car arrivals, car departures
- **Entities:** Cars that go through the gates. We could define two entity types, one for E-ZPass and one for cash payers. Alternatively, we could have one entity type and assign payment types as an attribute.

- **Resources:** Gates
- **Queues:** One for each gate
- **Attributes:** Car size and weight, fee payment mode. Many features could define cars (such as color, make, model, year, speed, and style) but we should only choose features as attributes that are going to influence the system's operation. For example, color is not a suitable attribute. However, payment mode is a suitable attribute because it will influence the service time at the gate. Cars with cash payments take longer to process than E-ZPass.
- **Clock:** Simulation clock that keeps track of time

Now that we have learned about building blocks of DES, we can explore its suitability, advantages, and disadvantages for modeling different systems.

LEARNING OBJECTIVE 9.2: EXPLAIN WHEN TO USE DISCRETE-EVENT SIMULATION

We learned that DES is a useful modeling tool for understanding complex and dynamic systems where the state variables change in discrete time points. DES offers flexibility and is a suitable choice when the system is complex or has a high level of detail (such as hospitals and complex networks). In addition, DES provides comprehensive outputs, meaning that users can define their own performance metrics and collect the desired statistics at the end of the simulation. Moreover, DES offers visualization tools and options. Often, users can include a system's floor plans into the simulation and visualize, track, or observe the movement of entities throughout the system. Visualization is an easy way to identify potential bottlenecks within the system. Also, DES can incorporate algorithms to optimize the distribution of resources based on given objectives and constraints. The combination of DES with optimization can be used for various applications, including scheduling, staffing, resource allocation, and capacity planning. Further, DES is a suitable tool for cost-effectiveness analyses. We can run what-if scenarios in a risk-free simulation environment and experiment with different options to identify the most cost-effective scenarios and predictive outcomes. For example, one popular application of DES is conducting cost-effectiveness analyses of different medications for given illnesses.

DES also has some disadvantages. DESs can be difficult to build, understand, and validate for complex systems. Additionally, building a reliable DES requires one to have data on all the details being modeled. Moreover, simplifying a system for modelling purposes might miss critical real-world factors and implications.

LEARNING OBJECTIVE 9.3: CREATE SIMPLE DISCRETE-EVENT SIMULATION MODEL

Before we learn about DES modeling in spreadsheet, it is worth noting the DES algorithm and its overall steps.

Discrete-Event Simulation Steps

A DES algorithm consists of four major steps: initialization, event scheduling, state update, and termination. In the initialization step, we define system boundaries (what is included and what is not); entities and their arrival or interarrival probability distributions, attributes, resources, and capacities; and service times (along with all initial conditions). In the event scheduling step, the algorithm maintains a full list of randomly generated future events that are drawn from the distributions and then processes them in chronological order. In the third step, the system state is updated when an event occurs. In the termination step, the simulation is concluded after a specified run time or other termination criteria (e.g., max number of entities).

Discrete-Event Simulation in Spreadsheets

Spreadsheets (e.g., Microsoft Excel) are effective tools that can be used to simulate fairly simple systems. In spreadsheet simulation, each row indicates an entity. We assume entities arrive chronologically, which is reflected by having sequentially numbered spreadsheet rows already available.

Assume we have a simple system with only one resource (i.e., a service). As we learn in Chapter 10, "Queueing and Scheduling," this system is called a single-server queue. If entities arrive at a faster rate than they leave, there will be a queue behind the server.

Consider an ED triage system in place for when patients arrive. Typically, the facility may employ a nurse (i.e., server, resource) that triages patients arriving to the ED. Patient arrival time and volume is often uncertain; however, we can use historical data to extract some patterns or empirical distributions about both. Similarly, the service time is uncertain, depending on patient needs and complexities. In this example, we show the use of Microsoft Excel to simulate the ED triage system and evaluate some of the performance measures about the process. The simulation process is shown in **Table 9.2**.

First, we list entities (i.e., patients). For demonstration purposes, we only show the first five entities in **Table 9.2**, but in real applications, the number of entities could easily reach into the hundreds or thousands of patients.

For each entity, we generate two random numbers from the desired distributions: one for interarrival time (column 2 in **Table 9.2**) and one for service time (column 3 in **Table 9.2**).

Note that Excel allows you to draw random numbers for a variety of distributions, including the uniform (0, 1) distribution. We can then convert them into desired distributions. The conversion process from a uniform distribution to another distribution is not always straightforward and might involve complex mathematical and statistical operations that fall beyond the scope of this course. However, students can use online calculators or other software to generate random samples from a desired distribution.

For instance, to draw a random number from an exponential distribution with $\lambda = 10$, we can generate a random number from a uniform (0,1) distribution using RAND function. Let us say the function RAND returns 0.83. Then, use the following equation to calculate the exponentially distributed random number:

$$-\frac{ln(1 - \text{RAND})}{\lambda} = -\frac{ln(1 - 0.83)}{10} = 0.177$$

To calculate the arrival time column, we cumulatively sum the interarrival times provided in sequence. This process begins with an initial time of zero (or a designated starting time if

TABLE 9.2 Discrete-Event Simulation of an Emergency Department Triage System

PATIENT	INTERARRIVAL TIME	SERVICE TIME	ARRIVAL TIME	SERVICE START TIME	SERVICE END TIME	WAIT TIME IN QUEUE	FLOW TIME	SERVER IDLE TIME
1	0	2	0	0	2	0	2	–
2	3	3	3	3	6	0	3	1
3	2	2	5	6	8	1	3	0
4	2	4	7	8	12	1	5	0
5	7	2	14	14	16	0	2	2

specified), and each subsequent arrival time is determined by adding the next interarrival time to the running total. For example, if the first patient arrives at time 0 and the first interarrival time is 3 minutes, the next patient's arrival time would be 0 + 3 = 3 minutes and so forth. This pattern continues until all arrival times are computed.

The service start time represents the earliest time a server can begin assisting a patient. For this to happen, two conditions must be satisfied: (1) the server must be available and ready, and (2) the patient must have already arrived. Therefore, the service start time for a given patient is determined as the maximum of the patient's arrival time and the previous service end time. This ensures that if a patient arrives before the server is ready, service cannot commence until the server is free.

The service end time is calculated by adding the service time for the current patient to their service start time. This marks the moment when service for the patient is completed, and the server becomes available for the next individual. Note that there is an underlying assumption that server is not allowed to pause and switch to a different patient when they start serving a patient (i.e., no preemption is allowed).

The wait time in the queue reflects how long a patient waits before receiving service. It is the difference between the service start time and the arrival time. If a patient is served immediately upon arrival, their wait time is zero. Note that wait time is a critical performance measure for any system. Once the wait time for each patient is calculated, we can calculate various statistics such as average wait time, maximum wait time, wait time range, and standard deviation.

Another key performance measure is the flow time (also referred to as the time in the system), which measures the total time a patient spends in the system, from their arrival until the completion of service. It is calculated as the difference between the service end time and the arrival time. Alternatively, we can sum service time and wait time in queue (why?).

Lastly, the server idle time quantifies the duration for which the server remains idle between two consecutive service operations. It is the difference between the current service start time and the previous service end time. If a patient arrives exactly when the server is ready, the idle time is zero (e.g., patients 3 and 4). Otherwise, any gap between the previous service end time and the current service start time represents server idle time.

Server idle time provides important information about system efficiency and utilization. It can be used for capacity planning, staffing, and resource management. Large idle times indicate low utilization and the need for better capacity planning.

In this example, the simulation terminated with the fifth patient at minute 16. One way to calculate the utilization of the triage nurse is to divide the total time that the nurse was working by the total simulation time. In this case, the triage nurse's utilization is $\frac{13}{16} = 0.8125 = 81.25\%$.

LEARNING OBJECTIVE 9.4: NAME SIMULATION SOFTWARE FOR COMPLEX DISCRETE-EVENT SIMULATION MODELS

Given the limitations of Excel in modeling complex systems, we use specific DES software to model complex real-world problems. Some of the popular software platforms for DES modeling are Arena, Simio, AnyLogic, and FlexSim. Each of these software packages offer different features and tools that require different syntax and rules. For example, AnyLogic includes the Process Modeling Library, a discrete-event simulation library that provides blocks for quickly simulating complex discrete-event systems. The AnyLogic software has online instructional examples with different levels of complexity, including a discrete-event simulation model of a bank office (https://anylogic.help/tutorials/bank-office/index.html), as shown in **Figure 9.1**.

FIGURE 9.1 Discrete-event simulation model of a bank office in AnyLogic.

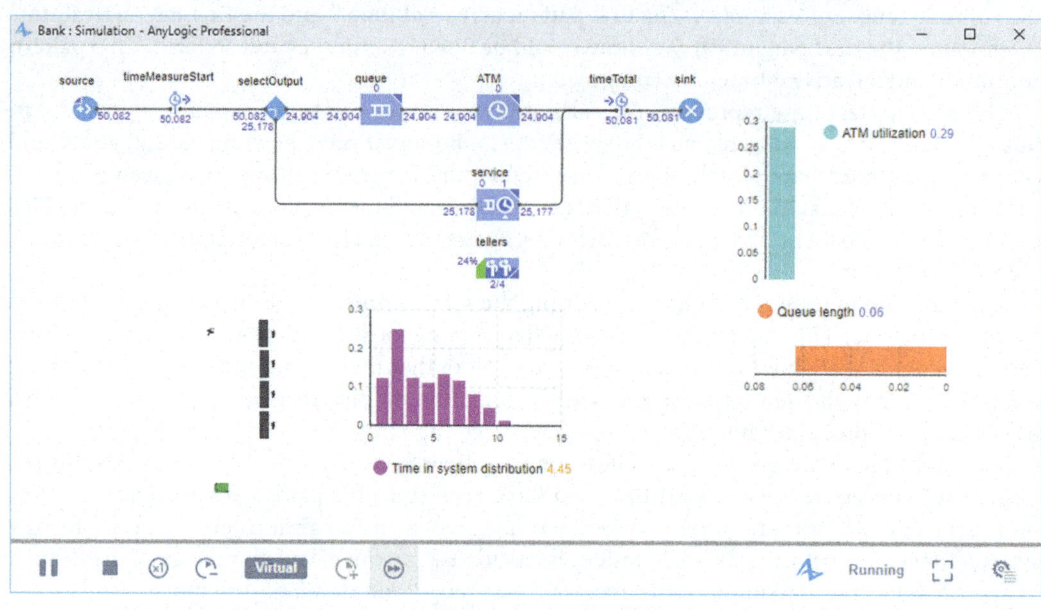

Source: The AnyLogic Company. (n.d.). *Bank office model.* https://anylogic.help/tutorials/bank-office/index
.html

The software provides a space to create a DES model by assembling and connecting prebuilt blocks that do different things. These models look similar to flowcharts where entities go through the chart in the same direction. We explore flowcharts in Chapter 18, "Project Management." Flowcharts are essential starting points in creating DES models. As you can see in **Figure 9.1**, each DES begins with a source block. The source block does the same random number generation and conversion steps as in Excel. We can specify the entity details and their probability distributions in the properties section of the source block. Any DES ends with a sink block, which basically disposes of the entities after they have been served. The sink block acts like the end or exit step in a flowchart. Anything between the source and sink blocks should come from your flowchart or logic model of the system. Once the simulation is completed, we can add plots and visualization to track performance measures in real time.

The Arena software has similar prebuilt blocks for modeling complex systems. **Figure 9.2** represents a simple single-server queue created in Arena. It begins with a create block (similar to source block in AnyLogic) and ends with a dispose block (similar to the sink block in AnyLogic). The process block is the main service with specific distribution that users can specify in its properties. Numbers under each block represent the number of entities that have passed through the block (i.e., counter). As the simulation proceeds, these numbers will begin to increase. The Arena software also offers visualization and plotting options that could be included within the

FIGURE 9.2 A simple single-server queue simulation created in Arena.

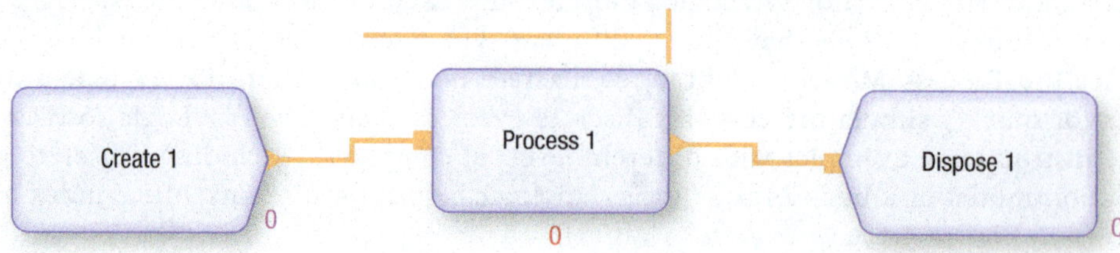

simulation model. At the end of the simulation, Arena automatically generates a detailed report of default and user specified performance measures, along with their statistics (e.g., half width, min, and max).

LEARNING OBJECTIVE 9.5: IDENTIFY THE APPLICATIONS AND POTENTIAL OF DISCRETE-EVENT SIMULATION IN HEALTHCARE MANAGEMENT

Most topics in healthcare operations management involve the flow of items or people through processes within a complex system. With the main goal of healthcare operations management to improve efficiency and reduce costs, the DES can play a critical role in addressing healthcare operations management challenges. Some of these applications include staffing, scheduling, patient flow management, and resource allocation.

Staffing

Staffing involves determining the right number and mix of personnel and skill sets needed to meet service demands efficiently. Staffing is a major challenge for hospitals and health systems due to its implications on total expenses, regulatory policies, availability of workforce, and retention and burnout issues, among others. Personnel and human resources make up the majority of expenses for health systems. Some states have mandatory policies for certain personnel types (e.g., nurse to patient ratios in the ICU). The use of part-time or per-diem personnel in healthcare is also very common due to shortages and budgetary constraints. Moreover, demand tends to fluctuate over time with the combinations of seasonality patterns, trends, and random variations. Hence, with so much variability on patient volumes and their needs and with so many influencing factors on the supply of medical care to patients, staffing remains one of the most important and challenging problems for all hospitals and health systems to solve.

Among different methods, discrete-event simulation is one of the popular tools to determine staffing levels in healthcare. With DES, we can model a complex system with the needed details and compare between different staffing scenarios. The base scenario usually assumes the current system with no intervention. Alternative scenarios could include variations in staffing levels, mix, or types. So, for example, would it be "better" (however you would like to define better) to have two part-time nurses instead of one full-time nurse in the ED? By increasing the number of ED nurses by 10%, how much will the average ED wait time and ED throughputs (e.g., number of visits, number of admitted patients, and length of stay) change? The DES can answer these questions with respect to costs and other performance measures of interest. In addition, DES can create a break-even point and justify the need for a specific staffing scenario.

Scheduling

Scheduling refers to determining the sequence and timing of tasks to be completed by resources (including human resources and equipment). Scheduling algorithms can determine the sequence and exact start time of various processes, for example, surgeries (tasks) within different operating rooms (resources).

Scheduling for some routine and repetitive processes, such as product assembly lines, is often more straightforward than those in healthcare because of the limited and shared nature of resources (e.g., beds, providers, and equipment) in healthcare and also the variability in service durations. Unlike routine tasks like providing vaccinations, some complex surgeries and procedures can vary widely among patients because of several factors such as surgeons' expertise, the preexisting conditions of patients, or other unknowns that are not clear until the process (surgery) is underway. On top of these, coordination among departments and different stakeholders (e.g., insurance companies, nursing home facilities, and diagnostic laboratories), the unpredictability of demand (e.g., ED patients), and the variability in patient preferences add additional layers of complexities to optimize scheduling policies.

In Chapter 10, "Queueing and Scheduling," we learn about some basic scheduling problems and algorithms; however, we need simulation tools to evaluate scheduling algorithms in complex systems. Once a complex system is modeled as a DES, various scheduling policies can be compared through simulation scenarios. How much will resource utilization, average patient wait time, and satisfaction change if we overbook patients for routine surgeries are the types of questions that DES can address.

Patient Flow Management

Operating with smooth patient flow throughout a system is a common goal for health managers. Doing so requires addressing bottlenecks and smoothing patient transitions between discharge and admission points. Many factors impede patient flow such as the variability in demand for care, resource limitations, and external factors such as the availability of beds in nursing homes or the discharge process within the hospital. Whether patient flow is a local issue within a single hospital unit or specific service line or a global issue throughout the hospital or even a care system, DES can be used to model the system and test various scenarios to achieve better patient flow.

Resource Allocation

Allocation and reallocation of resources in healthcare is not a one-time task. Bed management in hospitals, allocating ambulances for a region, and distributing vaccines or medical equipment are all examples of resource allocation that requires some level of balance between shortage risk and efficiency. Again, we can use DES to evaluate different allocation scenarios and quantify their impacts on efficiency and risk measures.

SUMMARY

This chapter provides a deeper understanding of discrete-event simulation due to its popularity in healthcare operations management. The chapter includes a brief overview of DES, its building blocks, and terminologies. The chapter lists some of the unique pros and cons of DES which provides further insights on when to use DES. The chapter also briefly explains how DESs work from the algorithmic perspective. It then provides general guidelines on how to use DES, both for simple systems and complex systems. The chapter concludes with a brief overview of broader applications of DES in healthcare operations management such as staffing, scheduling, patient flow, and resource allocation.

END-OF-CHAPTER RESOURCES

DISCUSSION QUESTIONS

1. What are the key building blocks of discrete-event simulation, and how do they interact?

2. How does discrete-event simulation differ from other simulation techniques, such as system dynamics or agent-based modeling?

3. How can discrete-event simulation improve decision-making in healthcare management?

4. How does the choice of parameters and assumptions impact the outcomes of a discrete-event simulation?

5. What real-world healthcare problems can be addressed using discrete-event simulation?

LEARNING ACTIVITIES

CourseConnect ›

To access self-assessment questions and interactive, competency-based learning activities for this chapter, visit www.springerpub.com/courseconnect. See inside front cover and tear-out card for CourseConnect details.

CHAPTER 10

QUEUEING AND SCHEDULING

LEARNING OBJECTIVES

10.1. Describe service systems and waiting lines using appropriate terms and concepts.

10.2. Analyze service systems and waiting lines using queueing theory.

10.3. Use queueing theory calculations to manage the relationship between waiting and the resources needed to provide service in different types of systems.

10.4. Identify scheduling problem components.

10.5. Solve single-server and identical parallel-server scheduling problems.

REAL-WORLD SCENARIO

Sumac MED-Care is an urgent care center. Analysis reveals that the average hourly arrival rate 4.0 per hour on weekdays during the 12-hour shift from 8 a.m. to 8 p.m. The current service rate is 6.0 patients per hour. The current staffing is one physician and one nurse. One receptionist is also available for patient registration, records maintenance, and billing. Sumac MED-Care is interested in applying queueing theory to analyze, on average, how long patients wait in the clinic and whether it could improve the flow by better aligning its resources.

LEARNING OBJECTIVE 10.1. DESCRIBE SERVICE SYSTEMS AND WAITING LINES USING APPROPRIATE TERMS AND CONCEPTS

We have all been there—waiting in line for service. Lines waiting for service are everywhere, including throughout healthcare. For example, laboratory specimens wait in line for processing. Bills wait in line for payment. Prescriptions wait in line for filling in a pharmacy. CT scans wait in line for interpretation. Patients wait to be seen by their primary care provider. Waiting in lines and healthcare today are ubiquitous. This chapter focuses on waiting lines and service systems and the quantitative models that can be used to balance the waiting time of units (e.g., people, laboratory specimens, bills, prescriptions) with the resources used to provide the service. Throughout this chapter, anything or anyone that waits in a line is referred to as a unit. The service provided to the unit is referred to as a unit of service. Most people find waiting lines, especially waiting lines they consider too long, somewhat obnoxious, as well as a contemporary fact of life. People generally do not like to wait. For the patient, waiting is nonproductive time and is referred to as idle time. From a service system perspective, however, a line represents a demand for service. As long as a line of units, such as people or patients, is present, the server has the ability to engage in productive activity, such as serving the (next) unit, patient, resident, or client. In situations that use lines, when no line exists, the server is idle until the next unit arrives. Idle servers are not productive elements of the organizations. Units, such as people waiting in line for service, suggest that a server is productive. If no unit is in line, the server is idle, just waiting for a unit to enter the line and proceed to be serviced. This last point is significant to your understanding of waiting lines. Servers, such as physicians, benefit from long patient waiting lines in their "waiting" rooms. When lines exist, the physician has no idle or nonproductive time between patients. When finished with one patient, the physician is able to immediately move on to the next patient in line. In other instances, waiting lines are not productive, such as with lab tests and diagnostics that may be highly time sensitive to helping patients. Providing a service requires and consumes resources. For example, filling a prescription requires a pharmacist's time as well as the supplies necessary to satisfy the demand expressed in the prescription. It also requires adequate space and, in some instances, specialized equipment. How long a specific unit, such as a prescription, waits in a line for service depends upon the number of pharmacists on duty to fill prescriptions as well as the time it takes the pharmacist to fill prescriptions that arrived earlier. In principle, adding more pharmacists and/or other resources can lower the time a unit waits in line. More pharmacists are able to process more prescriptions. Being able to process more units should lower the time any one unit has to wait in line for service. If, however, demand fluctuates and too many pharmacists are assigned, some will be idle and not engaged in productive activity.

Any service system has a finite (processing) capacity. Maybe one professor can grade five short papers per hour. Twelve minutes per paper or five papers per hour would be the (average) service rate of a system that relied upon one professor to grade short papers. As such, faced with a stack or line of 40 papers, it should take one professor 8 hours to process all the papers. Two professors should be able to complete the same task in approximately 4 hours, each devoting 4 hours to grading. Although the total amount of service time did not change, it remained at 8 hours; the time any one paper had to wait in line was shortened because all papers were graded in 4 hours. In other words, with one professor, the last paper in the line of stack had to wait 8 hours minus 12 minutes, or 7 hours and 48 minutes to be processed. With two professors, the last papers only had to wait 4 hours minus the 12 minutes necessary to process any one paper, or 3 hours and 48 minutes. By adding resources to the service system, such as adding an additional professor, the speed of the service system to process or serve units can be increased. A service rate (per hour) is defined as the amount of time it takes to provide service to one unit. In the previous example, the service rate per short paper was (on average) 12 minutes. Service systems, however, have a finite, not an infinite, capacity to provide a unit of service. In some instances, the limitation of the service system is a physical limit. A hospital with three surgical suites can perform only three surgical operations at any one time. If the demand for surgery is more than three at any one time, patients wait. Machines also have limitations. For example, the CT scanner may be technically capable of finite number of individual scans per hour, regardless of the staffing used to support the machine. In still other instances, management establishes a limitation of a service system based upon the number and type of servers assigned to the service system. By assigning one, in contrast to more than one pharmacist to the pharmacy, management has defined the service capacity of the pharmacy. If one pharmacist is able to fill 20 prescriptions per hour, assigning only one pharmacist to the pharmacy limits the pharmacy's ability to service prescriptions to no more than 20 prescriptions per hour.

Management needs to balance waiting time with the resources used to provide a service. Health administrators face a dual and potentially conflicting concern. On one hand, administrators are concerned about efficiency and worker productivity. Idle staff, machines, and surgical suites do not benefit the organization, its financial position, or its potential patients or clients. On the other hand, health administrators provide a quality service when it is needed. They want to minimize, for example, the amount of time a patient must wait for surgery, a laboratory test, or a specific treatment. Delay in providing a service is never therapeutic. Long delays may lead to a change or deterioration in the condition of the patient or a laboratory specimen awaiting a test. Although short delays are usually acceptable from a clinical perspective, the definition of what constitutes a long and or short delay is relative and circumstantial. Twenty minutes may constitute too long or an unacceptable delay for a special medical test or procedure, given the condition of the patient. Twenty minutes may, however, be a short or acceptable delay for a patient to be seen by the physician in an ambulatory care clinic. The clinical acceptability or unacceptability of the delay in the service system to provide the demanded (and needed) service varies based upon the specific service in question as well as other clinical and medical considerations. The client's acceptance of a delay also may affect a patient and participation in the service. For example, "too long a wait" as defined by a client, may decrease the demand for service. To have an efficient organization as well as efficient service systems and subsystems, managers must balance acceptable waiting times with the input resources used to provide the service.

This balancing can be referred to as "managing the service system." A system's arrival rate is the rate (per hour) at which a unit arrives for service. Upon arrival, a unit either waits for service or, if the service system is idle, is served immediately and experiences no waiting time. Most lines work using first in, first out (FIFO). Units that arrive first are serviced first. Some exceptions exist.

In some instances, service systems are managed using scheduling and appointment systems to predetermine when units arrive. For example, most physicians in private practice provide appointments to their patients. Most patient admissions to a hospital are scheduled by providing an appointment for a given day. Surgeons are provided appointments for using a specific surgical suite in the hospital. Providing an appointment attempts to minimize the wait for service by establishing a constant demand over time for a service that can be met within existing resource levels. In still other situations, special procedures are used to manage service systems. For example, in hospitals, a physician can order "stat" processing of a medical test, meaning that the test will be rushed to the laboratory and processed ahead of any other tests waiting service. In hospital EDs, patients are seen and evaluated and then placed in the service line based upon their immediate medical needs, not based upon the order in which they arrived for service. Referred to as medical triaging, in this type of service system, one's place in the service line is not established by the order of arrival. Thus, in a hospital ED, the order of units in the line is determined and redetermined every time another patient arrives based upon the new patient's medical need. A patient will remain last in line as long as patients with more pressing medical needs continue to arrive and demand service.

Many analytical models exist to assist the manager to analyze service systems and balance the capacity of the system to provide a unit of service with the time a unit must wait for service. In other words, quantitative models exist to help managers make decisions concerning the design and operation of waiting lines. Some of these models can be found in queueing theory, the formal study of waiting lines. Queue is the English term for a waiting line.

LEARNING OBJECTIVE 10.2: ANALYZE SERVICE SYSTEMS AND WAITING LINES USING QUEUEING THEORY

Queueing theory provides the ability to quantitatively describe lines, waiting, and the operative characteristics of a service system. Using this approach requires that the line and service system meet certain criteria. For example, units (e.g., patients, tests, and prescriptions) must arrive for service randomly; they are not scheduled. Also, when a unit arrives is not influenced by when previous units arrived or exited the system. The number of units waiting also must have no influence upon when a unit will arrive. If the average number of units that arrive in 1 hour is six, this does not mean that a unit arrives every 10 minutes. It means that in any 1 hour, six units on average will arrive. This is very different than one unit arriving every 10 minutes, even though both could be expressed as an arrival rate of six per hour. With an (average) arrival rate of six per hour, there is a probability that all will arrive at any one time during the hour. There is also the probability that each will arrive every 10 minutes. Random arrivals mean that probabilities govern when units arrive in the specified time period.

Another defining criterion is FIFO line behavior. FIFO means first in, first out, as a characteristic of how units wait in a line. In a FIFO situation, the order of service is determined by the order of arrival. FIFO is present when the order of arrival determines the order the service system services the unit. Using queueing requires channels and servers. Channels are the number of lines formed by the units. Supermarkets usually have many channels at the checkout stations. Some banks use one channel to feed multiple service windows or tellers. Channels are lines. Some systems are designed to have a single channel, and other systems are designed to have multiple channels. Servers provide the service. The checkout clerk in the supermarket is a server. The bank teller is a server. The physician in the walk-in ambulatory care clinic is a server. The pharmacist is a server. Sometimes a service team is composed of a number of healthcare providers (e.g., physician, nurse, and medical assistant) working together to provide the actual service. Some systems have one server or service team, whereas other systems have multiple servers or service teams. Common situations are one channel, one server and one channel, many servers. If waiting never occurs, then queueing theory is not appropriate. Queueing theory assumes that, on average, at least some of the units wait. This does not mean that every unit waits. It means that every unit, when it arrives for service, has some probability of waiting. Depending upon the situation, some or many may wait. In other words, the probability of a unit waiting for service is greater than zero. Wait is defined as the amount of time between when a unit arrives and enters the line or queue and when the unit begins to receive service.

Given these characteristics, analytical models can be used to analyze the operation of the line and assist the manager to make decisions concerning the line and service system. Any analytical model is intended to assist the manager make a decision, not to make the decision. Making the actual decision is the prerogative and role of the manager, not the analytical model or technique. At best, the model informs the manager and clarifies alternatives and implications. Other common terms and concepts from queueing theory are as follows:

- **Balking:** When a unit seeing the length of the line decides it is too long and refuses to enter the queue
- **Reneging:** When a unit waiting in line decides the wait has been too long and leaves the queue
- **Batching:** When more than one unit enters service at a time (e.g., family photo, well-child clinic)
- **Jockeying:** When the unit chooses one line and then decides another line is shorter and so changes queue

LEARNING OBJECTIVE 10.3: USE QUEUEING THEORY CALCULATIONS TO MANAGE THE RELATIONSHIP BETWEEN WAITING AND THE RESOURCES NEEDED TO PROVIDE SERVICE IN DIFFERENT TYPES OF SYSTEMS

Queueing theory uses the Poisson data distribution to describe arrivals to the service facility and the exponential data distribution—the inverse of the Poisson distribution—to describe service times. These are different than the binomial distribution. Arrivals and service times are random within the context of these two probability distributions. Based upon using these data distributions and specific formulae (**Table 10.1**), queueing theory can be used to estimate:

- The percent of the time that a service facility is idle
- The probability of a specific number of units in the service system
- The average number of units in the system
- The average time each unit spends in the system (waiting service time)
- The average number of units in the waiting line or queue
- The average time each unit spends in the waiting line
- The percentage of time or probability that an arriving unit will have to wait

TABLE 10.1   Queueing Theory Formulae: Parameters to Assess Waiting Lines

PARAMETER	SYMBOL	FORMULA
Service rate per hour	μ	
Arrival rate per hour	λ	
Probability (%) the service system is idle	P_0	$1 - \dfrac{\lambda}{\mu}$
Probability of *n* units in the system	P_n	$P_n = \left(1 - \dfrac{\lambda}{\mu}\right) \times \left(\dfrac{\lambda}{\mu}\right)^n$
Average number of units in the system	L	$\dfrac{\lambda}{\mu - \lambda}$
Average time a unit spends in the system	W	$\dfrac{1}{\mu - \lambda}$
Average number of units in line waiting	L_q	$\dfrac{\lambda^2}{\mu - \lambda}$
Average time (hours) a unit spends in line waiting	W_q	$\dfrac{\lambda}{\mu(\mu - \lambda)}$
Probability (%) a unit must wait on arrival	P_w	$\dfrac{\lambda}{\mu}$

This information, together with additional information on the cost of providing a service and patient waiting line limitations (e.g., space), provides the manager with ample information to analyze, design, and redesign waiting lines and associated service systems. A service "system" includes the line for service and the actual service facility. In a walk-in clinic, "system" includes the waiting room and the examination rooms used by the nurses and physicians to diagnose and treat the patient.

As stated, basic queueing theory uses a Poisson probability distribution to estimate the pattern in which units arrive for service. Studies generally indicate that the Poisson distribution is the most appropriate estimate of random arrival patterns. Unlike the binomial probability distribution, which is symmetrical and bell shaped, Poisson distribution has a long tail (on the right), and the distribution is not symmetric. Unlike binomial distribution, which gives equal probabilities to values on either side of a mean, Poisson distribution recognizes that random arrival rates cluster around mean but cannot be less than zero. Arrival rates also have a (low) probability of being much higher than the mean. The queueing theory models presented in this chapter are based upon the Poisson distribution being used to estimate the random arrival pattern.

Queueing theory also offers a probability distribution to describe service times. A service time probability distribution is needed to estimate how long it takes to provide a unit of service. The exponential probability distribution, unlike the binomial data distribution, suggests that service times will be greater than zero and more frequently short than long. It is important to note that the field of operations research indicates that using the Poisson probability distribution to describe and estimate random arrivals and the exponential probability distribution to describe and estimate service times is usually the "best" approach to use in modeling and analyzing waiting lines. It provides the most conservative estimates, that is, the longest waiting time. This does not mean that this model is always the best. In some instances, even these probability distributions fail to capture the essence of arrivals and service times. In such situations, other probability distributions are used or waiting line models are developed using computer simulations. This analytical model is predicated on a number of reasoned assumptions:

- The Poisson probability distribution is considered an appropriate representation of arrivals.
- The exponential probability distribution is considered an appropriate representation of service times.
- The lines to be analyzed are governed by FIFO.
- There is no balking, reneging, or jockeying.
- There are no batch services.
- The client population is infinite (i.e., sample with replacement).

Based upon these assumptions, queueing models are available to describe waiting lines based upon the number of channels (lines) and the number of servers. In general, as the arrival rate gets numerically closer to the service rate, the line will get longer while the idle time in the system will decrease. As the arrival rate gets numerically farther away (and less than) from the service rate, the line will get shorter but the idle time in the system will increase.

If the arrival rate is greater than the service rate, the queue will be infinitely long. In other words, all systems need to be designed with a service rate (per hour) greater than the arrival rate (per hour). As such, queueing theory provides the consequences when the service rate is higher than the arrival rate.

Single-Server, Single-Channel Queue Theory Model

This type of model has one server. To use this model requires estimating the expected number of arrivals per time period (mean arrival rate) and the number of services possible per time period (mean service rate). As stated, for any system to work, its service rate must be more than the arrival rate. Based on these rates the following parameters associated with a single channel single-server line can be estimated:

- The probability that the service system is idle (P_0)
- The average number units in the system (L)
- The average time a unit spends in the system (W; i.e., waiting + service time)
- The average number of units in the queue waiting for service (L_q)
- The average time a unit spends in the queue (W_q)
- The probability that a unit must wait (P_w)

These types of calculations and observations highlight the Poisson and exponential probability distributions at work and the type of trade-offs managers can consider. Any service system (usually) can increase its service rate by adding servers plus space, equipment, and other items needed to provide an additional service facility. Each of these costs can be estimated:

- Hourly wage rates can be used to estimate the cost of a service team.
- The cost of equipment can be estimated based upon its useful life, expressed in units of service and purchase operational costs or its rental costs.
- The cost of space can be estimated based upon operational and capital costs, expressed on a square-foot or market rental cost basis.

In this section, a single-server system is described using different service rates (e.g., service rate [μ] 4, 5, 6, 7, and 8 units per hour). Increasing service rates requires additional input resources.

The critical managerial question is the value associated with adding additional resources to the service system given characteristics of the service system. Consider the following example:

The combined cost per hour of a 1 MD and 1 RN service team for the clinic is $150 per hour. Using multiple examination rooms, this service team can service on average approximately seven patients per hour. If a PA is added to the team for an additional $12 per hour, the service team

TABLE 10.2 Performance Measures for Single-Server, Single-Channel Systems

Service rate per hour	4	5	7	8
Arrival rate per hour	3	3	4	4
P_0 (Probability of idle system)	25.00%	40.00%	42.86%	50.00%
L (Units in system)	3.00	1.50	1.33	1.00
W (Hours spent in system)	1	0.5	0.33	0.25
L_q (Units waiting)	2.25	0.9	0.76	0.5
W_q Waiting (hours)	0.75	0.3	0.19	0.12
P_w (Probability of wait)	75.00%	60.00%	57.14%	50.00%

can service on average up to eight patients per hour (i.e., 1 MD, 1 RN, 1 PA). If an additional RN is added to the team (i.e., 1 MD, 2 RNs) for an additional $30 per hour, the service team can service on average up to 10 patients per hour. Based on recent data, weekday arrival rates are estimated to be 5.3 patients per hour. Note that this rate fluctuates by time of day.

Considering **Table 10.2**, is it worth additional expense for additional staff to alter this system? To answer this question requires managerial judgment. The queueing theory model plus some basic cost estimates provide the manager with the information that is necessary to evaluate the situation and make this type of decision based upon the circumstance.

Multiple-Server, Single-Line Systems

Multiple-server systems have more than one server. They work differently than single-server systems. In a multiple-server system, when a unit gets to the head of the (single) line, the unit is served by the next available server. The actual formula for this analytical model is complex and is excluded here to avoid confusion. Similar to single-server, single-line queueing models are available to assess different server and line configurations. As the complexity of queueing models increases, so does the complexity associated with estimating associated line and waiting characteristics such as presented in the previous section on single-server, single-line models. For multiple-server systems, we recommend the use of a calculator that can be found online.

Recalling the previous example, it was stated that the cost per hour of a 1 MD, 1 RN service team for the ambulatory care clinic is $80 per hour. A team with 1 MD and 1 RN can service on average up to four patients per hour. Therefore, one team can be expected to average up to four patients per hour. Two teams can be expected to average up to eight patients per hour and so forth. If a PA is added to the team (i.e., 1 MD, 1 RN, 1 PA) for an additional $12 per hour, then each service team can service on average up to six patients per hour. If an additional RN is added to the original team (i.e., 1 MD, 2 RNs) for an additional $20 per hour, the service team can service on average up to eight patients per hour. The arrival rate is estimated to be three patients per hour. When an additional service team is added, costs also include expenses associated with the physical plant and equipment. For example, an additional service team may need additional offices, examination rooms, and/or treatment rooms. Additional equipment will be required so the new service team will not need to borrow from the original service team. The cost of adding a supplementary service team may be significantly different than adding salaries. For the example used, assume the estimate of these other costs is $5 per hour.

TABLE 10.3   Performance Measures for Ambulatory Care Clinic With Single-Server Model and Multiple-Server Models

Service rate per hour (μ)	4	5	6	7	8	9
Service teams	1	1	1	1	1	2
Arrival rate per hour (λ)	3	3	3	3	3	3
Staff cost per hour	80	92	92	100	100	165
P_0	25.00%	40.00%	50.00%	57.14%	62.50%	45.45%
L (units)	3.00	1.50	1.00	0.75	0.60	0.87
W (hours)	1.00	0.50	0.33	0.25	0.20	0.29
L_q (units)	2.25	0.90	0.50	0.32	0.22	0.12
W_q	0.75	0.30	0.17	0.11	0.07	0.04
P_w	75.00%	60.00%	50.00%	42.86%	37.50%	20.45%

Given the example used, the economic implications of different staffing levels for a single-server model can be compared with the economic implications of using two service teams. **Table 10.3** contains estimates concerning both types of service systems.

As this example continues to unfold, queueing theory calculations and costs estimates provide the manager the ability to examine line and system characteristics and, by adding cost estimates, consider different configurations of the service system, associated lines, and the economic implications associated with different configurations. **Table 10.3** contains sufficient information for the manager to use to do a comprehensive analysis of the walk-in ambulatory clinic example using the cited parameters. For example, if a manager wanted to minimize the probability that a patient wait when they arrive at the walk-in clinic, given the parameters cited in the example, two service teams would be used. The probability of waiting (P_w) is lowest under this option (P_w 20.45%). However, the cost of this option is the highest, at $165 per hour. If the manager wants to minimize costs, the best option would be to use a single-server system with a staffing configuration of 1 MD and 1 RN. Under this option, the cost per hour is $80. However, the probability of patient waiting (P_w) is the highest under this option (P_w 75%). Marginal costs and marginal benefits can be compared using the staff cost estimates included in **Table 10.3**.

Queueing theory models provide the manager with a rich and comprehensive ability to analyze and design service systems, including the evaluation of lengths of lines and the potential for waiting. Based upon the goals and objectives of the system, the manager uses this information to trade off economic considerations with service system characteristics and considerations in arriving at the preferred configuration.

Appointment-Based Systems

Most appointment-based systems used in healthcare resemble a single-server system. For example, a patient is given an appointment to see a specific physician, even though the physician may be one of many employed in a clinic. As a single-server system, appointment-based systems can be analyzed using the single-server queue theory model. Appointment systems fix the mean arrival rate but not necessarily the interarrival times. Note that an arrival rate of two units per hour means granting appointments every 30 minutes and an arrival rate of three units per hour means granting appointments every 20 minutes. An arrival rate of four per hour means granting

TABLE 10.4   Performance Measures for an Ambulatory Care Clinic With an Appointment-Based System

Service rate per hour (μ)	3	4	4	5	5
Arrival rate per hour (λ)	2	2	3	3	4
P_0	33.33%	50.00%	25.00%	40.00%	20.00%
L (units)	2.00	1.00	3.00	1.50	4.00
W (hours)	1.00	0.50	1.00	0.50	1.00
L_q (units)	1.33	0.50	2.25	0.90	3.20
W_q	0.67	0.25	0.75	0.30	0.80
P_w	66.67%	50.00%	75.00%	60.00%	80.00%

appointment every 15 minutes. The service rate (μ) is estimated in the same manner as estimated using the queue models (**Table 10.4**).

Using Queueing Theory for Staffing

A critical rule in queueing theory is that the arrival rate must be less than the system's service rate. The system service rate is the rate of the entire system, potentially made up of many servers providing "the service." In a single-server system, the system's service rate is equal to the service rate of the one server. In a multiple-server system, the system's service rate of the system is equal to the service rate of each server times the number of servers. Consider a clinic in which 280 patients arrived on average during the 7 hours the clinic was open. This would be calculated as an arrival rate of 40 patients per hour. Service time would be estimated to be the average minutes per patient per service team or server. This is a service rate of five patients per hour per server. If this was designed as a single-server system, with an arrival rate of 40 patients per hour and a service rate of five patients per hour, the system would create very long lines. To calculate the minimum number of servers needed so that the arrival rate, on average, is less than the system service rate, divide the arrival rate (40 per hour) by the service rate per server (five per hour). This yields the answer eight. With eight servers, the arrival rate (40 per hour) now equals the system's service rate (i.e., five patients per hour per server times eight servers results in a system service rate of 40 patients per hour). To be an efficient system, however, the system's service rate must be larger (not just equal to) the arrival rate. In this example, adding a ninth server could increase the service rate. With nine servers, the service rate is 45 patients per hour. As a system with nine servers, an arrival rate of 40 patients per hour, and a service rate of 45 patients per hour, appropriate calculations can be made to examine the characteristics of the system. Perhaps a tenth server will be desired. This is a general way to estimate the number of servers needed to staff a service system.

In situations in which arrival rates vary dramatically, such as by time of day or day of the week, the analysis needs to examine the system during its peak and slow times using the standard queueing theory calculations. The appropriate use of these models is dependent upon a series of assumptions involving the application of specific probability distributions. In instances in which these assumptions are not met, other approaches, such as computer simulations, must be used to develop and then use appropriate probability distributions that best fit the circumstances. Analytical models such as these can be used to analyze the operation of (waiting) lines and assist the manager in making informed decisions concerning the line and service system.

LEARNING OBJECTIVE 10.4: IDENTIFY SCHEDULING PROBLEM COMPONENTS

When there is a queue, entities in the system (e.g., patients, parts, procedures, and tests) can be processed based on FIFO or other policies. In healthcare, patients are usually served based on their acuity levels and other priority measures. These policies are determined using scheduling algorithms. Scheduling is sequencing (i.e., determining the order) with time elements. In other words, scheduling algorithms specify the order and start time of tasks. When the number of tasks is small, we can try different sequences and select the best order (for n tasks, total number of orders is n). However, this is not a feasible approach for most of the real-world problems. Scheduling algorithms consider the following components:

- Number of servers and their design
- Performance measures of interest
- Scheduling constraints and assumptions

Number of Servers and Their Design

Scheduling algorithms vary based on the number of servers and their placements throughout the system. The most basic system is a single-server system where there is only one server such as a nurse taking care of patient admissions to EDs. Slightly more complex systems are systems with parallel identical servers such as toll gates, grocery checkout stations, and airport security checkpoints that include multiple servers that each server perform the same identical task. A more complex system is a flow-shop system such as assembly lines that include multiple different servers positioned sequentially. Repetitive healthcare processes such as vaccination or routine checkups could be designed as a flow-shop system. More complex systems are job-shop systems that include different servers in different orders. In a job-shop system, customers (i.e., patients) go through different servers in different sequences such as patient flow in hospitals.

Performance Measures of Interest

Like any optimization problem, scheduling algorithms require objective functions that are usually in the form of minimization or maximization. Objective functions could be a single performance measure such as minimizing average wait time, minimizing maximum tardiness, minimizing average flow time, or a combination of performance measures. We usually assume that arrival time (a), duration or processing time (p), and due date (d) of tasks are given. We can then calculate some of the common performance measures for a given schedule as follows:

- c (completion time) = s (start time that is determined by the scheduling algorithm) + p
- f (flow time) = $c - a$
- MS (makespan) = maximum c among all tasks
- T (Tardiness) = maximum $\{0, c - d\}$

Scheduling Constraints and Assumptions

To simplify scheduling problems, we often make some assumptions about the system and tasks being scheduled. These assumptions, in a way, are constraints of the problem that limit the size and complexity of the solutions. For instance, we usually assume that task durations (p)

are deterministic (not stochastic). This is a strict assumption because task durations are rarely known in real-life examples. Another assumption is about the setup time. Setup time is the time it takes to set up the task before starting it such as cleaning a bed before assigning a patient to it. We usually assume setup times are zero or fixed (so could be added to the duration time). But in real life, setup times are usually sequence dependent. Depending on the most recent task, the setup time can be longer or shorter. Another assumption is about whether preemption is allowed or not. If preemption is allowed, we can pause the ongoing task and switch to a different task (usually higher priority task), then resume the initial task. For simplicity, we usually assume that preemption is not allowed. In other words, once we begin a task, we should complete it. The list of assumptions could be a long one, depending on the specific problem and application area.

LEARNING OBJECTIVE 10.5: SOLVE SINGLE-SERVER AND IDENTICAL PARALLEL-SERVER SCHEDULING PROBLEMS

For a single-sever scheduling problem with the assumptions of no setup time, no preemption, and deterministic processing time, arrival time, and duration, we can use various algorithms to optimize various performance measures.

Shortest Processing Time

Scheduling based on shortest processing time (SPT) in a single-server system with the aforementioned assumptions will minimize average completion time and average flow time. The SPT sorts all tasks based on durations (or processing time) in ascending order. In other words, priority is given to tasks that can be completed quickly.

Example: Schedule the following imaging tasks on an x-ray machine so that the average flow time is minimized (**Table 10.5**).

Since it is a single-sever scheduling problem (where server is the x-ray machine), we can use the SPT rule. The optimal sequence is T5, T2, T3, T1, T4, and T6. We can use Gantt chart to visualize the schedule with start and end times (**Figure 10.1**).

Under each task, numbers represent the completion time of the corresponding task. For instance, task 5 starts at time zero and is completed at time two. Immediately after, task 2 starts and is completed at time five. Maximum completion time is 27, which is the MS. It turns out that for a single-server scheduling problem, any sequence has the same MS of 27.

TABLE 10.5 Single-Server Scheduling Example

TASK	T1	T2	T3	T4	T5	T6
Arrival time	0	0	0	0	0	0
Duration (min)	5	3	4	6	2	7

FIGURE 10.1 Gantt chart for the SPT rule.

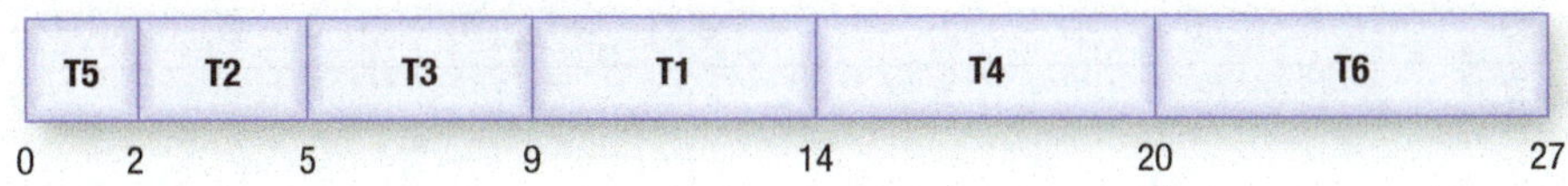

SPT, shortest processing time.

Earliest Due Date

We use earliest due date (EDD) rule to minimize maximum tardiness or average tardiness (i.e., late) in single-server systems. A task is considered tardy if it is completed after the designated due date. The number of time units that the task is delayed is the tardiness. For example, if a task's due date is 3 but gets completed in day 5, its tardiness will be 2 days. The EDD sorts all tasks from the smallest to largest due dates. In real-life examples, we use EDD without noticing it. For example, to avoid submitting assignments late, students usually tackle the one with the earliest deadline first. If due dates represent expiration date of healthcare products (e.g., medications, blood packages), the EDD will result in minimum waste.

Example: Schedule the following imaging tasks on an x-ray machine so that the average tardiness is minimized (**Table 10.6**).

Given the performance measure of interest, we should use the EDD rule to sequence the tasks. The optimal sequence is T1, T4, T2, T3, T5, and T6. The following Gantt chart represents the task start time and completion times based on the EDD rule (**Figure 10.2**).

We can calculate the average tardiness based on the individual tardiness for each task as shown on **Table 10.7**. Thus, the average tardiness is $21/6 = 3.5$.

TABLE 10.6 Single-Server Scheduling Example With Due Dates

TASK	T1	T2	T3	T4	T5	T6
Arrival time	0	0	0	0	0	0
Duration (min)	5	3	4	6	2	7
Due date (min)	5	9	10	7	18	25

FIGURE 10.2 Gantt chart for the EDD rule.

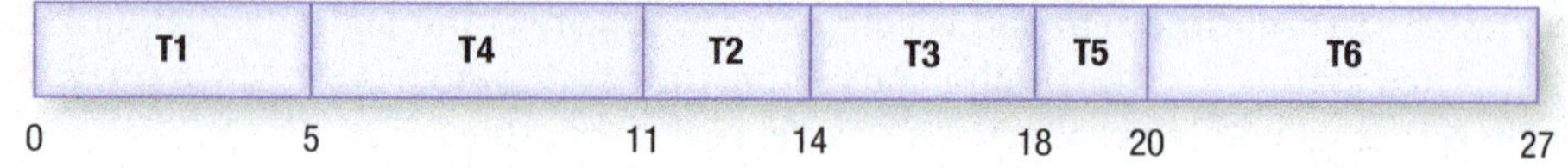

EDD, earliest due date.

TABLE 10.7 Single-Server Scheduling Example With the EDD Rule

TASK	T1	T2	T3	T4	T5	T6
Arrival time	0	0	0	0	0	0
Duration (min)	5	3	4	6	2	7
Due date (min)	5	9	10	7	18	25
Completion time	5	14	18	11	20	27
Tardiness	0	5	8	4	2	2

EDD, earliest due date.

Parallel Identical Servers Scheduling Problems

Scheduling tasks on parallel identical servers such as toll gates, grocery checkout stations, or multiple identical x-ray machines are similar to single-server scheduling with the exception of minimizing the MS.

We use the SPT rule to minimize average flow time or average completion time to determine the sequence of tasks and assign tasks to the least busy server each time. Similarly, we use the EDD rule to minimize the average tardiness. Once the sequence of tasks is determined by the EDD, the tasks are assigned to the least busy servers.

To minimize the MS, we use largest processing time (LPT) rule. In other words, we order the tasks from the largest to smallest (i.e., opposite of the SPT rule) and start assigning them to servers based on their least busy times. An everyday example of the LPT rule is packing a car trunk with large bags and smaller items. By loading the large items first, we leave room to fit the smaller items into the remaining spaces more efficiently.

SUMMARY

This chapter introduces key concepts and terminology used to describe service systems and waiting lines, with an emphasis on applications in healthcare. We have also presented queuing theory as a foundational tool to analyze service systems. Queuing theory provides a structured approach to evaluate and manage the balance between customer wait times and the resources required to meet service demands. The chapter offers calculations that help quantify performance and guide decision-making. In addition, we have outlined the components of scheduling problems and demonstrated how to solve them in both single-server and identical parallel-server systems. Together, queuing and scheduling methods provide healthcare managers with a practical framework for optimizing resource use and reducing inefficiencies in service systems.

END-OF-CHAPTER RESOURCES

DISCUSSION QUESTIONS

1. How do service systems and waiting lines impact customer satisfaction and business efficiency?
2. What are the key factors that influence waiting times in a queueing system?
3. How do unpredictable customer arrivals impact service system design?
4. What challenges arise when scheduling services for single-server versus parallel-server systems?

LEARNING ACTIVITIES

CourseConnect ▶

To access self-assessment questions and interactive, competency-based learning activities for this chapter, visit www.springerpub.com/courseconnect. See inside front cover and tear-out card for CourseConnect details.

CHAPTER 11

INVENTORY AND SUPPLY CHAIN MANAGEMENT

LEARNING OBJECTIVES

11.1. Explain different components of supply chains.
11.2. Describe different forms of inventory.
11.3. Explain different functions of inventory.
11.4. Select and perform appropriate inventory management methods for a given problem.

REAL-WORLD SCENARIO

Northfield Health System, which includes three hospitals and 12 outpatient and specialty clinics, serves a large, diverse region with a population of over 200,000 people. During a recent global pandemic, Northfield faced significant and unprecedented challenges. As the virus spread rapidly across the community, the health system experienced a sudden surge in demand for essential medical supplies, including personal protective equipment (PPE), ventilators, and high-demand medications. This increased demand led to critical stockouts of essential items, particularly for high-use medications and PPE. The pandemic disrupted the entire healthcare supply chain, impacting Northfield's ability to procure necessary supplies. Lockdowns, workforce shortages, and heightened demand across the country caused severe strain on distribution networks, leading to delayed shipments and national shortages. For several months, Northfield Health System struggled to access medications and equipment that were previously readily available. Learning from these challenges, Northfield Health System recognized the need for a robust, flexible, and resilient supply chain model that could withstand future disruptions.

A supply chain refers to a broad network of companies and stakeholders that are involved in delivering a finished product or service to customers. Supply chain management is a field that aims to improve efficiencies, costs, quality, and reliability of supply chains. A key component of any supply chain is its inventory that runs through the chain.

This chapter reviews supply chain components, inventory types and functions, and inventory management models that are used in health services administration.

LEARNING OBJECTIVE 11.1: EXPLAIN DIFFERENT COMPONENTS OF SUPPLY CHAINS

Supply chain refers to the chain of activities that are involved to get from raw materials and products to final users and customers. Supply chain management is a field that aims to improve efficiency, costs, quality, and customer satisfaction within supply chains.

To better coordinate and manage the flow of materials, information, capital, and labor through the supply chain, we divide supply chains into different components and functions such as planning, sourcing, manufacturing or service, logistics and distribution, return management, and inventory management.

Planning

In planning, organizational strategies are planned to match the supply with demand. At minimum, planning requires demand forecasts, supplier and inventory information, and production or service capacities.

Sourcing

Once production or service is planned, sourcing is needed to manage the relationship with suppliers. It includes identifying vendors, establishing contracts with selected vendors and suppliers of raw materials or needed parts, and monitoring their performance and quality.

Manufacturing or Service

Manufacturing or service refers to transforming the raw material to finished goods or services. It can include a sequence of different operations such as production, assembly, painting, inspecting, packaging, and quality control.

Logistics and Distribution

Logistics and distribution deals with the movement of finished products to customers and end users. This part of supply chain includes transportation, warehousing, and order fulfillment.

Return Management

Modern supply chains include return management to handle product returns, recalls, and customer complaints.

Inventory Management

Inventory management deals with balancing the risks and costs of holding inventory of raw materials and items. Holding too much inventory increases the costs, while holding too little inventory increases the shortage risk. Inventory management is present in every component of the supply chain, from sourcing to logistics and return management. Inventory management is usually viewed as a core of any supply chain.

In addition to these functions, supply chain in healthcare requires functions to manage risks, while meeting regulatory constraints. Risk management is essential in healthcare supply chains to fill the gaps among connected chains of players throughout the network. If you trace a healthcare product from its origin (i.e., raw material) all the way to the point of care at the patient's bedside, you can highlight numerous transition points (e.g., suppliers to producers, producers to distributors, distributors to facilities, facilities to hospitals, and hospitals to medical teams) throughout this journey. Any transition point in healthcare supply chain makes the entire chain vulnerable and introduces additional gaps throughout the chain.

Risk management becomes a key in global supply chains. Supply chains could be disrupted by external and global events like natural disasters, pandemics, wars and conflicts, and political or policy reforms. In globally connected supply chains, a subtle disruption in one point could spread through the network and affect the entire chain.

There are key steps to reduce these risks in healthcare supply chains. By diversifying suppliers and vendors in different ways (e.g., size, location, and type) and sourcing them closer to end users (e.g., hospitals and clinics), much of the risks related to shortage and disruptions could be managed. Moreover, real-time and accurate inventory management can enhance transparency across the supply chain and trigger immediate actions when shortage is expected. Given the central role of inventory management in supply chain management, we spend the rest of this chapter on this topic.

LEARNING OBJECTIVE 11.2: DESCRIBE DIFFERENT FORMS OF INVENTORY

Inventory can flow throughout the supply chain in different forms. More common inventories are raw materials and finished goods. However, inventory also includes work-in-process (WIP), in-transit items, and maintenance-repair-overhaul (MRO) items. Each of these represents a category of inventory that could include hundreds or thousands of subtypes.

Raw Materials

Raw materials refer to materials that are not being processed to their final product. Raw materials are rarely used directly in services because they require additional processing to transform them into final products. In healthcare, examples include utilities like water and gas, powders and liquids, and medicinal chemicals that are used directly or in combination with other materials. Raw materials are more commonly used in manufacturing. These materials include natural resources such as oil, gas, lumber, and steel sheets that are used to produce the final product.

Finished Goods

Finished goods refer to items or products that are being fully processed and produced and ready for being used. These items represent a majority of inventory in wholesale and retail stores. For example, malls and grocery stores carry finished goods in large varieties and quantities for sale. Hospitals and healthcare systems also carry large amounts of finished goods. For example, a specific medication, as a category of finished goods inventory, may include over tens or hundreds of subtypes, varying on the packaging size, dosage, active ingredients, and manufacturer.

Work In Process

WIP represents items or materials that fall between raw materials and finished goods. These are incomplete and partially processed items that require further processing to become a finished good. The WIP inventory is a significant portion of inventory in both manufacturing and service systems. While having some level of WIP could act as a buffer inventory to smooth out the system under congestion, WIP is generally viewed as an undesired type of inventory. Thus, systems with lower WIP are more efficient and less costly. Imbalanced manufacturing systems, where stations run in different pace, result in higher WIP throughout the system. In healthcare, patients that are being served could be viewed as partially completed services or WIP. Having too many patients because of bottlenecks and slower services could increase the number of patients being served (i.e., partially completed services or WIP). In an efficient healthcare system, patient flow is smooth, resulting in lower WIP throughout the system. Since WIP is spread over the system, measuring and quantifying WIP is not as straightforward as raw materials and finished goods. Therefore, it is viewed as a hidden and often overlooked inventory.

In-Transit Inventory

In-transit inventory refers to all items and materials that are in transit to the system. Usually, buyers pay in advance for the in-transit inventory and retain ownership, while sellers remain accountable for the safe and timely delivery of the in-transit inventory. Delayed shipping and transportation times and less visibility throughout the delivery process can make it difficult to accurately measure and track the in-transit inventory. Examples of in-transit inventory in healthcare include home healthcare supplies that are in transit to the system or leaving the system to patient homes.

Maintenance-Repair-Overhaul

The MRO inventory refers to all items, tools, supplies, and equipment that are used for maintenance, repair, and operation of the business. Examples include office supplies, cleaning supplies, safety tools like gloves, and spare parts that are owned by the system. The MRO is essential for smooth operation of any business in the face of disruptions and outages. The amount of MRO inventory is directly related to the size, type, and risk level of the system. Larger organizations, with lower levels of risk tolerance, invest more on MRO inventory; however, the rule of thumb is to have about 1.5% of replacement asset value (RAV) as MRO inventory. In simple terms, the RAV is the total cost (TC) of rebuilding the business or system from scratch. As such, if a hospital's RAV is $500M, total value of MRO inventory should be around $7.5M.

LEARNING OBJECTIVE 11.3: EXPLAIN DIFFERENT FUNCTIONS OF INVENTORY

Inventory management is a key component of manufacturing and service supply chains. In manufacturing, inventory is needed to ensure smooth production processes. In service systems, such as healthcare, inventory is closely related to service quality and reducing the shortage risks. For instance, hospitals need to have a certain level of inventory for each blood type as a safety measure. Beyond the key function of inventory, which is reducing the shortage risks, it has also other functions and benefits related to purchasing, finance, forecasting, and sales. Due to breadth and depth of inventory across the supply chain, the relative importance of its functions and benefits could vary. Hence, it is important to understand these functions and their relative importance for each unique situation.

Inventory can affect purchasing decisions, finance, and relationships with suppliers. Often, purchasing raw materials, items, and equipment in higher quantities results in cheaper price per unit, known as quantity discount, or economies of scale. More tangible examples of quantity discount are in retail stores where customers can take advantage of higher discounts for purchasing in higher quantities. Thus, one of the key functions of inventory is to take advantage of quantity discounts. We can buy more at cheaper price per unit and hold it over time. In addition, purchasing in higher quantitates reduces the purchasing frequencies and associated administrative costs.

Another function of inventory is to absorb temporary spikes in demand. The increase in forecasted demand due to external and environmental changes (such as closing hospitals or specific service lines in the region) can inform inventory decisions.

Inventory can be used as a hedging technique against price increase or price fluctuations. Expectation of price increase for raw materials, items, and equipment can increase the inventory levels.

In addition, inventory is sometimes inevitable for seasonal products and items that are available only during certain seasons. Examples include agricultural products and seeds that are not available throughout the year. In healthcare, seasonality refers to seasonal demand for healthcare services such as flu vaccination that requires prior planning and inventory management.

Sometimes, inventory is required to meet regulatory requirements. In healthcare, minimum inventory levels might be required to meet certain regulations.

Example: Consider a hospital pharmacy that carries various medications for patients visiting the hospital. Inventory in this pharmacy is mostly in the form of finished goods (i.e., medications) that are ready for sale. Various functions of inventory include the following:

- **Reducing shortage risk:** The pharmacy carries inventory and safety stock of critical medications and supplies to meet demand spikes.

- **Improving patient satisfaction:** The pharmacy identifies patient demands based on past discharge prescriptions and carries popular medications in order to improve convenience for discharged patients.

- **Economies of scale:** The pharmacy purchases popular medications with longer shelf lives in larger quantities in order to reduce the price per unit.

- **Meeting regulatory requirements:** The hospital can leverage the pharmacy's inventory to meet certain regulatory requirements for medication inventories.

- **Hedge against price increase:** The pharmacy purchases medications with volatile or seasonal prices when they are cheaper.

- **Meeting seasonal demands:** Before fall and winter, the pharmacy purchases flu vaccines and antiviral medications to prepare for seasonal demand increase for these items.

Depending on the main goal of inventory management and relative importance of inventory functions, different inventory management methods can be used. Some of these methods are discussed here.

LEARNING OBJECTIVE 11.4: SELECT AND PERFORM APPROPRIATE INVENTORY MANAGEMENT METHODS FOR A GIVEN PROBLEM

Inventory management is concerned with balancing the costs and risks associated with inventory levels. The ultimate goal of inventory management is to have the right quantity of products or items, at the right time and place, for the right users. Some inventory management models like economic order quantity (EOQ) and newsvendor models aim to find the right quantity for purchasing inventories, while other models like reorder point (ROP) aim to find the right time for purchasing inventories. While just-in-time inventory management aims to eliminate unnecessary inventories, ABC analysis aims to embrace the inventory issue but categorizes them into different importance levels. As such, each inventory management model is designed to achieve a certain goal that is driven by the inventory's primary function. In practice, it is rare to use a single inventory management technique or model; instead, a collection of them is used. We review some of these popular inventory management models and techniques in the following sections.

Just-In-Time Inventory Management

From Lean's perspective, holding too much or unnecessary inventory is viewed as a waste. Inventory requires capital to purchase, hold, and maintain. To minimize the use of inventory, lean approach offers just-in-time technique that aims to eliminate the need for unnecessary inventory (see Chapter 5, "Quality and Process Improvement"). Although the just-in-time technique reduces inventory costs, it is not always a suitable or feasible technique. Just-in-time inventory management is suitable for flexible systems with stable demands. Systems with just-in-time inventory management should have reliable suppliers to ensure short turnaround times. In healthcare, the just-in-time technique could be used when the demand is known in advance such as elective surgeries. This way, hospitals can plan and coordinate the inventory needs with suppliers and downstream units like the postanesthesia care unit (PACU) and ICU.

Consignment Inventory Management

In consignment inventory management, suppliers retain ownership of the product until it is sold or used. The supplier is called consigner, and the user or seller is called consignee. Consignment inventory management offers advantages to both consignees and consigners. Consignees do not need to pay for the items, enabling them to manage their financial risks and opportunity costs. Unsold or unutilized items remain until used or returned to consigners after the agreed-upon duration. For perishable or seasonal items, the duration is usually after the expiration or season (e.g., returning unsold summer outdoor furniture to suppliers after the summer).

On the other hand, consigners get higher visibility and larger platforms to increase their sales. Examples in healthcare include perishable items like medication supplies or seasonal products like vaccines.

First In, First Out and Last In, First Out

First in, first out (FIFO) and last in, first out (LIFO) are two different inventory management methods that are adopted from scheduling and queueing theory. FIFO functions similar to daily lines and queues that we see everywhere; whoever joins the line first will be served first. FIFO as an inventory management tool implies that the first arrived item (i.e., oldest items) should be used first. FIFO is more common in businesses with perishable items like grocery stores, pharmacy stores, and restaurants.

LIFO, on the other hand, is the exact opposite of FIFO. The functionality of LIFO is similar to stacking plates. When you need a plate, you simply pick the top one (i.e., the most recent plate that was stacked).

Hence, in LIFO, the newest item will be used first. LIFO is more common when it is physically more convenient to do so, like picking plates from a stack or picking filled prescriptions from stacked packages.

The LIFO method is also used in industries where inventory costs tend to increase over time, such as in energy or healthcare. With LIFO, companies prioritize the sale of their most recently acquired (and often more expensive) inventory. This approach better aligns the cost of goods sold with current revenues, which can provide a more accurate representation of profit margins during inflationary periods. Additionally, because the cost of the most recent inventory is typically higher, LIFO can result in lower reported taxable income, which helps defer taxes and conserve cash flow.

Drop-Shipping

In drop-shipping, sellers do not carry any inventory. Instead, a third-party supplier owns the inventory. After any sale, suppliers ship the items to the buyer. Drop-shipping is not common for manufacturing and service businesses. It is more common for online or sales businesses that do not require any inventory. While drop-shipping can reduce costs associated with inventory, it can decrease the seller's control over inventory and harm the relationship with customers. In healthcare, drop-shipping could be an effective inventory management for vendors and online stores that function as a middle party between suppliers and health systems. Another example is for delivering patient needs such as durable medical equipment (e.g., wheelchairs, walkers) and respiratory equipment (e.g., oxygen tanks, ventilators) to their homes through a third-party supplier.

Cross-Docking

In cross-docking, sellers ship the inventory to customers immediately after receiving it from suppliers, without processing or storing it. Cross-docking is suitable for perishable items with limited shelf life like seafoods, vegetables, and medications. Cross-docking requires precise coordination with suppliers and customers.

Perpetual and Periodic Inventory Management

Sales or consumption of products should be monitored closely over time to make replenishment decisions in order to avoid shortage risks. The monitoring frequencies can be continuous (i.e., in

FIGURE 11.1 Inventory curve for perpetual inventory management.

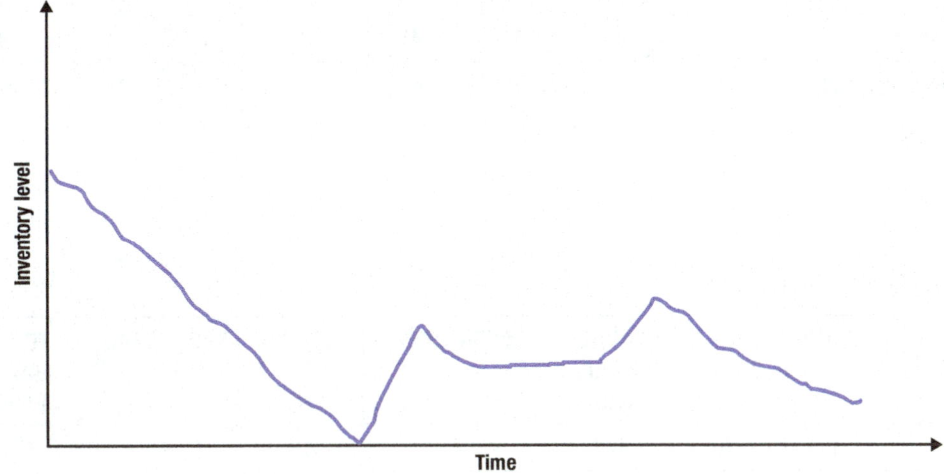

real time) or discrete at certain time periods (e.g., every week). The former method is called perpetual inventory management, and the latter is called periodic inventory management. Perpetual inventory management usually uses barcoding or similar technologies to track and update the inventory levels in real time. Hence, it is more suitable for important or more expensive items.

We use inventory curves to visualize the inventory level over time. **Figure 11.1** shows a sample inventory curve with perpetual monitoring. The curve starts with initial inventory level then continues to decline with a fixed or varying slope which is the same as the demand rate. If demand is higher, the decline will be steeper. When inventory is being replenished, the inventory level starts to go up. When the curve reaches zero, it means there is no inventory in the system (i.e., stockout). To avoid this situation, we normally have a certain level of inventory as safety stock.

Periodic inventory is usually suitable for small systems with limited items that are easier to track manually at certain periods. A complex system, like large hospitals, may utilize a combination of perpetual and periodic inventory management to track different items with different importance and values. Relative value of items is usually determined using ABC analysis.

ABC Analysis

ABC analysis is an inventory classification method that classifies items or products based on their value and volume into three classes: A, B, and C. Within this method, class A includes a few types of items or products that account for majority of the inventory capital. These could be a few but expensive items like medical equipment or items that are inexpensive but kept in large quantities like medication supplies that overall end up consuming most of the inventory capital. Often, about 10% to 20% of items fall in this category and account for more than 50% to 60% of the total inventory purchase costs. Class C is the opposite of class A which includes a larger number of products, about 50% to 60%, that account for 10% to 20% of the total inventory capital. Any item that does not fall in either of these categories is considered a class B item.

The ABC analysis is used to prioritize inventory management efforts on more important items and products. Thus, ABC analysis is not an inventory management method by itself, but it informs inventory management policies to focus more on important items and products. Using ABC method, health organizations can identify the most important items and use perpetual inventory management on those items. Similarly, they can identify the least important items and use periodic inventory management on them. For these reasons, ABC analysis is usually performed before inventory management models.

TABLE 11.1 Annual Demand and Item Costs

ITEM	1	2	3	4	5	6	7	8
Annual Demand	34	12	19	4	51	9	104	29
Unit Cost ($)	5	9	41	43	76	100	1	5

TABLE 11.2 ABC Analysis

ITEM	DEMAND	UNIT COST	ANNUAL DOLLAR VALUE	CLASSIFICATION	% ITEMS	% OF TOTAL DOLLAR	% TC FOR EACH CLASS
5	51	76	3,876	A	13	62	62
6	9	100	900	B	25	14	27
3	19	41	779			12	
4	4	43	172	C	63	2.7	11
1	34	5	170			2.7	
8	29	5	145			2.3	
2	12	9	108			1.7	
7	104	1	104			1.66	

TC, total cost.

Example: A small clinic uses the following eight items in its operation. Annual demand and unit cost for each item is given in **Table 11.1**. Run the ABC analysis, and plot A, B, and C on a graph where the horizontal axis represents the percentage of items and the vertical axis represents the percentage of total annual dollar value.

As shown in **Table 11.2**, we calculate the annual dollar value for each item by multiplying the annual demand and unit cost. We then sort the items based on the annual dollar value. For example, item 5, with the annual dollar value of 3,876, represents the most important item. We then look for drastic shifts in the annual dollar value to identify items that belong to class A. The change from 3,876 to 900 is relatively large, so we only assign item 5 in class A. Next significant drop is between 779 and 172. Thus, we label items 6 and 3 as class B. All other items belong to class C. This rule might not work if annual dollar values do not represent significant changes. On that case, we can use the suggested rule of thumb where class A includes 10% to 20% of items that include 50% to 60% of the total dollar values. Columns 6 and 7 provide these percentages that align with our classes. Class A includes only item 5, which represents about 13% (1/8) of items. It includes about 62% of total dollar values as shown:

$$\% \ of \ total \ dollar \ value \ for \ class \ A = \frac{3,876}{total \ annual \ dollar \ value \ of \ all \ items} = \frac{3,876}{6,254} \approx 0.62 \times 100 = 62\%.$$

We can plot these classes to visualize the relative volumes and values of each class as shown in **Figure 11.2.**

FIGURE 11.2 **ABC analysis visualization.**

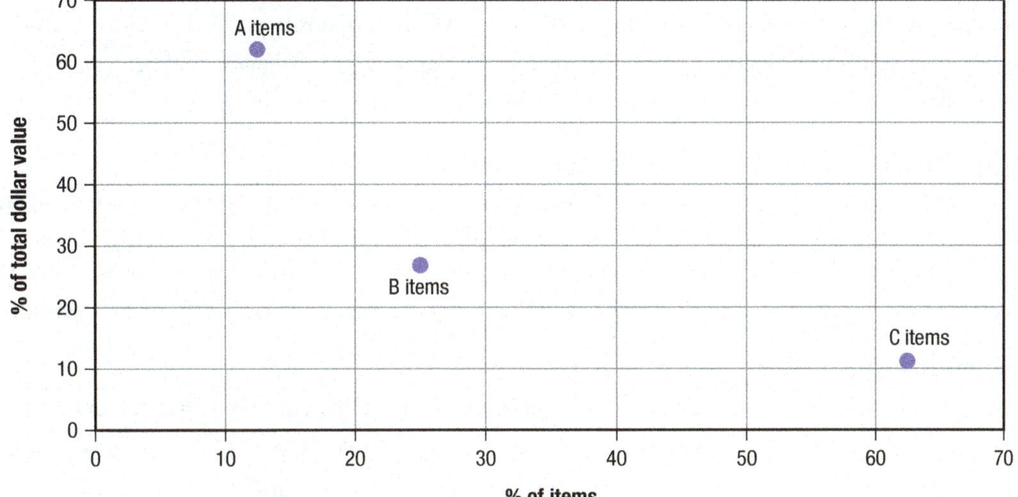

Economic Order Quantity Model

One of the challenges in healthcare inventory management is determining the order quantity and ordering time for different units and items such as medications, surgical supplies, and equipment parts. The main challenge in inventory management relates to uncertainties involved in demand and delivery times. Ordering too many items will increase the holding cost, while ordering too little will increase the order frequency and ordering costs. Some inventory management models attempt to determine the optimal order quantity and frequency that minimizes the TC. Often, the TC consists of inventory holding cost, ordering cost, and shortage cost. These are usually expressed as annual costs. Thus, annual TC would be the sum of annual inventory holding cost, annual ordering cost, and annual shortage cost.

EOQ is a classic model to determine the optimal order quantity (Q) such that the total annual cost is minimized. Under EOQ, we assume that the annual demand for the item is constant and known (shown by parameter D). Similarly, we assume that the lead time is also constant and known. Lead time is the time that it takes for items to arrive once they are ordered. Additionally, we assume that ordering cost (shown by parameter S) and holding cost (shown by parameter H) are constant and known. The ordering cost is the sum of all expenses related to fulfilling each order such as shipment costs, inspection costs, and packaging costs. Therefore, each time that we order, we incur $\$S$. The holding cost is the sum of all expenses related to holding one unit of the item for 1 year (such as rent, insurance, utility bills, and protections). Thus, holding 2 units of the item for 1 year will cost $\$2H$.

Annual Shortage Cost in Economic Order Quantity

Under EOQ, the annual shortage cost is zero because with known and constant lead time and demand, we can easily avoid shortage and stockout. Therefore, the annual shortage cost is eliminated from the annual TC.

Annual Ordering Cost in Economic Order Quantity

We can express the annual ordering cost in terms of order quantity (i.e., Q). Intuitively, if we order in large quantities, we should be able to reduce the ordering frequency and costs. So, the relationship should be inverse.

Under EOQ, we incur \$S for each order. The total number of times that we order is A $\frac{D}{Q}$. For example, suppose the annual demand is 1,000 units and order quantity is $Q = 100$ units. We need to order 10 times to meet the demand. Therefore, the annual ordering cost will be $\frac{D}{Q}S$. We can verify that the relationship between annual ordering cost and Q is in fact the inverse.

Annual Holding Cost in Economic Order Quantity

We can also express the annual holding cost in terms of order quantity, Q. If we order too much, we can expect to have higher holding cost. Therefore, increasing Q should result in higher annual holding cost. Under EOQ, we incur \$H to hold each unit for 1 year. The average amount of inventory that we hold every year is, $\frac{Q}{2}$ which is equal to the area under the inventory curve. Therefore, the annual holding cost will be $\frac{Q}{2}H$.

Suppose $D = 1,200$ and $Q = 300$. The average inventory for EOQ curve is $\frac{Q}{2} = 150$. It is straightforward to verify this using the inventory curve shown in **Figure 11.3**. We have four triangles. Area of each triangle is $\frac{1}{2}(base \times height) = \frac{1}{2}\left(\frac{3}{12} \times 300\right) = \frac{300}{8}$. Therefore, the total area under the inventory curve is, $4 \times \frac{300}{8} = 150$ which is the same as $\frac{Q}{2}$.

Note that in the EOQ curve, slope represents the demand rate. Since demand is constant and fixed, slopes are all equal. When inventory levels hit zero, it comes right back to Q level.

Annual Total Cost in Economic Order Quantity

The annual TC is the sum of annual shortage cost, annual ordering cost, and annual holding cost. Thus,

$$TC(Q) = \frac{D}{Q}S + \frac{Q}{2}H$$

We can show that the TC is minimized when $\frac{D}{Q}S = \frac{Q}{2}H$. We can solve this equality equation for Q that minimizes the TC, which is $Q = \sqrt{\frac{2DS}{H}}$.

FIGURE 11.3 EOQ inventory curve.

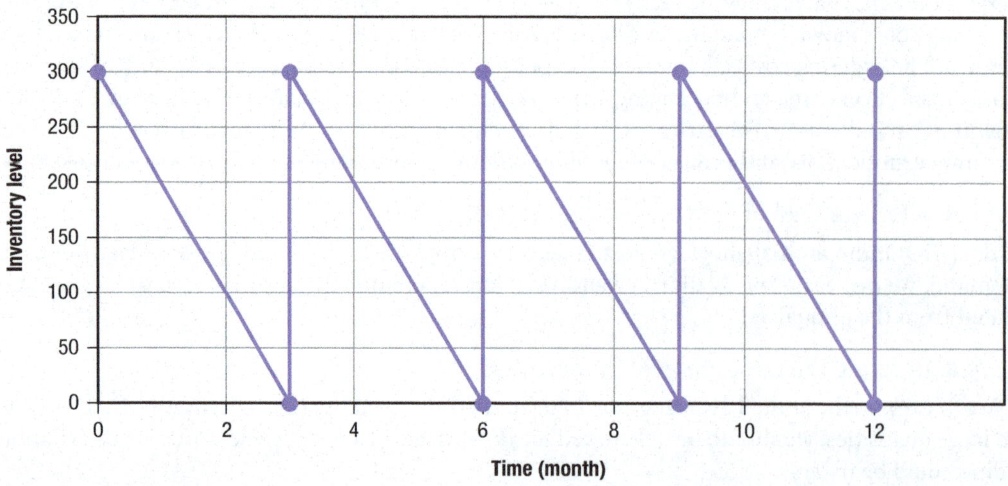

EOQ, economic order quantity.

Example: A pharmacy store is interested in managing its mask inventory using EOQ model. The store sells 100 masks per week. Ordering cost is $104, and holding cost is $1. Assuming there are 52 weeks per year, determine the optimal order quantity using EOQ.

In order to use EOQ, we need to calculate annual demand which is D = *weekly demand × number of weeks per year* = $100 \times 52 = 5,200$.

We can then use the formula to determine the Q.

$$Q = \sqrt{\frac{2DS}{H}} = \sqrt{\frac{2 \times 5,200 \times 104}{1}} = 1,040 \text{ masks.}$$

Safety Stock

Usually, some level of inventory is kept as a safety stock to reduce the risk of shortage and stockout. It functions similar to saving money as emergency funds. Although EOQ assumes a constant demand, in reality, demand is never constant. In healthcare specifically, external and unforeseen events, such as outbreaks, and natural hazards can increase the demand unexpectedly. In these situations, having some level of safety stock can absorb the increased demand. Safety stock is usually expressed as SS which is a fixed number of units that we would like to keep all the time. Thus, inventory diagram for EOQ should shift SS units upward to reflect this change. If $SS = 50$ for the example earlier, we can modify the inventory diagram as shown in **Figure 11.4**.

Reorder Point

While EOQ answers the question of "how much to order?", it does not answer the "when to order?" question. To answer the latter, we need to consider the lead time. If lead time is zero (meaning, you will receive your order instantly), we can reorder when the inventory level reaches zero. However, the lead time is usually nonzero. Therefore, ordering when the inventory is empty will result in shortage and stockout. One way to avoid shortage is to order exactly to lead time before the inventory hits zero. For example, suppose the lead time in **Figure 11.5** is 1 month. We can then order $Q = 300$ at months 2, 5, 8, 11, and so forth. This way, we will receive the order exactly when the inventory level reaches zero.

Although this approach works, it is not convenient to keep track of time to determine the timing of orders. Alternatively, we can reorder when inventory reaches a certain level. On **Figure 11.6**,

FIGURE 11.4 EOQ inventory curve with safety stock.

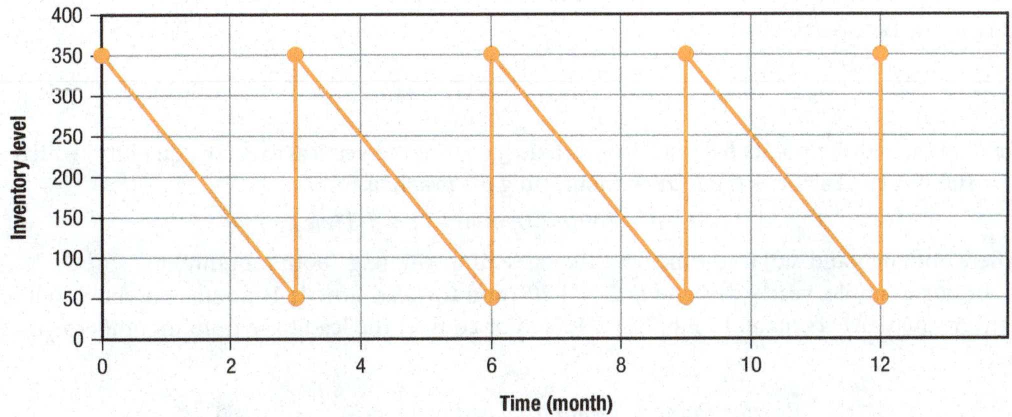

EOQ, economic order quantity.

FIGURE 11.5 EOQ inventory curve with reorder points over time axis.

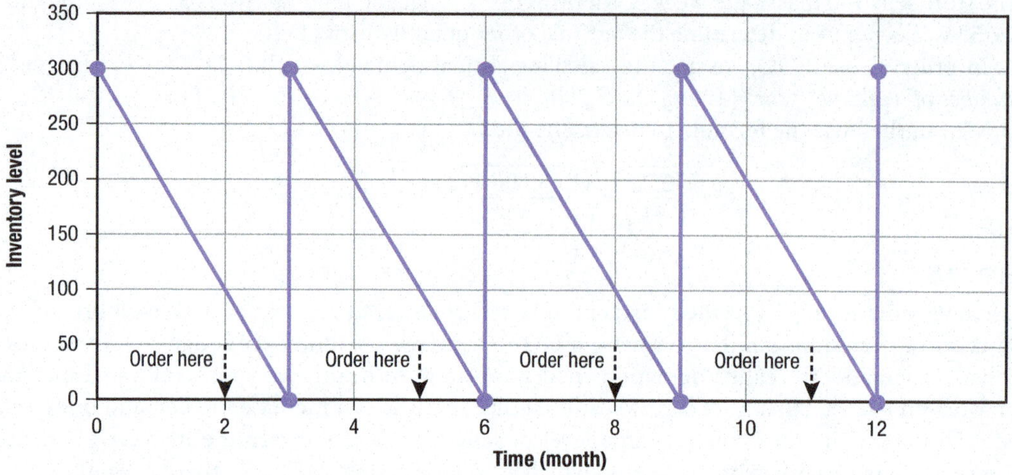

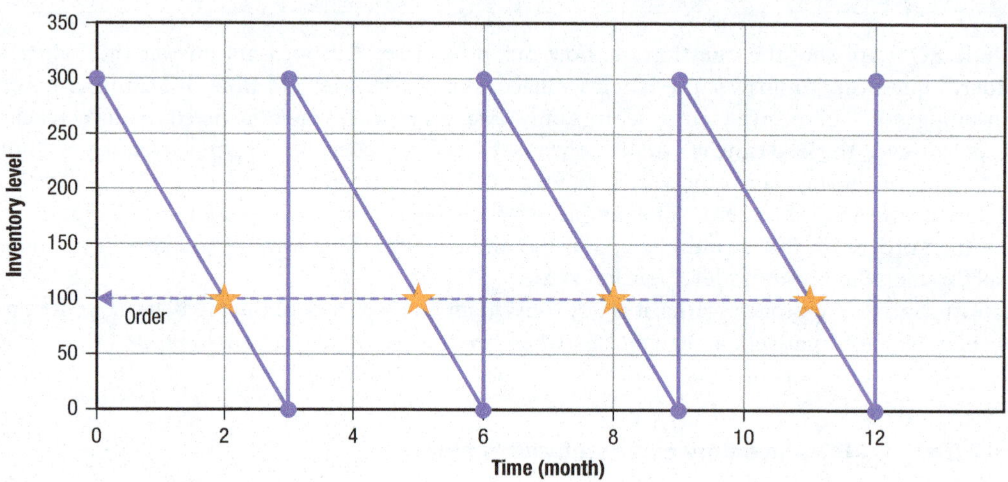

EOQ, economic order quantity.

FIGURE 11.6 EOQ Inventory curve with reorder points over quantity axis

EOQ, economic order quantity.

we map the reorder points from horizontal axis (i.e., time) to vertical axis (i.e., quantity) which is $Q = 100$. We can calculate the ROP without using the graph as follows:

$$Reorder\ Point = Demand \times Lead\ Time$$

where both demand and lead time have the same time unit (e.g., both monthly).

In our example, yearly demand is $D = 1{,}200$ and the lead time is 1 month. We should either convert the yearly demand to monthly demand or convert the lead time from monthly to yearly unit.

$$Reorder\ Point = Demand \times Lead\ Time = \frac{1{,}200}{12} \times 1 = 100$$

If there is safety stock in the model, we add the *SS* to the previous equation:

$$Reorder\ Point = Demand \times Lead\ Time + SS$$

Newsvendor Model

In some cases, replenishment and reordering during the selling period is not allowed. You have only one shot to order for the entire season. The season could be a year, quarter, month, week, or a day. The newsvendor model is also suitable when the value of the item diminishes over time such as perishable items like medication supplies, vaccines, blood banks, food, and fresh produce. Ordering too much or too little can result in costs. In this model, demand can be expressed with a probability distribution rather than a constant number.

For example, consider a newsvendor who sells newspapers throughout the day. The newsvendor should buy a certain number of newspapers at the beginning of the day. If the newsvendor ends up not selling all the newspapers, there will be some leftovers. Their value at the end of the day will be minimal, known as salvage value.

If the newsvendor runs out of newspapers, then there will be unmet demand and lost profit. Given the uncertain demand for newspapers, how many newspapers should be purchased at the beginning of the day so that the expected costs of shortage and overage are minimized?

To determine the optimal order quantity, we need to calculate the cost of underage and overage. Suppose that the newsvendor buys each newspaper for c and sells to p. The salvage value of each leftover newspaper is s. Usually $s < c$, meaning the salvage value is lower than the item cost. Cost of overage, C_o, is the cost of each leftover newspaper. Thus, $C_o = c - s$. Similarly, cost of underage, C_u, is the cost of unmet demand. For each unmet demand, we lose a potential profit. Thus, $C_u = p - c$.

We define critical fractile as $CF = \dfrac{C_u}{C_u + C_o}$ that tries to balance the overage and underage costs.

The CF is always a positive number between 0 and 1 that represents the cumulative distribution of the demand for the order quantity. In other words, the area under the demand distribution from negative infinity to the order quantity should be at least CF. This rule applies to both discrete and continuous probability distributions.

Example: A hospital blood bank needs to decide how many units of a specific blood type (say A negative) to order and store each month. Blood is perishable, meaning it has a limited shelf life (about 1 month for red blood cells), and the demand is uncertain (normally distributed with the mean of 8,000 units per month and the standard deviation of 500 units).

The challenge is balancing the cost of overordering (blood expiring and incurring additional cost for compost) with the cost of underordering (running out of blood and being unable to meet patient needs).

Each blood unit costs $200. Each used blood unit results in $1,000 revenue. Each expired blood unit requires an additional $22 to safely compost.

Determine the number of blood units that the hospital needs to order each month.

Given $c = 200$, $p = 1,000$, and $s = -22$, we can calculate underage and overage costs as follows:

$$C_o = c - s = 200 - (-22) = 222 \text{ and } C_u = p - c = 1,000 - 200 = 800$$

We then calculate the critical fractile as $CF = \dfrac{C_u}{C_u + C_o} = \dfrac{800}{800 + 222} \approx 0.783$

Using a Z table for standard normal distribution, we find $z = 0.78$ for 0.783. Thus, the optimal order quantity would be $x = z.\sigma + \mu = 0.78 \times 500 + 8,000 = 8,390$ units.

Example: Using the same assumptions on the previous example, now we assume that demand has a discrete probability distribution (**Table 11.3**).

TABLE 11.3 Discrete Probability Distribution for Demand

DEMAND	PROBABILITY
700	0.1
750	0.15
800	0.45
850	0.2
900	0.1

TABLE 11.4 Discrete Probability Distribution for Demand and Cumulative Probabilities

DEMAND	PROBABILITY	CUMULATIVE PROBABILITY
700	0.1	0.1
750	0.15	0.1 + 0.15 = 0.25
800	0.45	0.1 + 0.15 + 0.45 = 0.7
850	0.2	0.1 + 0.15 + 0.45 + 0.20 = 0.90
900	0.1	0.1 + 0.15 + 0.45 + 0.20 + 0.10 = 1

To determine the optimal order quantity, we need to calculate the cumulative probabilities as seen in **Table 11.4**.

For $CF \approx 0.783$, the minimum nearest cumulative probability is 0.90 which corresponds to $x = 850$. Thus, we order 850 units.

SUMMARY

Here, we have presented an overview of supply chain components and management techniques to improve efficiency, costs, and quality throughout the chain. We have then focused on one of the key components of supply chains, inventory. We have introduced different forms of inventory with specific healthcare examples under each category then overviewed different functions of inventory in practice. Lastly, we have introduced a broad range of inventory management models and techniques and discussed their advantages and disadvantages for various applications. We have concluded the chapter by introducing quantitative inventory management models such as EOQ, ROP, and newsvendor model and their uses cases in healthcare.

END-OF-CHAPTER RESOURCES

DISCUSSION QUESTIONS

1. Explain how do the different components of a supply chain interact to ensure efficiency and responsiveness?

2. Discuss the advantages and disadvantages of various forms of inventory (e.g., raw materials, work-in-progress, and finished goods)?

3. How do supply chain disruptions (e.g., pandemics, natural disasters, and geopolitical issues) impact inventory strategies?

4. What are the key challenges businesses face in managing inventory effectively?

LEARNING ACTIVITIES

CourseConnect ▶

To access self-assessment questions and interactive, competency-based learning activities for this chapter, visit www.springerpub.com/courseconnect. See inside front cover and tear-out card for CourseConnect details.

FORECASTING AND PREDICTION

CHAPTER 12

FOUNDATIONS OF FORECASTING

LEARNING OBJECTIVES

12.1. Describe the concept of forecasting as a managerial tool.
12.2. Describe the difference between analytic and nonanalytic forecasting.
12.3. Understand the assumptions of analytic forecasting.
12.4. Describe the limitations of forecasting and the challenges forecasting presents.

REAL-WORLD SCENARIO

The director of University Health Services for Northern College, a large liberal arts college in the northeast, is tasked with preparing for the upcoming academic year. Northern College Health Services serves undergraduate and graduate students who live both on and off campus with a broad range of primary care services. In recent years, visit volume has been increasing, both during the academic year and the summer months. At times, the staffing and supply resources of the College's Health Services have become strained. They have decided that it would be best to attempt to forecast upcoming visits to Heath Services to better anticipate resource demands. They would like to understand the type and precision of each type of forecasting available to them. As director, they have heard anecdotal stories of increased workloads from staff over the past 6 months. They believe there has been an increase in visits but would like to quantify these claims and attempt to understand if their own expert intuition of volume is a good substitute for a more analytic forecast.

LEARNING OBJECTIVE 12.1: DESCRIBE THE CONCEPT OF FORECASTING AS A MANAGERIAL TOOL

A forecast is an attempt to predict the future. Such attempts, however, are usually guesses of some form, given that no one can see into the future or predict it with certainty. Managers are not clairvoyant. They do not employ crystal balls or use fortune tellers as consultants. And although predictive modeling is making great strides to better predict medical outcomes with upwards of 90% accuracy in some cases, even the best current artificial intelligence cannot predict the future with 100% certainty. Any lottery that builds with no winners can attest to that.

Yet managers must anticipate the future to prepare for it. In fact, it is a primary requisite of most managerial positions. Budgets are based upon forecasts. The number and type of employees is based on present and future service demands. Hiring and reductions in staff are based upon forecasts, and the health preparedness of vaccines and disease burden are all anticipations of unknown future events.

Any forecast is, at best, an imprecise estimate. Few forecasts will be completely accurate, and so most contain some degree of inherent error. The challenge faced by managers and analysts is to minimize this error; or otherwise stated, managers must try to minimize the difference between what is predicted and what happens. Or more simply put, the goal is to be incorrect or off by the least amount.

Take a simple example. Let us note "F" as the forecast that was made yesterday of today's temperature and "TEMP" as today's actual temperature. The only way F can equal TEMP (F = TEMP) is if the forecast was correct, or else we get a revised formula that accounts for the difference of the two or error, "E," where "E" is the positive or negative error of the forecast.

If today's temperature was forecasted to be 65 degrees yesterday and the actual temperature today is 65 degrees, then the error in the forecast would be zero. However, if yesterday's forecast for today's temperature was 80 degrees, not 65 degrees, then F = (TEMP − E), where the error (E) would be 80 − 65 or 15 degrees.

Managers are interested in methods that can minimize the error included in all forecasts. The challenge with forecasting is to strive for accuracy and produce a "best" forecast, or one that employs the least amount of error. However, not all error is created equally. Error can be thought of as comprising both systematic error, which can be controlled for by the appropriateness and precision of the forecasting technique being used, and random error, which is inherent in every forecast. Think of error as having two parts: one that is within some control to estimate and one that is completely random and out of any control to estimate.

In our real-world example, if the director of health services did not account for the seasonal trends in visit volume to Northern College's Health Services, they would be allowing systematic error to bias the forecasting estimates. At the same time, even if they account for this variation, it is still possible that they could see a spike in visit volume over the summer months, for example, which could be entirely owing to random chance. This would be an example of random error, and there would be no way to predict its occurrence. The goal of all managers is to control for systematic error while being aware that random error is unpredictable and always possible.

LEARNING OBJECTIVE 12.2: DESCRIBE THE DIFFERENCE BETWEEN ANALYTIC AND NONANALYTIC FORECASTING

As the chapter title implies, forecasting is both an art and a science. To that end, there are two branches of forecasting: analytic, or statistical forecasting, and nonanalytic forecasting, often called judgmental, genius, or expert forecasting. Both have their merits and limitations.

Nonanalytic Forecasting

Judgment forecasting does not strictly imply making decisions based on intuition, although this can be the case. Most forms of this type of forecasting are both less accurate than analytic forecasting and can be very labor intensive depending on the forecasting need. For example, the Delphi method is a systematic method to collect opinions—usually from experts—and use these opinions in multiple round-robin cycles to arrive at a forecast that captures the essence of all the individuals (e.g., experts) used in the forecasting exercise. This type of effort may be good for forecasting a phenomenon that is relatively new or for which there is little existing data, but it is not something one would use to predict the annual inventory for a services organization, for example.

Other examples of judgment or genius forecasting can be found in multiple forms—these can be found online or on television outlets when noted "experts" forecast the outcome of a certain situation, such as what stock performance will be, who will be wearing what next season, what sports team might make what trade or perform better or worse, or what the new year will bring.

This chapter is not devoted to this type of forecasting. Except for the Delphi method, all forms of judgment forecasting are based upon individual opinion. Obviously, sometimes the individual will be right and other times wrong. And, as we will repeat, being wrong is almost always the outcome given no one can predict the future. It is important to remember that the challenge in forecasting is to *minimize the error* inherent in all forecasts. Judgment forecasting is often used to forecast far-off events that defy other approaches.

For example, consider an assignment to forecast the year when a cure will be available for dementia. The only reasonable and logical approach would be to examine the literature on progress and then to identify either one or multiple experts and ask their opinion(s) on this question. The hypothesis is that the error in their forecasts will be less than the error in other forecasts because they are experts and have greater knowledge of this area than others. Before leaving judgment forecasting, it is important to note that sometimes, the forecasting problem requires the use of judgment forecasting, such as with the example involving the dementia prediction. Judgment forecasting is still forecasting, even though it can be highly judgmental and not based upon mathematical models.

LEARNING OBJECTIVE 12.3: UNDERSTAND THE ASSUMPTIONS OF ANALYTIC FORECASTING

In contrast to nonanalytic forms of forecasting, analytic forecasting attempts to be more systematic and precise. This usually entails a mathematical approach to analyzing data to predict future outcomes and trends. Most forecasting problems faced by the health services manager can be accomplished using some form of analytic forecasting. Analytic forecasting methods are typically based on one of two assumptions.

1. The past is a reliable predictor of the future.
2. The future can be predicted based on knowable cause-and-effect relationships.

Assumption A: The Past Can Predict the Future

This assumption is founded on the idea that future events are related to what has occurred in the past and is the most common of the assumptions used in forecasting. Under this assumption, analytic approaches are used to examine past and present events and extend or extrapolate the values of these past events forward. In using analytic approaches based upon this assumption, managers count on the past being a valid and reliable predictor of the future.

This assumption needs to be thoroughly considered by health services managers who use analytic forecasting approaches. For example, if the assignment is to forecast the number of patient days a hospital will generate (or produce) in the following month, basing the forecast on past patient-day production or generation seems appropriate because the past may be a reasonable predictor of the future. Examine the data in **Figure 12.1**. By a quick visual scan, if asked to predict the next month's visits, most would place the forecast near 100. This, however, would be a visual judgment forecast. Instead, there are methods to mathematically use past data to predict

FIGURE 12.1 Patient days by month.

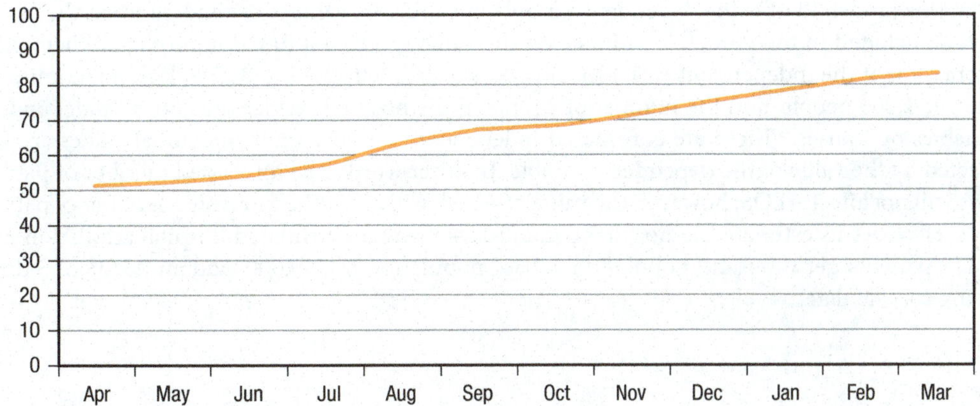

the future within some range of certainty. One question that first must be answered is how far back should past data be included in making the forecast? Another is, how far into the future can and should one forecast given the data at hand? What if, for example, you were asked to forecast hospital patient days for the next 10 years? Ten years is a very long time in the future, and many unknown variables could affect the accuracy of such a distanced forecast. Given the ambiguity associated with such a long-time interval, most health services managers would be very reluctant to base a 10-year forecast solely upon past data.

Chapter 13, "Time Series Forecasting Techniques," explores forecasting methods that are based on this assumption. The methods examined are as follows:

- Extrapolations using averages
- Moving averages as forecasts
- Exponential smoothing in forecasting

Assumption B: The Future Can Be Predicted Based Upon Cause and Effect

Many forecasting approaches are based upon cause and effect and are known as causal models. The models used in this category of forecasting attempt to capture the primary factors that are believed to cause (therefore the name causal) or influence the future. For example, consider a forecast of the number of patient days to be generated by a hospital: Patient days can be considered as the "effect." Using the number of patient days forecasted (PD-f), a conceptual and analytic cause-and-effect model can be constructed. Based on the knowledge that patient days are a function of both admission and average length of stay (ALOS), we get:

Equation 12.1

$$PD\text{-}f = ALOS \times Total\ admissions$$

where ALOS is the average length of stay for patients in the hospitals (in days) and total admissions is the number of patients to be admitted into the hospital next year. This requires that we project admissions next year. To do this, examine the admissions calculation formula:

Equation 12.2

$$Admissions = Hospital\ admission\ rate\ per\ 1{,}000\ people \times$$
$$the\ Number\ of\ people\ in\ the\ hospital\ service\ area$$

Substituting Equation 12.2 for admissions in Equation 12.1 allows us to develop a cause and effect forecast model:

Equation 12.3

$$PD\text{-}f = ALOS \times (Hospital\ admission\ rate\ per\ 1{,}000\ people \times$$
$$the\ Number\ of\ people\ in\ the\ hospital's\ service\ area)$$

In this model, PD-f is the dependent variable, meaning its value is dependent upon the causal factors included in the model. It will take on the value given to it based upon the mathematical interaction of the independent variables. It is the model's "effect." The ALOS, hospital admission rate per 1,000 people, and the number of people in the hospital service area are all independent variables or "causes." These are considered independent because their individual values are not affected by the value of the dependent variable. In other words, the forecasted number of patient days will not affect ALOS; however, the value of ALOS will affect the forecasted number of patient days. Here, let us estimate the hospital patient days using an estimated hospital admission rate of 118 patients per thousand population, a base population of 250,000, and an ALOS of 5 days. Doing so, calculate:

$$\text{PD-f} = ALOS \times (\textit{Hospital admission rate per 1,000 people} \times$$
$$\textit{the Number of people in the hospital's service area per 1,000 people})$$
$$= 5.0 \times (118 \times 250)$$
$$= 5.0 \times 29{,}500$$
$$= 147{,}500 \text{ patient days}$$

In this example, the hospital admission rate per 1,000 was estimated based upon known characteristics of the population. The number of people in the hospital's service area was also estimated using known census data and knowledge of patient origin. Here, each independent variable in the model could be quantified and used to solve for the number of patient days. Usually, the dependent variable is to the left of the equal sign in any equation and the independent variables are to the right of the equal sign. This is sometimes also called equational modeling and is the foundation for regression modeling, covered in Chapter 15, "Seasonality and Other Model Considerations." It can also be expanded to other predictive models, which we mention. One example would be attempting to model what predicts the risk of contracting influenza. As one can imagine, there are numerous variables, called independent variables, that could lie on the right-hand side of that equation. Examples include time of year, age of person, contact with others through work or school, virulence of the influenza for that year, prior health and comorbidities, vaccination status, and so forth.

Sensitivity Analysis

As in the previous example, the cause-and-effect forecast often must be based on estimates of some kind. In this example, estimates of population in the hospital's service area were calculated. However, these estimates may be off. To address this, you may wish to conduct an analysis using more than one estimate of future population. This is called a sensitivity analysis. Sensitivity analysis allows the manager to examine the cause-and-effect relationship while determining the impact a change in one or more independent variables will have on the dependent variable.

Using the previous model, involving hospital patient days and an estimated hospital admission rate of 118 patients per thousand population, with a base population of 250,000 and an ALOS of 5 days, we projected 147,500 patient days. However, if we estimate the population to be 10% less than the previous estimate $(250{,}000 - (250{,}000 \times 0.1) = 225{,}000)$, that our ALOS also decreased by 10% to 4.5 days, and that our admission rate will decrease 10% to 106.2 admissions per thousand, then our new forecast would be:

$$\text{PD-f} = 4.5 \times (106.2 \times 225)$$
$$= 4.5 \times 23{,}895$$
$$= 107{,}527.5 \text{ patient days}$$

This represents a 27% decrease in the forecasted number of patient days from the original estimate.

Sensitivity analysis examines multiple "what if" questions to determine which variable in the model has the most power to change the overall answer or forecast. It is also used to determine the overall effect of changes in specific variables. For example, in the previous example, the value of each variable was adjusted downward by 10%. The overall effect of those adjustments was a 27% decrease in the forecasted number of patient days. In reality, any or all the variables could be adjusted—something that healthcare managers must take care to do thoughtfully.

Using Epidemiology in Forecasting

Epidemiology produces many rates that can be incorporated into various types of forecasting methods. Epidemiologic information is critical when the manager or policy analyst must forecast the need for health and medical care. Epidemiology is usually considered the science that describes and analyzes the presence and spread of disease in populations and the need for health and medical care. It is usually defined as the distribution and determinants of health-related events (HREs) in human populations and the social and economic determinants of health. If managers or policy analysts know who has disease, injuries, pregnancies, and so forth and the risk factors associated with these, they can more accurately design service systems to either treat HREs or prevent them through risk reduction.

Forecasting with use rates appears simple but requires a high degree of caution because of changes in the population over time, especially with respect to age and socioeconomic status. Rates include the following:

- Birth rate
- Fertility
- Mortality rate
- Crude death rate
- Cause of specific mortality rate
- Infant death rate and other age-specific rate
- Morbidity rate
- Incidence rate
- Prevalence rate

At this point, it is important to realize that whenever epidemiologic rates are used to forecast, care must be taken to adjust the rates so that approximate equality is achieved in demographic variables involving age, gender, race, income, and other factors thought to have a significant influence on death and disease. For example, if the national crude annual death rate were 8.7 deaths per 1,000 people, this rate could not be applied to a specific community or market area until it was adjusted or modified based upon demographic variables. This is known as adjusting or normalizing rates to some base population or group. The demographic variables used to calculate the national rate must be matched with the demographic variables in the population being forecasted. If the average age in the nation is 35 and the average age in a specific community is 28, using the national average of 8.7 deaths per 1,000 people would grossly overestimate the number of anticipated deaths because of the age discrepancy between the national rate and the demographic composition of the specific community. Rates must be age adjusted.

Adjusting rates to match demographic variables is a challenge when use rates are used in forecasting. National use rates also include utilization rates of health and medical services. Examples include the following:

- Hospital discharges per 100 or 1,000 people
- Average length of stay
- Rate of hospital occupancy
- Average daily census of hospitals
- Average number of visits to a physician's office per year per person

Again, whenever rates are used, the demographic characteristics represented in the national rate must be matched with the equivalent demographic characteristic in the population being forecasted. It is also important to consider that use rates themselves change over time; they are not static.

LEARNING OBJECTIVE 12.4: DESCRIBE THE LIMITATIONS OF FORECASTING AND THE CHALLENGES FORECASTING PRESENTS

Forecasting is an attempt to predict the future, the unknowable. In this sense, it is much akin to guessing. And like guessing, there are levels of reasoning about any prediction. Data and information about the past and about known relationships among variables can help inform reasoning, and forecasting can be approached systematically and thoughtfully. In this sense, forecasting is scientific; it is governed by rules and conventions. Being proficient at forecasting requires a sound understanding of these rules and conventions and how to use them. Developing a forecast that minimizes systematic error requires a high level of proficiency, judgment, and common sense. Thus, forecasting is also an art form. Science is unable to provide health services managers with explicit rules to govern these judgmental aspects of forecasting. Experience, organizational knowledge, strategic context, and application help develop the manager's ability to use forecasting as an art.

Just doing the math correctly does not always make for a good forecast. Inputting data and using software programs and modeling algorithms for forecasting are important and convenient steps to analysis. However, it is the preparation of the forecasts, understanding the assumptions made about the estimates, and the collection of the data that distinguish the accuracy of these methods. The manager/analyst is responsible for minimizing forecasting errors. The primary test of any forecast is whether it has minimized the systematic error. Often, managers forecast using multiple techniques to determine which forecast provides the least error using historical data. Each forecast should teach the manager something. Expert forecasters use multiple methods and continue to ask themselves what each method has taught them about the overall forecast as well as the phenomenon under study.

The number one rule of forecasting is to always plot the data on a graph. If the assignment is to forecast the number of inpatient admissions or clinic visits, plot all the historical data. Also plot the variables that might influence them. This will illustrate any association that might exist and can assist the manager in developing the appropriate forecast.

Examine **Figure 12.2**. Here, the manager has plotted the data and then used three different techniques to forecast the future. Each utilized a different technique, covered in the following chapters, based upon the foundation of the past predicting the future to arrive at a forecasted number of patient days. The reason for doing this is to attempt to minimize systematic errors. To do this, they would forecast the past or use known historical data to examine how accurately each method compared with what occurred. Similar answers using different methods should add some confidence. Very different answers using different methods should suggest the existence of method bias—one or both methods are biasing the forecast based upon some inherent assumption and should force the manager to proceed with caution. When faced with the need for a forecast, use as many methods as possible.

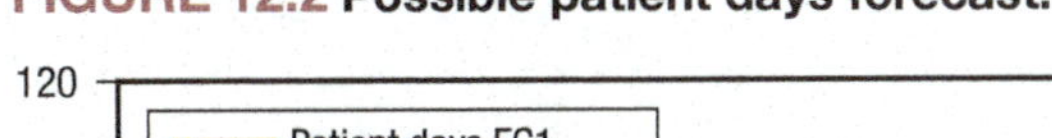

FIGURE 12.2 Possible patient days forecast.

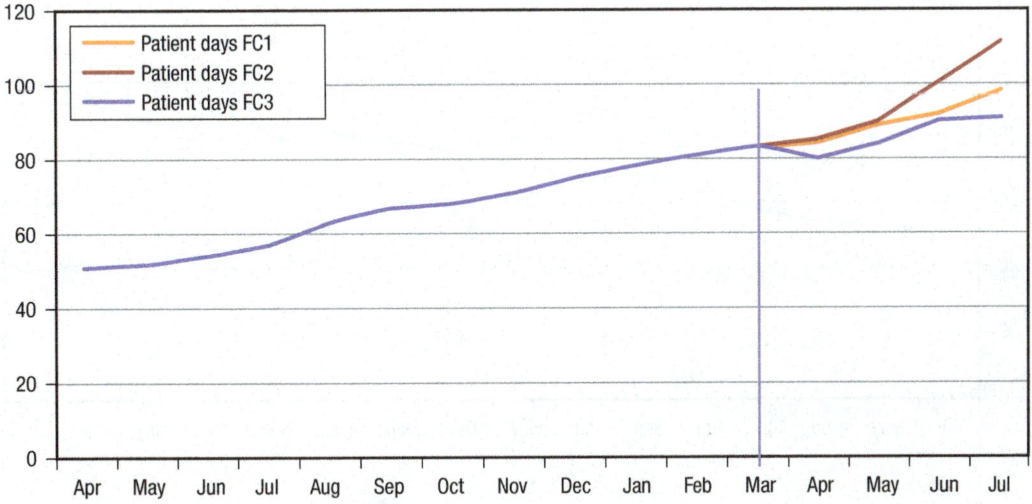

Analytic forecasting does involve mathematics. If forecasting were just math, however, then mathematicians and actuaries—not managers—would prepare forecasts. Forecasting requires that managers know their data. A classic example in which this is relevant to health services managers involves the use of months in forecasting. Sometimes, it is important to realize that months have a different number of days. For example, February usually has 28 days and March has 31 days. Also, be aware that different months have different numbers of weekdays, Saturdays, and Sundays. Sometimes the different numbers of days by month and the ratio of weekdays to weekend days can have a strong impact on what is being forecasted. For example, one recent July had 31 days, of which 23 were weekdays and 8 were weekend days. In contrast, March of that year had 31 days, of which 21 were weekdays and 10 were weekend days. These types of minor changes in the number and type of days per month can create artificial variation in data that can be minimized. Managers are responsible for knowing their data and adjusting as needed.

Forecasting also requires knowledge of the phenomena being forecasted. This includes knowing how one variable drives another. Any form of forecasting is a reasoned judgment made by a manager after a series of thoughtful considerations. Examine **Figure 12.3**, which presents a scenario for what could occur regarding future patient days. In this example, none of the three forecasts accurately predicted what was to occur. There could be many reasons for this. One could be that the spike in volume was simply owing to random chance. This is random error, and no amount of analytic consideration will help adjust for it. However, it is more likely that the jump in patient days results from some form of cause and effect. Perhaps a large organization relocated a major office with many employees to the area, or another competing facility ceased or downsized operations. Managers must know their data but also be aware of its context, which is the nature of the work of the organization and the external environment. Managers should be able to choose the appropriate variables to use in cause-and-effect models.

There are also other limitations to forecasting techniques. As stated, managers need to be careful not to extrapolate their forecasts too far into the future. Doing so may overestimate the ability of past trends to continue. The COVID pandemic completely uprooted all assumptions about the past predicting the future, at least for some time.

FIGURE 12.3 Actual data compared to forecast.

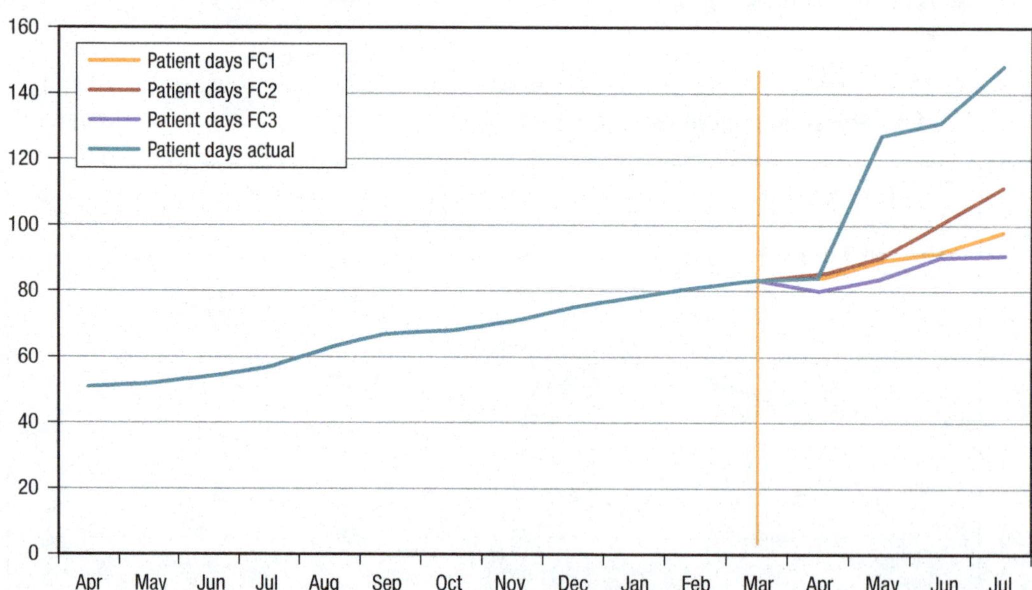

In the final analysis, managers are responsible for their forecasts. The future, not the manipulation of formulae, will indicate whether the forecast was accurate. When asked to prepare a forecast, managers are expected to use recognized methods and generate forecasts that are logical and reasonable given the state of existing knowledge and data. If, in the future, it is found that the forecast was highly inaccurate but reasonable, given the available information possessed at the time the forecast was prepared, most organizations will understand the high degree of inaccuracy. If, however, in the future, a forecast was found to be highly inaccurate because the manager failed to consider certain information or methods, then it may be appropriate to question the competence of the manager.

The following questions should be considered when forecasting:

1. What (variable) is being forecasted?
2. What answers are needed from the forecast?
3. What variable(s) are associated with the variable being forecasted?
4. What information is available or will be needed to be made available on these variables?
5. What is known about the relationships regarding the phenomena being forecasted?
6. To what degree are the variables associated (i.e., correlated)?
7. How far into the future does the forecast need to go?
8. What is the overarching strategy objective being met by the forecast?

SUMMARY

This chapter introduces forecasting and how it is used in health services administration. Forecasting is one of the primary tools used by managers to plan for how organizations will position themselves and operate in the near and long term. It can be used to predict volume of services, supply of inventories, and salary expense; make revenue projections; and much more.

Forecasting is also both an art and a science. There are many different methodologies that can be employed to forecast. The two primary types of forecasting are analytic and nonanalytic. Nonanalytic forecasting consists of judgment, genius, or expert forecasting. This method relies on personal knowledge and individual experience to predict the future. Although intuitive in nature, this method is also less analytic and more susceptible to systematic error. Analytic forecasting can include a number of mathematically based techniques that rest on one of two assumptions: the past predicts the future, and cause-and-effect relationships exist between operational and environmental variables. Predicting the future from the past is a method that is most often used in forecasting and requires examining visual and mathematical trends in the data to extrapolate into the future. Although these are explained in the next two chapters, this requires putting values or weights on the data, both in terms of how much to value the past relative to the future and how to consider the relationship or correlation between two or more variables.

Managers are also encouraged to use multiple techniques on historical data to examine which technique is more accurate at predicting what occurred. This is a process of minimizing the systematic error of the forecasting model. Utilizing sensitivity analysis and confidence intervals can help to create an understanding of the potential impact of the assumptions made and to place limits around your predictions. Managers also need to be cautioned that all forecasts have their limitations. The amount of historical data to consider, the length of time into the future one predicts, and unforeseen events can all affect the accuracy of any forecast. At best, forecasting is a gamble, a guess. However, by using proven analytic methods and sound reasoning, a good health services manager can provide a thoughtful forecast within a scope of confidence. What is important is that any forecast be done comprehensively and transparently.

END-OF-CHAPTER RESOURCES

DISCUSSION QUESTIONS

1. Think about some of the things we need to forecast in the health services industry.
   a. What kind of timeframes are needed both for past data and into the future?
2. What is the role of uncertainty when thinking about forecasts?
3. What would be helpful for a manager to have or know when trying to assess how much faith to put in a forecast?
4. What are the important elements of a forecast that managers should either present or request when conveying forecasts?

LEARNING ACTIVITIES

CourseConnect ➤

To access self-assessment questions and interactive, competency-based learning activities for this chapter, visit www.springerpub.com/courseconnect. See inside front cover and tear-out card for CourseConnect details.

TIME SERIES FORECASTING TECHNIQUES

LEARNING OBJECTIVES

13.1. Examine the role of time intervals in forecasting models.

13.2. Examine guidelines for length of future forecasts.

13.3. Understand forecasting based on average change, average percent change, and confidence intervals.

13.4. Understand weighted forecasting models by using moving averages.

13.5. Understand weighted forecasting models by using exponential smoothing.

13.6. Be able to select between forecasting models based upon the calculated mean forecast error.

REAL-WORLD SCENARIO

Mo Adel, the senior administrative analyst at Northern University Health Services, must determine the staffing and resource needs for the system's outpatient and walk-in services clinic for the upcoming year. They have collected monthly visit volume for the past 60 months. After meeting with the university admissions office, they do not predict any stark increases in enrollment to the University; however, this is only a short-range projection. They are also uncertain how useful data from more than 5 years in the past are to projecting volume into the future as the student population has grown and services have changed in that time. Mo wants to be sure that their forecast is accurate enough to project resource needs into the near future but also flexible enough to anticipate changes in the external environment.

Remember that all forecasting is essentially future telling, and all future telling requires some basic assumptions. The methods that are described in this chapter are based upon the assumption that the past (and present) can predict the future—or that whatever trends we have seen thus far will continue in some way. These forecasts are termed naive models in that they only recognize the past (and current) state into a forecast. They are naive to the potential for small or major changes in the contexts that gave rise to the forecasts. In our real-world example, this might include a dramatic and unexpected enrollment into the college that results in an influx of students seeking care. In real life, think of the COVID-19 pandemic.

Being naive does not make these models inappropriate to use in forecasting. Usually, naive models are used when detailed information on the near past is available, and the need is to forecast the near future. For these purposes, they can be quite effective. Caution, however, must be taken when extending these forecasts too far into the future or relying too heavily on past data. Careful consideration should also be given to any trends within historical data, such as seasonality factors, and adjustments made when forecasting ahead. Sometimes, even identifying these trends becomes challenging, which is why forecasting is as much art as science. A good analyst will carefully take time to consider *why* and *when* things occur or be able to see patterns in the data—remember Chapter 3, "Statistical and Analytical Foundations."

LEARNING OBJECTIVE 13.1: EXAMINE THE ROLE OF TIME INTERVALS IN FORECASTING MODELS

Time intervals define forecasts. It is essential that forecasts be prepared in the same time interval as the historical data. For example, if the historical data are expressed in weeks, the forecast should be expressed in weeks. If the historical data are expressed in years, the forecast should be expressed in years and not in months, weeks, or days. In contrast, if the historical data are expressed in days, it is acceptable to express a forecast in a larger time interval such as weeks, months, or years. Remember, time is a continuous variable.

Assessing trends within time intervals is also essential. The primary goal of any forecast is to minimize the *systematic error* associated with the forecast. Systematic error is usually some element that is causing an effect in what we are trying to predict that goes unaccounted for. Seasonality is one example. Some systematic error can be minimized by critically examining the historical data and determining whether the time intervals are useful for future prediction. For example, if Mo Adel would like to forecast the number of visits to the outpatient clinic at Northern University Health Services for the month of September, they must determine *if* the number of visits that occurred in June, July, and August should be used in the forecast. Given that the student population in these summer months is quite different than the student population in September, when many more students are back on campus, it may not be prudent to include only these months in their forecast or at least make some adjustment for them.

In this example, previous Septembers are likely to have greater predictive power when forecasting the next September. In other words, June, July, and August are not equal to September in that the phenomenon being forecasted (e.g., clinic visits) is fundamentally different in these summer months than in September, October, or November, when the campus is fully populated. Thus, the forecast is dependent upon a seasonal trend.

Using equal time intervals can also refer to the length of the time interval. Some months have a different number of weekdays and weekend days and an unequal number of days. In some situations, failure to recognize this may artificially distort the forecast.

Further, a day may not be a day. The number of clinic visits may (naturally) vary by day of the week. For example, the urgent care clinic may be closed Saturdays and Sundays or have shorter hours on weekend days than on a weekday. Utilization may be higher on certain days of the week, especially those days after a day the clinic was closed, such as a Monday. Although any forecast will have some degree of time interval distance, the challenge is to minimize the excess error in the forecast and achieve time intervals that are as equal as possible.

LEARNING OBJECTIVE 13.2: EXAMINE GUIDELINES FOR LENGTH OF FUTURE FORECASTS

The first guiding principle of forecasting is to always plot the data visually. Doing so with the historical data provided by Mo Adel would quickly reveal the seasonal downtrend during June, July, and August (**Figure 13.1**).

Visually examining the data can show linear trends in the data, be they positive or negative. It can also provide clues that could be signal points to analysts for investigation when possible. Perhaps the change was a one-time shock that could not be anticipated, or perhaps it is an event that reoccurs systematically over time, such as a reimbursement policy, an administrative policy, or simply a holiday. When plotting the data, the x-axis is used to plot time and the y-axis is used to plot whatever other variable we are interested in.

Second, the forecast's length should not exceed one third the historical data's length. If you have 24 months of historical data, then the forecast should be no longer than 8 months, or one third of 24. If 6 weeks of historical data exist, the forecast should be no longer than 2 weeks into the future. This is a convention provided as a guide, not as a rule. It is important that the length of

FIGURE 13.1 Outpatient visits to university health services—prior year.

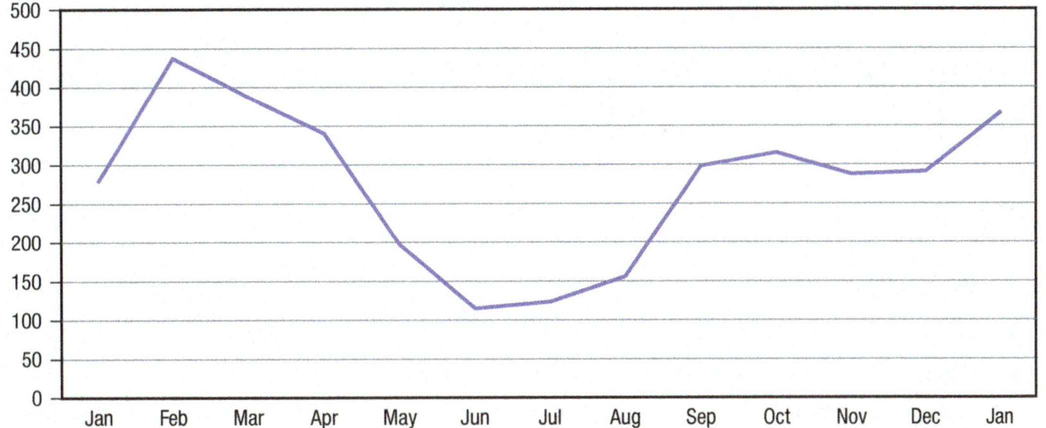

the forecast be appropriate given the historical data. Forecasting the next 5 to 10 years based upon 2 or 3 months of past data, regardless of the approach used, would be inappropriate.

Another guiding principle of forecasting is to be conservative. Being conservative requires an understanding of what is being forecasted and how important the estimate is to the organization. A commonsense approach here is to remember that *all* forecasts are most likely going to be wrong. No one can predict the future with complete certainty. The goal with forecasting in uncertainty is to be as *less wrong* as possible.

For example, it may be important to know whether it is worse to be 10% or 20% high or 10% or 20% low with a forecast. It is better to provide a high forecast for a hospital's need for blood, as being out of blood supply is unacceptable and compromises the health of patients. Conversely, it is better to provide a low forecast for the number of hospital inpatient days because that forecast is used to establish budgets, and it is usually easier to add temporary staff than reduce core staff. Yet other things may have more of an error buffer to them, such as how many hours are needed to staff the hospital valet or how many open parking spaces are acceptable on a Tuesday (if one would even devote time to such an analysis).

Forecasts should be sensitive to the positive and negative implications associated with being off—either high or low—from what actually occurs. Some forecasting techniques permit the calculation of a standard deviation and thus confidence interval (CI) associated with the forecast. As shown in Chapter 3, "Statistical and Analytical Foundations," 1.96 standard deviations above and below the forecasted mean provides a 95% CI of where the actual future value will fall. In some instances, setting the forecast to 1.96 standard deviations above the mean will provide a conservative forecast. Other times, setting the forecast to 1.96 standard deviations below the forecasted mean may be more conservative. Sometimes, calling the forecast at the 50% level (forecast mean) is also the conservative approach. In this chapter, we give examples of each. Again, knowing the implications of being high or low with a forecast is essential to an accurate and effective forecast.

A final guiding principle is that forecasts should be *transparent*. This means all assumptions and calculations used in any forecasting technique should be clearly stated and replicable. If you provide a forecast that weighs data based more on current observations than historical ones, this, as well as the degree of weighting applied, should be provided with the forecast. This is especially important when the forecasting methods are being used and reviewed by others, be they higher level managers, executives, or boards of directors. Many of these individuals may not understand the intricacies of the methods used but will want to be able to make comments and/or approvals based on them. Being transparent allows them to solicit helpful input on your forecasting techniques but also ensures that if some unexpected event should occur, the assumptions and process used to forecast were openly discussed and understood.

LEARNING OBJECTIVE 13.3. UNDERSTAND FORECASTING BASED ON AVERAGE CHANGE, AVERAGE PERCENT CHANGE, AND CONFIDENCE INTERVALS

▶ VIDEOS FOR LEARNING OBJECTIVE 13.3

- Video 13.1 Average Change

- Video 13.2 Average Percent Change

- Video 13.3 Confidence Interval and Comparison Table

As the name implies, time series techniques identify a historical trend and base the forecast upon extending this trend into the future. At least three approaches can be used to do this: (1) extrapolation based upon average change, (2) extrapolation based upon a CI, and (3) extrapolation based upon average percent change. For this section, we use the data in **Table 13.1** on patient days.

Before using any mathematical technique, the data must be plotted. Examining Figure 13.2, the data plot or cloud of data suggests a linear relationship with a positive slope. One method to extend or extrapolate this historical trend to forecast the number of births for April would be to use a ruler to draw a straight line that "best fit" the historical data plot. This would entail trying to draw a line centered among the data points. Doing so, however, is prone to error unless the line is mathematically derived, which we explore in Chapter 14, "Linear Regression Forecasting." The methods described here provide more systematic methods for forecasting these data.

TABLE 13.1 Visits to University Health Services

MONTH	VISITS
January	279
February	437
March	387
April	340
May	197
June	115
July	123
August	156
September	298
October	315
November	287
December	291
January	366

FIGURE 13.2 Plot of visits to university health services.

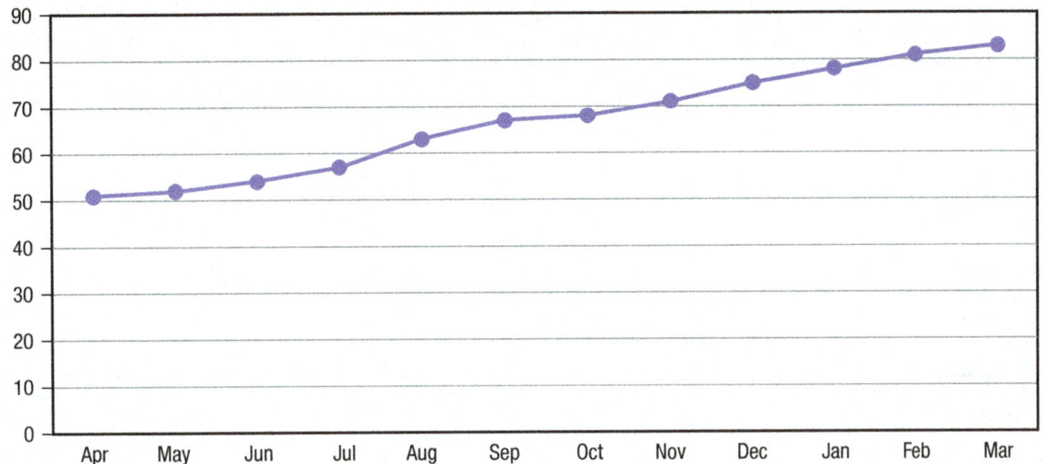

If the data plot looks random, or like a cloud of data points without any evident linear relationship, one should decompose the time series data. This means examining groupings of the data in pieces and then regrouping it, a technique called clustering. For example, multiple years of Januarys, multiple years of Februarys, and so forth can be examined to see if this method of plotting the data presents a different picture. One might also try composing the data by adding months together to create quarters (3-month periods) or group data by days, weeks, months, or any other relevant time period to the organization or external environment. As manager, you must attempt to construct the data in a manner that will best lend itself to forecasting.

Let us consider the data in **Table 13.1** and try to forecast the next 4 months. There could, in fact, be multiple futures. **Table 13.2** shows three potential forecasts for these months.

Examined graphically, we get **Figure 13.3**. Any of these potential futures are indeed possible and feasible. And yet, so are others. Perhaps something unexpected occurs and patient days spike, such as in **Figure 13.4.**

Forecasting Based on Average Change

Equation 13.1: Formula for Average Change

Forecast month (FM) = Average of the data + (Midnight of the data × Average charge)

This approach to forecasting requires examining the month-to-month change that occurs in the data. **Table 13.3** includes 6 months of births data for a community hospital and how much each month varied from the previous month. You will note that most months increase, while June decreased two births from May's total births. To forecast using Average Change, we first need to calculate the month-to-month changes in the data and then compute the average of these changes by totaling up the column of the changes and dividing by the number of data points, here 5. Note that there are 6 months of data, but because we are taking the change from month to month, there are only 5 points of change.

Also note that month-to-month change is calculated in whole terms, not its absolute value. Once the average of the month-to-month change has been derived, a forecast of births for June can be prepared. The basis for this forecast is the mean or average level of births experienced over the history of the available data. This approach ensures that no single value artificially distorts the forecast.

TABLE 13.2 Forecasts for the Next 4 Months

	FC1	FC2	FC3
April	51	51	51
May	52	52	52
June	54	54	54
July	57	57	57
August	63	63	63
September	67	67	67
October	68	68	68
November	71	71	71
December	75	75	75
January	78	78	78
February	81	81	81
March	83	83	83
April	**84**	**85**	**80**
May	**89**	**90**	**84**
June	**92**	**101**	**90**
July	**98**	**111**	**91**

FIGURE 13.3 Plot of next 4 months forecasts.

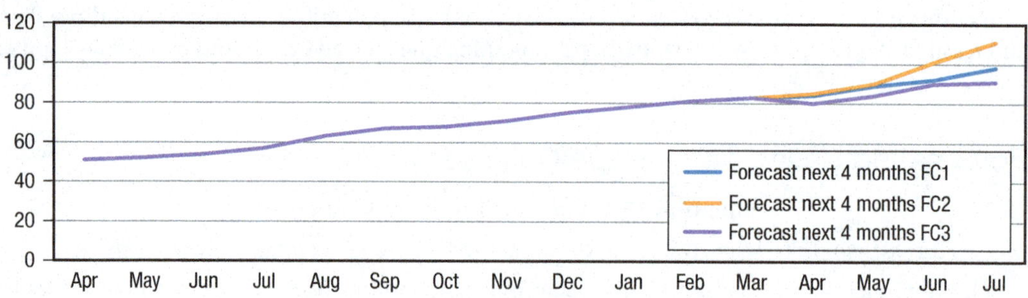

FIGURE 13.4 Plot of next 4 months forecast with outlier.

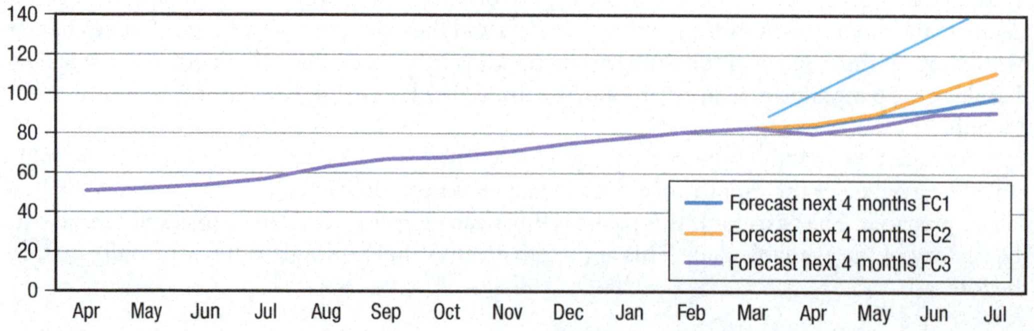

TABLE 13.3 Average Change Forecast

	NUMBER OF BIRTHS	CHANGE IN BIRTHS
January	77	
February	81	4
March	83	2
April	85	2
May	87	2
June	85	–2
Total	498	
Average	83	1.6
Mid Point		3.5
FM July = 83 + (3.5 × 1.6) =		88.6

FM, forecast month.

TABLE 13.4 Average Percent Change Forecast

	NUMBER OF BIRTHS	CHANGE IN BIRTHS	CHANGE IN BIRTHS
January	77		
February	81	4	5.19%
March	83	2	2.47%
April	85	2	2.41%
May	87	2	2.35%
June	85	–2	–2.30%
Total	498		
Average	83	1.6	2.03%
Midpoint		3.5	
FM July = 85 + (85 × .0203) =		88.6	**86.73**

FM, forecast month.

Continuing with Equation 13.1, we also need to find the midpoint *number of data points* for the data. This is not the same as the median (the statistical midpoint value of the data), discussed in Chapter 3, "Statistical and Analytical Foundations." The midpoint used here is a measure of how much data is being used. For this example, the data's midpoint is 3.5, or the data point between the third and fourth data points. To determine the midpoint, the data must be arranged from either lowest to highest or the reverse. The midpoint becomes $\frac{(n + 1)}{2}$.

For this example, the midpoint of the data distribution is $\frac{(6 + 1)}{2}$ or 3.5. **Table 13.4** shows the calculation of these elements.

Now that we have all the information, we can calculate the average change forecasted for July:

Forecast Month (FM) = Average of the data + (Midpoint of the data × Average Change)
$$\text{FM July} = 83 + (3.5 \times 1.6)$$
$$= 88.6$$

or 89 births rounded into real terms, as there is no such thing as .6 of a birth. See Video 13.1 on calculating average change using Excel.

Forecasting Based Upon Using Average Percent Change

Equation 13.2 Formula for Average Percent Change

Forecast month (FM) = Most recent data point + (Most recent data point × Average % change)

Extrapolation based on average percent change builds upon that based on average change by calculating the percent change in births from month to month. **Table 13.4** shows the data to include the percent change in births from month to month. A common mistake in calculating the percentage change is juxtaposing the numerator and denominator. A rule of thumb when dealing with time series data is to remember to take the change between time periods (future-past/past). We can also take the change from month to month first (future-past) and then divide that by the most recent past time period. We are assuming that the future data will continue to increase or decrease at a constant rate (the average % change), so we simply apply that rate to our last point of data. Here that is the month of June, so once we calculate the average rate of change to be a positive 2.03%, we increase the number of June births by this amount. Now we can calculate the average change of births by percentage:

Forecast month (FM) = Most recent data point + (Most recent data point × Average % change)
$$\text{FM July} = 85 + (85 \times .0203)$$
$$= 86.73$$

or, again, 87 births rounded into real terms, as there is no such thing as .73 of a birth. See Video 13.2 on how to calculate the average percent change using Excel.

Forecasting Based on a Confidence Interval

Equation 13.3 Forecasting Using a 95% CI

Forecast month (FM) = Average of the data ± (1.96 × Standard deviation) for a population or average of the data ± (1.96 × Standard Deviation) for a sample of the data

As the name implies, this method uses a CI to forecast. It is important to remember that 1.96 standard deviations above and below the mean represents a 95% CI. Revisit Chapter 3, "Statistical and Analytical Foundations," for a more detailed discussion of CIs and distributions. A forecast based upon this method can be 95% confident that the future value being forecasted will fall within the interval constructed, here the number of future births.

The benefit of using a CI forecast is that you can be more confident in your ability to accurately forecast the future period within a range. The caution is that as your confidence level increases, the accuracy with which you can predict lessens. This is the fundamental nature of CIs in that as confidence increases, so does the size of the interval. It is possible to construct a 100% CI, which is simply the entire range of possible values. As the interval narrows, the level of confidence drops.

Using CIs as forecasts becomes helpful to the manager in many ways. One is when precision is not the primary motivation for forecasting. If, for example, the manager wishes to forecast visit volume for staffing purposes, knowing that at each level of staffing (e.g., adding one additional staffing unit) allows for moderate flexibility in volume to be handled. Thus, a team of one nurse practitioner, one nurse, and one physician can see between 1 and 20 visits, but adding another nurse practitioner increases that volume to 35. If the manager forecasts using a CI for the coming month and finds the interval to be 21 to 34 visits, they can accurately construct an adequate

TABLE 13.5 Forecasting Based on a 95% Confidence Interval

	NUMBER OF BIRTHS		
January	77	UCL	90.01
February	81	LCL	75.99
March	83		
April	85		
May	87		
June	85		
Total	498		
Average	83		
Standard deviation sample	3.58		

LCL, lower control limit; UCL, upper control limit.

staffing plan. Another value CIs provide is when they are analyzed within the context of the other forms of forecasting, which is explored later in the chapter.

To use CI forecasting as an approach, the standard deviation and/or standard error is used. If the historical data represent the entire set or population of all data and not a sample of the data, the standard deviation can be used. If, however, the historical data are only a sample of data, the standard deviation of the sample is used, which is simply the standard deviation divided by $n - 1$. An example of a sample of historical data would be in attempting to develop a forecast of future births for a state based on only a sample of data from select hospitals. If the forecast is for just one hospital using that hospital's data, the standard deviation will suffice. A more complete description of calculating the standard deviation as well as standard error appears in Chapter 3, "Statistical and Analytical Foundations."

Table 13.5 shows the calculation for extrapolation based on a 95% CI. Here, the standard deviation is 3.58, reflecting that we only have 6 months of data, so we would use the function for a standard deviation of a sample. CIs also have two values because they represent a range. These are the upper control limit (UCL) and the lower control limit (LCL). This is also why the formula reads plus AND minus. For this example, to find a 95% CI for July births, we take our mean of the data or 83 and both add it to and subtract from it the sum ($1.96 \times$ standard deviation or 3.58). This leads to $83 + 7.01$ or 90 and $83 - 7.01$ or 76. We would then write this as: FM July, 95% CI (76–90).

Comparing Forecasting Techniques

At this point, it is important to compare the different forecasting methods for July births given the available data and using the different approaches as shown in **Table 13.6**.

Although each technique yields a different estimate, collectively, the techniques provide sufficient information to venture a forecast. Choosing a technique is not an attempt to determine which

TABLE 13.6 Comparison of Forecasting Methods

METHOD	Forecast Value(s)
Average change	89
Average % change	87
95% confidence interval	(76–90)

provides the correct forecast for the next time frame. Each technique or method provides a "right" answer. These forecasts provide the manager with data on which to select a forecast, which may or may not be the exact forecast provided through them. Forecasting requires judgment, not just the ability to solve mathematical formulas. In other words, forecasting is an art as well as a science.

In retrospect, each of these basic methods is based upon different properties of the data used in the forecast. Each assumes a certain degree of linearity in the data and an inherent relationship between time (as the independent variable) and births (as the dependent variable) that has a positive or negative slope. For example, the level of births forecasted for July, in one instance 89, is higher than the actual number of births recorded for June (i.e., 85).

Although helpful in forecasting, these three techniques may be too simple for most applications. These techniques mask variability in the data. In the example used, some of this natural variability is based upon a different number of days per month. These methods also distill the data using the average or average percent change calculations. Except for the CI approach, each method assumes that the forecast will be based on the theoretical line that best represents the past data. Therefore, these methods are offered as a starting point for forecasting, not as definitive methods that can be relied upon exclusively to provide a relevant forecast. Video 13.3 shows how to calculate a forecast using a 95% confidence interval and present a comparison table using Excel.

LEARNING OBJECTIVE 13.4: UNDERSTAND WEIGHTED FORECASTING MODELS BY USING MOVING AVERAGES

 **VIDEO FOR LEARNING OBJECTIVE 13.4**

- Video 13.4 Moving Averages

Because historical data often vary, sometimes considerably, it is helpful to utilize a technique that does not tend to mask the inherent variability of the data, as do the methods we have covered so far. Moving averages correct for this and provide a method to examine the variability in the data and use this pattern of variability in constructing a forecast.

To demonstrate moving averages, the data in **Table 13.1** have been revised by adding more historical data (July–December) and changing one of the original historical data points (March

TABLE 13.7 Live Births January to June

MONTH	NUMBER OF BIRTHS
July	68
August	79
September	81
October	55
November	71
December	60
January	77
February	81
March	63
April	85
May	87
June	85

FIGURE 13.5 Monthly births plotted.

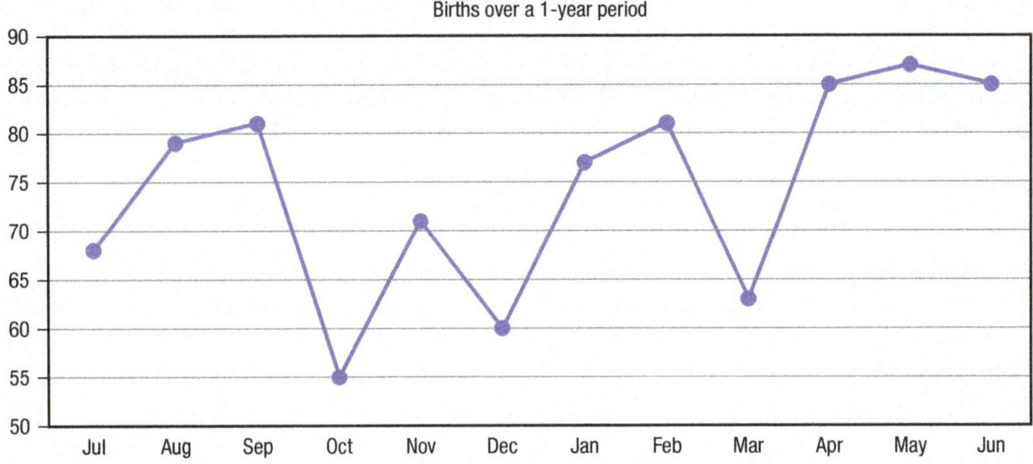

TABLE 13.8   Live Births January to June $n = 2$ Moving Average

MONTH	NUMBER OF BIRTHS		
	Actual	**FV ($n = 2$)**	
July	68		
August	79		
September	81	73.5	$= \dfrac{68 + 79}{2}$
October	55	80	$= \dfrac{79 + 81}{2}$
November	71	68	
December	60	63	
January	77	65.5	
February	81	68.5	
March	63	79	
April	85	72	
May	87	74	
June	85	86	

FV, forecast value.

from 83 to 63). These data are restated in **Table 13.7**. **Figure 13.5** is the plot of the data included in **Table 13.8**. Note that the scale of the y-axis used in this historical data plot has been selected to magnify the variability of the historical data.

Using a moving (time period to time period) average to forecast is a method that first examines the variability in the historical data and then provides the ability to mathematically "smooth or soften" the historical variability in search of an underlying trend. The first step is to choose some time period over which to calculate the moving average. Simply put, the assumption is that some grouping of previous time periods (months, years, etc.) might better predict the upcoming time period. The problem is we do not know how many. Is 2 months a good predictor of the third? 3 months? 8 months? This is why we must do some calculating using multiple groupings of months to assess which is a better predictor.

To designate our time period, here months, we will use n. Here, n can represent any number of time periods, such as a 2 month ($n = 2$), 3 month ($n = 3$), 4 month ($n = 4$), or any n we choose given the availability of historical data. The steps to developing a moving average forecast are as follows:

1. Select an n (n must be >1). Because 12 months of historical data are included in **Table 13.8**, n could be 2, 3, 4, 5, 6, 7, 8, 9, 10, or 11. To begin, we will start with $n = 2$.

2. Calculate the n-period moving average, again starting with the oldest data and working forward.

In this example, we would start with July, our first data point, and use $n = 2$, so we would average the first two historical months, July and August. This means that our first averaged forecast would be for September. The forecast for September, using a 2-month moving average, is $\dfrac{(July + August)}{2}$. We would then carry this forward, averaging August and September to get October. The forecast for October, using a 2-month moving average, is then $\dfrac{(August + September)}{2}$. Continue to do this with all the historical data. **Table 13.9** shows this.

The FV stands for the forecast value and the $n = 2$ refers to the use of 2 months of averaging. As we stated, however, we do not know if 2 months of data is a superior predictor to 3 months or 4 or 5. Thus, we must use each and create averaging for those n's as well. **Table 13.9** shows this.

Notice that each set of forecasts steps down as we average more data. This is also the reason that the largest n one can use when using moving averages is the total number of data points minus one. Here that is 11 or 12 − 1. Using all 12 months would simply produce the average of

TABLE 13.9 Live Births January to June n's 2 to 8 Moving Average

MONTH	NUMBER OF BIRTHS							
	Actual	FV						
		$n = 2$	$n = 3$	$n = 4$	$n = 5$	$n = 6$	$n = 7$	$n = 8$
July	68							
August	79							
September	81	73.5						
October	55	80.0	76.0					
November	71	68.0	71.7	70.8				
December	60	63.0	69.0	71.5	70.8			
January	77	65.5	62.0	66.8	69.2	69.0		
February	81	68.5	69.3	65.8	68.8	70.5	70.1	
March	63	79.0	72.7	72.3	68.8	70.8	72.0	71.5
April	85	72.0	73.7	70.3	70.4	67.8	69.7	70.9
May	87	74.0	76.3	76.5	73.2	72.8	70.3	71.6
June	85	86.0	78.3	79.0	78.6	75.5	74.9	72.4

TABLE 13.10 Moving Average $n = 2$ with FEs

MONTH	NUMBER OF BIRTHS		
	Actual	FV ($n = 2$)	FE
July	68		
August	79		
September	81	73.5	7.5
October	55	80.0	25.0
November	71	68.0	3.0
December	60	63.0	3.0
January	77	65.5	11.5
February	81	68.5	12.5
March	63	79.0	16.0
April	85	72.0	13.0
May	87	74.0	13.0
June	85	86.0	1.0

FE, forecast error; FV, forecast value.

the data, which, as we mentioned earlier in this chapter, is a viable but highly naive method of forecasting.

Now, we have a series of forecasts for the past months but still have the problem of how to forecast the future. Let us continue to assume our goal is to forecast the next July. We must have some mechanism to compare these groups of averages to select which is "best." To do this, we need to determine how effective our forecasting methods are. Although we cannot know what the future will be, we have our historical data, and we have already created forecasts for events that have occurred. Looking at the table and visually comparing our actual data to the forecasts, you can see we were most often a bit off in one way or another. This is the forecast error, or FE, and it is the mechanism we will use to compare our forecasts. Examine **Table 13.10** which only shows our $n = 2$ forecast. We have added a new column for FE which is simply the actual data for a given time period, here September minus our forecast for September. Note that we have to start with September because we could not forecast for July or August using $n = 2$.

Table 13.11 expands this to show $n = 2$, 3, 4, and 5 moving averages and FEs. Now that we have both the actual historical data and a forecast based on these n months, we can compare the accuracy of those forecasts using the FEs in absolute terms by taking their average. Why absolute terms? Because we are interested in how close we were to what really happened. We do not really care if it was high or low—both were off. Remember the goal with forecasting is always to be *less wrong*, or to **minimize error.**

The FE gives us a month-by-month picture of variation in the data and allows us to calculate the total and, more importantly, the average FE.

The absolute error is calculated by summing the FE columns. The mean forecast error (MFE) is calculated by taking the average of the FE columns. The "best" interval n is selected based upon the minimum MFE value, which is simply the overall forecast that predicted the historical data with the minimum amount of error.

TABLE 13.11 Moving Average with *n*'s 2 to 8 with FEs

MONTH	Actual	FV (n = 2)	FE	FV (n = 3)	FE	FV (n = 4)	FE	FV (n = 5)	FE
July	68								
August	79								
September	81	73.5	7.5						
October	55	80.0	25.0	76.0	21.0				
November	71	68.0	3.0	71.7	0.7	70.8	0.3		
December	60	63.0	3.0	69.0	9.0	71.5	11.5	70.8	10.8
January	77	65.5	11.5	62.0	15.0	66.8	10.3	69.2	7.8
February	81	68.5	12.5	69.3	11.7	65.8	15.3	68.8	12.2
March	63	79.0	16.0	72.7	9.7	72.3	9.3	68.8	5.8
April	85	72.0	13.0	73.7	11.3	70.3	14.8	70.4	14.6
May	87	74.0	13.0	76.3	10.7	76.5	10.5	73.2	13.8
June	85	86.0	1.0	78.3	6.7	79.0	6.0	78.6	6.4
Total FE			105.5		95.7		77.8		71.4
Average FE			10.55		10.63		**9.72**		10.20

FE, forecast error; FV, forecast value.

Looking at **Table 13.11**, we can see that when averaging 4 months of data, the forecasts have the lowest average error than the other methods, 9.72. The other methods were above 10. This means that when averaging 4 months of previous data, the next month's forecasts were off 9.72 births on average. Again, not perfect, but no forecast is. It is simply the forecast that was closest to what actually happened.

Next, we can conduct the important task of forecasting the future. To forecast July, the previous 4 months of values would be averaged (those for March, April, May, and June). This produces a forecast of 80.

Once a specific month is forecasted (e.g., July 80), insert it in the "actual" column on the worksheet and continue to calculate the moving average as shown in **Table 13.12**. Note, however, that the forecast becomes dampened as it moves forward. This means the forecast is likely to be further from the actual (i.e., observed) value as it extended further into the future. This is because the forecast is actually based on averages.

Once the forecast is extended beyond the selected *n*, in this case *n* = 4, you can see in **Table 13.13** that the entire forecast is based upon calculated, not observed, values. Therefore, a general convention when using moving averages is that forecasts must include at least one actual data point. For example, with an *n* = 4, we can only forecast four periods into the future.

Moving averages provide the ability to recognize the variability in time series data and use the pattern of variability to construct an appropriate forecast. Unlike previous methods, moving averages also provide the ability to extend the forecast some number of time intervals into the future, depending on the number of historical months used in averaging. Video 13.4 shows how to calculate a moving average forecast using Excel.

TABLE 13.12 July Forecast Using $n = 4$

MONTH	NUMBER OF BIRTHS	
	Actual	**FV ($n = 4$)**
July	68	
August	79	
September	81	
October	55	
November	71	70.8
December	60	71.5
January	77	66.8
February	81	65.8
March	63	72.3
April	85	70.3
May	87	76.5
June	85	79.0
July FV		**80.0**

FV, forecast value.

TABLE 13.13 Forecasting Forward Using $n = 4$

MONTH	NUMBER OF BIRTHS	
	Actual	**FV ($n = 4$)**
July	68	
August	79	
September	81	
October	55	
November	71	70.8
December	60	71.5
January	77	66.8
February	81	65.8
March	63	72.3
April	85	70.3
May	87	76.5
June	85	79.0
July FV	**80.0** ←	**80.0**
August FV	**84.25**	
September FV	**84.06**	
October FV	83.33	

FV, forecast value.

LEARNING OBJECTIVE 13.5: UNDERSTAND WEIGHTED FORECASTING MODELS BY USING EXPONENTIAL SMOOTHING

▶ VIDEO FOR LEARNING OBJECTIVE 13.5

- Video 13.5 Exponential Smoothing

Examination of the data in **Table 13.7** shows that the numbers of births start at 68 births in July and end with 85 births in June. The data suggest that the future will more likely involve numbers toward the higher levels (i.e., 90) than lower numbers (i.e., 68). In other words, it seems appropriate to base a forecast more on the most recent data than on the older data if some type of linear trend is believed to exist. Exponential smoothing provides a technique to take these types of considerations into account. To smooth and thereby minimize the effect of this fluctuation in the forecast, the initial step is to select a smoothing constant (SC). The SC is a weighting factor that influences the degree the forecasted value (F) and the observed value (O) for a past period influence one another in calculating the forecast for a future period. The SC must be between 0 and 1.00, or 0% and 100%, and typically SCs are only used up to .5 as weights beyond 50% are unadvisable. Exponential smoothing uses the following general formula:

Equation 13.4: Formula for a Smoothing Constant Forecast

$$FV = \left(SC \times O_{t-1}\right) + \left[\left(1 - SC\right) \times \left(F_{t-1}\right)\right]$$

where:

SC = the smoothing constant (a number between 1 and 0)
FV = the forecast for next period in the future
O_{t-1} = the observed value for the last or most recent period at time minus 1
F_{t-1} = the forecasted value for the last or most recent historical period

This formula indicates that the forecast for the next period will equal the observed value for the most current time period (O_{t-1}) times the SC plus the forecast for the most recent historical period (FV_{t-1}) times 1 minus the SC. For example, if a forecast for hospital patient days for this past month (FV_{t-1}) was 550 patient days and the observed (actual) number of patient days (O_{t-1}) was 525, the next month's forecast using an SC of .3 would be:

$$FV = \left(SC \times O_{t-1}\right) + \left[\left(1 - SC\right) \times \left(FV_{t-1}\right)\right]$$
$$= (.3 \times 525) + [(1 - .3) \times 550]$$
$$= (157.5) + (.7 \times 550)$$
$$= 157.5 + 385$$
$$= 542.5 \text{ patient days}$$

Note that in this type of forecast, there is an expected value based upon a weighted average of two variables, the most recent actual value, and a forecast. The SC is a weighting factor that influences the degree to which a forecasted value and the observed value (O) for a past period influence one another in calculating the forecast for a future period. This last example combined 30% (0.30) of the observed value for a previous month with 70% (0.70) of the forecasted value for previous month to calculate the forecast for the future month.

Table 13.14 shows our birth data from the previous examples and demonstrates forecasting using .01 as the SC. This places 10% of the weight on the actual data from the previous month and 90% on the forecast. You may realize, however, that we do not yet have a forecast to start with. For this reason, we must start forecasting in the *second* time period and assume the forecast for the second time period is the actual data from the first time period (see **Table 13.14**). This step is then

TABLE 13.14 Exponential Smoothing With a Constant of .1

MONTH	NUMBER OF BIRTHS		
	Actual	**FV (SC = .1)**	
July	68		
August	79	68	
September	81	69.1	$= (.01 \times 79) + (.09 \times 68)$
October	55	70.3	
November	71	68.8	
December	60	69.0	
January	77	68.1	
February	81	69.0	
March	63	70.2	
April	85	69.5	
May	87	71.0	
June	85	72.6	

FV, forecast value; SC, smoothing constant

repeated for the next month or time period, taking .1 and multiplying it by the observed data at $t - 1$ and adding to .9 multiplied by the forecast at $t - 1$.

Once we have completed this for a .1 SC, it can be repeated for other SCs. Again, the convention is to only use constants up to .5. What can also be calculated at this point, similar to our moving averages example, is an FE or FE. This will again enable us to choose the SC with the lowest average error. **Table 13.15** shows these calculations.

Examining **Table 13.5,** we can see that the SC for .3 and the SC for .4 yield the same FEs or 10.71 on average. At this point, either one would be acceptable to use, or the analyst could run another forecast using an SC of .35 and .45 to see if they would result in a lower FE (doing so, in fact, produces a minimally smaller FE for the SC = .3 of 10.70, making these realistically similar).

This forecasting technique presents certain challenges. An SC must be determined using systematic methods. This is done in much the same way as it was for moving averages. By using historical data, a forecast can be generated and its accuracy determined using the FE. By using multiple SCs, the FEs, summarized by the MFEs for each SC (.1, .3, .5, etc.), can be compared and a forecast of minimum error selected or that which generate the lowest MFE. The next step is to forecast into the future once an appropriate SC is selected. For this example, we will choose SC = .3.

Table 13.16 shows how we begin to do this. We can create an FV for July by taking .3 multiplied by the actual value for June (85) and add that to .7 multiplied by our forecasted value for June (78.3), giving us 80.28.

An obvious problem now occurs when we try to forecast further. We have no actual value for July. To counter this, we simply reverse what we did when we began this forecasting method but instead now move the forecasted value for June over to become the new "actual" value for July. See again **Table 13.16.** Once done, we can then conduct a new forecasted value for August and repeat the process. At this point, you may be thinking, but does that not create forecasts based on forecasts? The answer is yes. And it leads us to our second rule for forecasting which is that we

TABLE 13.15 Exponential Smoothing Using Multiple SC

MONTH	Actual	NUMBER OF BIRTHS									
		SC = .1		SC = .2		SC = .3		SC = .4		SC = .5	
		FV	FE	FV	FE	FV	FE	FV	FE	FV	FE
July	68										
August	79	68	11.00	68	11.00	68	11.00	68	11.00	68	11.00
September	81	69.1	11.90	70.2	10.80	71.3	9.70	72.4	8.60	73.5	7.50
October	55	70.3	15.29	72.4	17.36	74.2	19.21	75.8	20.84	77.3	22.25
November	71	68.8	2.24	68.9	2.11	68.4	2.55	67.5	3.50	66.1	4.88
December	60	69.0	8.98	69.3	9.31	69.2	9.21	68.9	8.90	68.6	8.56
January	77	68.1	8.91	67.4	9.55	66.4	10.55	65.3	11.66	64.3	12.72
February	81	69.0	12.02	69.4	11.64	69.6	11.39	70.0	11.00	70.6	10.36
March	63	70.2	7.18	71.7	8.69	73.0	10.03	74.4	11.40	75.8	12.82
April	85	69.5	15.54	69.9	15.05	70.0	14.98	69.8	15.16	69.4	15.59
May	87	71.0	15.98	73.0	14.04	74.5	12.49	75.9	11.09	77.2	9.79
June	85	72.6	12.39	75.8	9.23	78.3	6.74	80.3	4.66	82.1	2.90
Total FE			121.44		118.79		117.85		117.81		118.37
Average FE			11.04		10.80		10.71		10.71		10.76

FE, forecast error; FV, forecast value; SC, smoothing constant

TABLE 13.16 Exponential Smoothing Forecast Using SC = .3

MONTH	NUMBER OF BIRTHS	
	Actual	**FV (SC = .3)**
July	68	
August	79	68.0
September	81	71.3
October	55	74.2
November	71	68.4
December	60	69.2
January	77	66.4
February	81	69.6
March	63	73.0
April	85	70.0
May	87	74.5
June	85	78.3
July FV	78.3	80.28
August FV	80.3	79.68
September FV	79.7	79.86
October FV	79.9	79.80

FV, forecast value; SC, smoothing constant.

should never forecast forward more than one third of our original data. So, if we have 12 months, the furthest we should forecast forward is 4 months or 12/3. You will also note that as we do move forward into the future, this method as well as moving averages slowly remove the variability from the data, and thus all future forecasts will begin to dampen or converge to a single point. See Video 13.5 for how to calculate an exponential smoothing forecast using Excel.

LEARNING OBJECTIVE 13.6: BE ABLE TO SELECT BETWEEN FORECASTING MODELS BASED UPON THE CALCULATED MEAN FORECAST ERROR

Both moving averages and exponential smoothing approaches attempt to soften the variation in past data searching for a master trend and use this master trend to forecast. Moving averages do this by calculating grouped or pooled averages. A two-period ($n = 2$) moving average steps through the data in units of two. It calculates averages based upon every consecutive 2-month period. A three-period moving average does the same in groups of three. Exponential smoothing does not group data together in different combinations (e.g., $n = 2$, 3, 4, or 5). Instead, it bases a forecast on different weighted monthly calculations, with less weight placed on observations based further in the past. An SC of .3, for example, bases 30% of the forecast on the actual level of the preceding time period and 70% on the forecast for the previous entire time period. Changing the SC to .5 bases a forecast equally (i.e., 50% and 50%) on the actual and FVs for the preceding time period. Both moving averages and exponential smoothing are mathematical approaches used to soften the time-period to time-period variability in time series data to determine an underlying trend.

Methods other than using MFE do exist as a basis for selecting specific forecasting models. Many software packages have adjustments for seasonality of the data. Others use the standard error and select the specific forecasting model with the lowest standard error. Doing so provides for a slightly more specific measure of inherent variation in the data.

What is most important for analysts and managers when interpreting forecasting measures is to relate the forecast to the context of the data and remember the assumptions of how the forecast mechanism works.

One method is that we could compare the MFE across both moving averages and exponential smoothing techniques. It would be acceptable to take that with the lowest MFE and forecast forward. But again, context matters. Recall that in our example, the SCs .4 and .3 both yielded MFEs within .01 of each other. Here, we are measuring the number of births; therefore, in essence, when rounded to whole births, using an SC of .3, .35, or .4 and moving averages for $n = 2$ and $n = 3$ return equally accurate forecasts. In this instance, a level of specificity to the hundredths is not required. Had this been a financial forecast, however, the hundredth place would have an impact, as a difference of a few cents when carried across the entire organization's service volume can amount to large amounts of expense or savings.

Also note how variability is handled. Average change and average percent change rely on the idea that some underlying trend in past variation will continue. With average percent change, this is made explicit by taking the average historical percent change and simply bringing it forward. A 95% CI, on the other hand, is typically "right" but not very "accurate." This means we will get a good sense of where the future will fall, but the range of values could be either quite large as to not be helpful or narrow enough to provide some strategic meaning. Our final two methods dampen variability, so if one has volatile historical data (wide fluctuations from time period to time period), then this may be helpful for a short-term forecast, but those forecasts will begin to converge together the further one estimates forward.

SUMMARY

Forecasting, regardless of method, requires a knowledge of what is being forecast and how the assumptions of forecasting may or may not apply. When there is variability in the data, using a linear forecasting method may not be as appropriate as using a moving average approach where the variability is captured more closely or an exponential smoothing method which flattens out the variability. If not discernable trend is present, a simple method based on averaging in combination with a CI may yield a more accurate or actionable result. Comparing the MFE across methods in one way to assess historical fit with the data. That all said, forecasting is as much art as science, and other factors such as seasonality and other considerations may come into play. We explore these in greater detail in Chapter 15.

END-OF-CHAPTER RESOURCES

DISCUSSION QUESTIONS

1. What are some of the assumptions of using average change and average percent change as forecasting tools?
2. Think about the comparison forecasts presented in **Table 13.6**. Now pick a final best guess forecast. How did you use the information from each of these to come up with your forecast. Discuss your reasoning.

3. What are some of the assumptions of moving averages when forecasting? When are these useful and when are they not? For what types of data or phenomena?

4. What are some of the assumptions of exponential smoothing and SCs when forecasting? When are these useful and when are they not? For what types of data or phenomena?

LEARNING ACTIVITIES

CourseConnect ▶

To access self-assessment questions and interactive, competency-based learning activities for this chapter, visit www.springerpub.com/courseconnect. See inside front cover and tear-out card for CourseConnect details.

LINEAR REGRESSION FORECASTING

LEARNING OBJECTIVES

14.1. Examine the foundations and components of the regression model.
14.2. Test the validity of the underlying assumption of linearity in the data.
14.3. Examine the use of time as an independent variable in linear regression forecasting.
14.4. Use regression residuals to develop a best forecast based upon mean forecast error.
14.5. Construct confidence intervals around regression forecasting estimates.

REAL-WORLD SCENARIO

After finding the model with the lowest mean absolute forecast error (MFE) given the methods in Chapter 13, "Time Series Forecasting Techniques," Mo Adel would like to develop and examine a series of regression forecasting models. Because they believe that there could be an underlying linear trend, regression forecasting techniques can be highly suitable. Using the data available to them, they will attempt to construct a line of best fit to the historical data or portions of it.

Regression analysis, often called ordinary least squares regression, or simple linear regression, derives from the basic algebraic notions of linearity between a set of variables, the simplest being that between two variables, X and Y. One way to examine these two variables is through correlation, in which an association or lack thereof is determined between the variables (see Chapter 3, "Statistical Foundations"). Regression models, however, take this idea further by examining the potential existence of a linear relationship between X and Y. Once established, such a relationship can be used to predict the change in Y as X also changes.

The purpose of this chapter is to apply linear regression to forecasting. The regression model is sufficiently robust to be used in many management applications. Regression is used as a type of predictive model and is the foundation for more advanced types of prediction.

The function of predictive models is to understand the relationship between factors that could be related to that which we want to predict. Some of these may be hypothesized, meaning they are apparent in our thinking, and at other times, they may be hidden. The type of regression we will use here will be the hypothesized type and will start with the simplest form of a predictive model.

Simply put, a model is a replication or simplification of reality. For example, a painting can be considered a model because it describes some reality at a point in time. Although some models are merely descriptive, such as a painting, others, like regression, can be predictive.

Generally, models are not given; they must be constructed. For example, a healthcare administrator may need to know the relationship between the number of inpatient days and the number of staff hours. Managers in ambulatory care may need to know the relationship between the number of clinic visits and number of laboratory tests ordered and/or performed. Managers in nursing homes may want to know the relationship between staff hours and measures of quality of care. Managers of medical device services may wish to know the relationship between hours of use and request for repairs. Knowing these types of relationships provides managers the ability to predict the number of staff hours given forecasted hospital inpatient days for next year, the number of laboratory tests given anticipated clinic visits for next month, the levels of patient quality in the nursing home given the anticipated number of staff hours for the next 3 months, or the number of replacement parts and labor required per medical device sold. Regression analysis provides the tools to construct these types of models in algebraic form.

The difficulty with constructing models is that care must be taken to be as thoughtful as possible about the components of the model. The components are simply other things, typically variables, that we also have measurements for, such as number of staff, dollars spent, total population, a count of other diseases patients may be diagnosed with, and so on. Further, no model is perfect and should not be taken as fact. There are two reasons for this. One is that it is rarely possible to fully understand all the variables that create a given phenomenon. For example, if we try to create a model that determines the number of lab tests our hospital runs, we will quickly find ourselves with a very long list of contributing factors. These could be elements such as the number and severity of the patients, the number of accidents, the severity of the allergy season, the number of bee stings, and so forth. Even if we could measure and predict each of these things, which we cannot, our model would be too complex to be useful.

This does not mean that all models are useless. Models may be constructed to include those elements that are both contributors to what we are trying to predict and those that we can accurately measure.

The second reason is that even when a useful model has been determined, the variables used and the relationships between them are often situational and open to change. For example, the relationship between the number of inpatient days in a hospital and the number of staff hours is different from hospital to hospital and can change over time due to technology or the population being served.

For this reason, the models we create will also have a measure of mathematical predictive probability—or, more simply put, the likelihood of being accurate.

Some regression models are constructed using historical data. As with other methods, they utilize the primary assumption of the past being an accurate predictor of the future. Because of this, one needs to be confident that this is a sound assumption. Conversely, if a fundamental change has occurred, historical data may be less effectual for prediction and the model flawed.

LEARNING OBJECTIVE 14.1: EXAMINE THE FOUNDATIONS AND COMPONENTS OF THE REGRESSION MODEL

The purpose of simple linear regression analysis is to construct an appropriate but simple mathematical relationship between two or more *continuously measured* variables. Once established, the formula can be used to predict levels of the dependent or Y variable, given values of the X or independent variable(s). Although regression can be used to examine the relationship of many independent variables (X_1, X_2, X_3, etc.) on some dependent variable Y, this chapter restricts attention to the simple linear model using only one predictor or X variable.

In regression analysis, Y is used to represent the dependent variable; the value Y takes on depends on the value of X. The X variable is the independent variable; as it changes, so too does the value of Y. Expressed algebraically as Equation 14.1, this simple relationship is the foundation for all regression modeling.

The linear regression model is usually expressed as:

Equation 14.1

$$Y = b_0 + b_1 X$$

where b_0 is the Y intercept and b_1 represents the slope.

Some students may recall the intercept is that point where $X = 0$ or where the line crosses the X axis. You might also recall that this formula looks something like that for a straight line: $Y = mX + B$.

In the line formula, B is the intercept and m is the slope and their places are flipped, but the two formulae are, in fact, identical.

A regression model establishes the best fit between a straight-line equation and the available data which describes a relationship between X and Y. This also requires that we believe some sort of correlation exists between our X variable and our Y variable.

Let us look at an example. Consider a set of data taken from a laboratory over 8 weeks that examines the number of lab tests performed and the number of total clinic visits. **Table 14.1** shows this data. We also need to develop some hypothesis of relationship so we can assign one of the variables, the X and one the Y so that we can say that we believe that lab tests and clinic visits are correlated. To examine this, we could create a scatterplot as in **Figure 14.1**. One could likely eyeball the plot of the data and imagine any number of lines that would "fit" these data. **Figure 14.2** shows some of these. However, we would ideally want to develop a line that minimizes the distance of each data point to the line we develop. Why? Because if we use this line to forecast into the future, all future points will be linear, or on the line. For this reason, the line is quite similar to

TABLE 14.1   Clinic Visits and Lab Tests by Week

WEEK	CLINIC VISITS (x)	LAB TESTS (y)	VISIT (y/x)
1	65	105	1.62
2	67	125	1.87
3	62	110	1.77
4	68	120	1.76
5	71	140	1.97
6	65	135	2.08
7	61	95	1.56
8	75	130	1.73
Average	66.8	120	1.79

FIGURE 14.1 Scatterplot of Table 14.1.

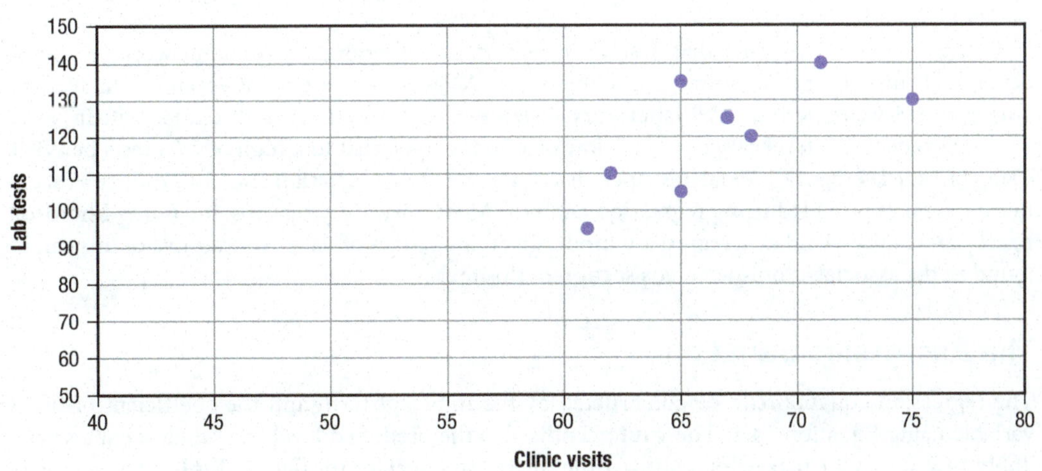

FIGURE 14.2 Scatterplot of Table 14.1 with potential trend lines.

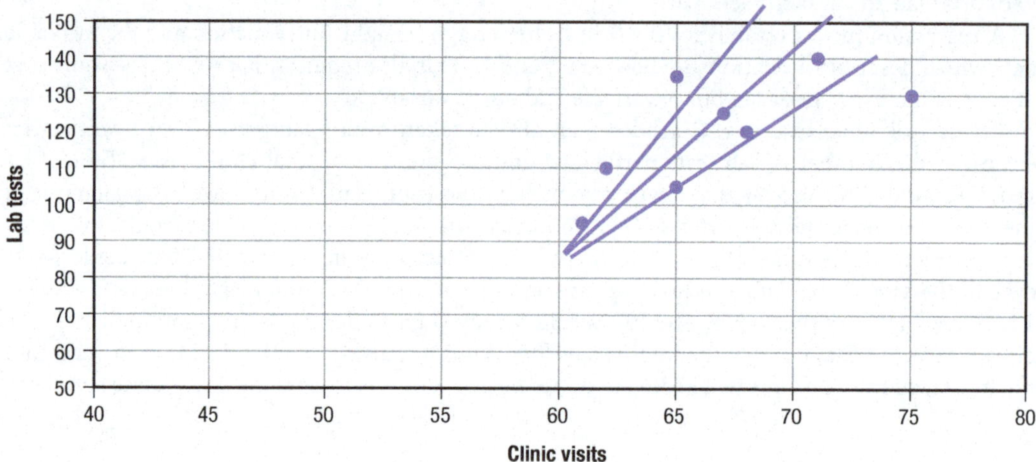

our MFE from Chapter 13, "Time Series Forecasting Techniques." The points are real. The line is the forecast. Therefore, the distance from any point to the line is error.

Prior to doing this, we need to hypothesize which variable predicts which. Here, we only have two possibilities. We believe either that lab tests predict clinic visits or that clinic visits predict lab tests. Let us assume that patients do not get preorders for lab tests and that all lab orders originate while they are at the clinic (this is not always the case, but we will assume it here). If this is the case, then it should be safe to assume that the higher the number of visits, the more likely there would be a greater number of lab tests. So, just as we did in Chapter 3, "Statistical Foundations," we could create a set of hypotheses. One might be correlational or that clinic visits are positively correlated with lab tests and then test against our null hypotheses of no difference using the Pearson correlation test. Testing this relationship is always a good first step in linear regression and something we will cover in more detail later in this chapter. A second would be that one variable (X) has some predictive relationship to the other (Y).

Mathematically, creating and fitting a regression line relies upon the least squares method to determine the straight line that best (but not necessarily perfectly) establishes the equation representing the relationship between X as the independent variable and Y as the dependent variable. This method minimizes the distance between the line developed using the regression model and the actual X and Y data points.

Examine again **Table 14.1** that describes the number of laboratory tests per week (Y) as the dependent variable and the number of clinic visits (X) as the independent variable. On average, during this 8-week period, 1.79 laboratory tests were performed for each clinic visit. In some weeks, however, this level ranges from a low of 1.56 tests per visit to a high of 2.08 tests per visit. Using just the average of 1.79 lab tests per visit might mask this variation and not produce as accurate a model as provided using regression analysis. Most software programs, including Microsoft Excel, can readily calculate a regression model given the ranges of data. An example of this can be found in the associated online videos section of this text.

The Regression Equation

The regression equation can be constructed by the intercept term and the coefficient of the X variable using Equation 14.1. The y intercept is also the predicted level of y when x equals zero. **Table 14.2** shows the regression output using Microsoft Excel for the data in **Table 14.1**, where we try to predict the number of lab tests using the number of clinic visits.

TABLE 14.2 Regression Output of Clinic Visits and Lab Tests

SUMMARY OUTPUT								
Regression Statistics								
Multiple R	0.714097387							
R^2	0.509935078							
Adjusted R^2	0.428257591							
Standard error	11.78353631							
Observations	8							
ANOVA								
	df	*SS*	*MS*	*F*	*Significance F*			
Regression	1	866.8896321	866.8896321	6.243275793	0.046612991			
Residual	6	833.1103679	138.851728					
Total	7	1,700						
	Coefficients	*Standard error*	*t stat*	*p value*	*Lower 95%*	*Upper 95%*	*Lower 95.0%*	*Upper 95.0%*
Intercept	−40.73578595	64.46369147	−0.631918294	0.550743189	−198.4727566	117.0011847	−198.4727566	117.0011847
Clinic visits (x)	2.408026756	0.963729267	2.498654797	0.046612991	0.049866191	4.766187321	0.049866191	4.766187321

ANOVA, analysis of variance; *df*, degrees of freedom; MS, mean square; SS, sum of squares.

Here, we see that the intercept is −40.74 rounded. The X variable coefficient, or b_1 term, is rounded 2.41. This gives us the regression equation Lab Tests = (2.41 × Clinic visits) – 40.74. From this, we can input any number of clinic visits to estimate the corresponding number of lab tests predicted by our model. So, for example, if we believe there would be 70 clinic visits in the next month, we expect to see approximately 128 lab tests using the equation, Lab Tests = (70 × 2.41) − 40.74. Obviously, this is an estimate. In fact, the likelihood of there being exactly 128 lab tests given 70 clinic visits is quite small. However, before we can address the issue of accuracy of our prediction, we have another consideration. The regression line is that which minimizes the distance from the line to the X and Y variable points. It assumes that there is some linearity between these variables. To do this, we need to explore the regression output a bit more fully. The next section examines this assumption more closely and describes how to test to ensure it is correct before using a regression equation to forecast.

LEARNING OBJECTIVE 14.2: TEST THE VALIDITY OF THE UNDERLYING ASSUMPTION OF LINEARITY IN THE DATA

What do we mean when we say that we assume there is linearity in the data? Well, if we examine a scatterplot of two variables, such as that in **Figure 14.3**, we could no doubt consider one or more possible lines or perhaps no line at all that might be drawn to best fit the data. In examples such as this, the data often have a cloudlike appearance, where a discernible pattern or relationship is difficult to estimate. In fact, the line of best fit here could potentially be a horizontal line or vertical line. The problem in dealing with horizontal or vertical lines is that their slopes are either zero in the horizontal case or undefined in the vertical case. When using regression, we are primarily concerned with slopes that are potentially zero. This would mean that no matter what value X had, Y remains the same. This is not a good predictive equation to use for forecasting because regardless of what happens to the x variable, your prediction will also always be the same.

For example, if our regression formula were to be $y = 111 + 0x$, y would be a constant, 111, regardless of whether $X = 1$, or 100, or any number. Therefore, before using the line that our regression output provides to describe the relationship between X and Y, a statistical test must be performed to determine whether the predicted slope is not, in truth, zero.

If we examine our previous example, Excel calculated the equation of $y = −40 + (2.41x)$ or $y = 2.41x – 40$ for the data we provided it. Since this slope was calculated based on only a sample of data and not all lab tests and clinic visits, we need to test whether the slope is truly different from zero or a result that we got just by chance.

FIGURE 14.3 Birth by year plot with trend line.

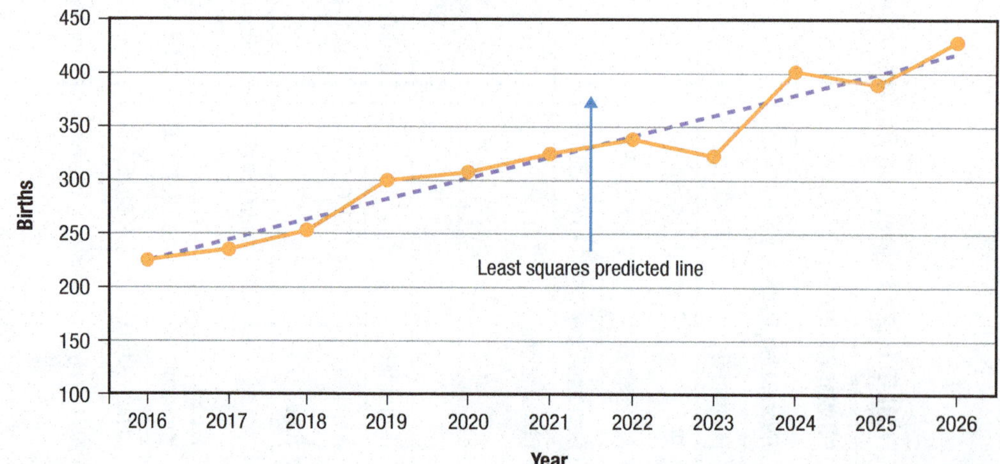

TABLE 14.3 *p* Value Subset from Table 14.2 Output

	COEFFICIENTS	STANDARD ERROR	*t* STAT	*p* VALUE
Intercept	−40.735786	64.46369147	−0.63191829	0.550743
Clinic visits (x)	2.40802676	0.963729267	2.498654797	0.046613

Many techniques exist to test a regression line. Here, we will use our regression output further, which tests whether, at a 95% level of confidence, the slope of the regression line is other than zero. The test statistic we will use is the t statistic which you will remember from Chapter 3, "Statistical Foundations." The question we are asking is "What is the likelihood that the predicted slope of our regression line actually equals zero in reality?" Our statistical hypotheses are as follows:

H_0: There is no difference between the calculated slope and zero, otherwise put,

$b_1 = 0$ (This is the null hypothesis.)

H_a: There is a difference between the calculated slope and zero, otherwise put,

b_1 does NOT $= 0$

Because we have collected a sample of historical data, it is possible that in reality, there is no true linear relationship between X and Y—that is, that we would fail to reject H_0, the null hypothesis. Thankfully, the information we need to make this assessment is readily available in our regression output. **Table 14.3** is a subset of **Table 14.2** focusing on the output we want. Here, we see two columns: one labeled t stat and one labeled p value. The t statistic is the value of t derived from the regression equation. The p value is the probability of that t statistic given the appropriate t distribution. As with any probability value, we need to identify an alpha value that we will use as a "cutoff" for determining when to reject our null hypothesis. Here, we have said we will use a 95% level of confidence to assess if the slope is nonzero to reject the null or an alpha of .05. This is also the default for Excel and most statistical programs.

Thus, if our p value is <.05, we can be 95% confident our slope is not zero, and we may use this regression model for prediction. In **Tables 14.2** and **14.3**, our t statistic is 2.499 and our p value is .047 rounded. Because .047 is <.05, our alpha value where we created our decision rule for rejecting the null hypothesis, H_0, we can reject the null hypothesis that the slope is statistically zero and use this regression equation as a forecasting tool. If the calculated p value had been >.05, the appropriate decision would be to fail to reject the hypothesis that the slope could in fact be zero and we would have to discard the previously calculated regression equation as unusable.

Following this process provides us the ability to conclude whether the calculated regression equation is a valid expression of the relationship portrayed in the data.

LEARNING OBJECTIVE 14.3: EXAMINE THE USE OF TIME AS AN INDEPENDENT VARIABLE IN LINEAR REGRESSION FORECASTING

 VIDEO FOR LEARNING OBJECTIVE 14.3

- Video 14.1 Using the Regression Function in Excel

For many practical purposes in healthcare, using linear regression to forecast often requires that time be the independent or X variable. Time can be expressed in any appropriate unit such as days, weeks, months, or years. We often may want to know if a certain volume of services is increasing or decreasing over time in a predictable way, for example. To simplify calculations and provide equal units, it is important to express time intervals in small numbers. For example, instead of using actual years, such as 2025, 2026, 2027, and so forth as the X variable, the year

TABLE 14.4 Births by Year

Year	RENUMBERED (x) Year	Births (y)
2016	1	225
2017	2	236
2018	3	253
2019	4	300
2020	5	308
2021	6	325
2022	7	338
2023	8	323
2024	9	403
2025	10	390
2026	11	430

would be numbered and time intervals of one integer are used, such as 1, 2, 3, and so forth. This reflects the equal lengths of each as being 1 year. This is the assumption of having two continuous variables to work with. An example of the aforementioned analysis is provided in Video 14.1, "Using the Regression Function in Excel."

This may produce slightly skewed estimates when dealing with months because some months are of different length in days. However, it works well with days, weeks, and years because the subunits within those larger time units are generally of equal length.

Consider the data in **Table 14.4** and the graphed data with least squares line in **Figure 14.3**. Here, the x values are the numeric intervals for x and will be first graphed and then entered into the Excel regression function. As you can see from **Figure 14.3,** there appears to be a visible upward trend in the relationship of the X and Y variables, but again we need to test the slope of least squares line inherent in the data. **Table 14.5** shows the regression output for the data in **Table 14.4**. The intercept is calculated at 202.8 and the slope as 19.7. This gives the line equation: $y = 202.8 + 19.7x$.

However, we still need to test the potential that the slope is actually zero. Looking at the high-lighted t statistic and the p value of the t statistic, we find that $p < 7.6018$ E-07. The E-07 means that there is actually 7 preceding decimal places to this number, so the full number is 0.00000076018. This is far below our cutoff of .05 for being 95% confident of a nonzero slope. This further allows us to reject the null hypothesis that there is no difference between the calculated slope and zero with a 95% level of confidence. Given that the regression model is useful, it can be used to forecast births (y).

Forecasting Forward Using Linear Regression

To forecast using a regression equation, we use our regression line. Remember that all future values will fall on this line. So, to forecast, we simply plug future values of x into the equation and solve for the corresponding predicted values of y. **Table 14.6** shows 3 months of forecasted data.

TABLE 14.5 Excel Regression Output of Table 14.4

SUMMARY OUTPUT

Regression Statistics

Multiple R	0.970228266							
R^2	0.941342889							
Adjusted R^2	0.934825432							
Standard error	17.19205243							
Observations	11							

ANOVA

	df.	SS	MS	F	Significance F			
Regression	1	42,689.9	42,689.9	144.4340814	7.6018E-07			
Residual	9	2,660.1	295.5666667					
Total	10	45,350						
	Coefficients	*Standard Error*	*t stat*	*p value*	*Lower 95%*	*Upper 95%*	*Lower 95.0%*	*Upper 95.0%*
Intercept	202.8	11.11758094	18.24137832	2.0414E-08	177.6502846	227.9497154	177.6502846	227.9497154
Year	19.7	1.639197882	12.01807312	7.6018E-07	15.99187677	23.40812323	15.99187677	23.40812323
Equation: $y = 202.8 + 19.7x$								

ANOVA, analysis of variance; *df*, degrees of freedom; MS, mean square; SS, sum of squares.

TABLE 14.6 3 Months of Birth Forecasts

	RENUMBERED (*x*)		
Year	Year	Births (y)	
2016	1	225	
2017	2	236	
2018	3	253	
2019	4	300	
2020	5	308	
2021	6	325	
2022	7	338	
2023	8	323	
2024	9	403	
2025	10	390	
2026	11	430	
2027 (*f*)	12	*439.2*	
2028 (*f*)	13	*458.9*	*Forecasted values*
2029 (*f*)	14	*478.6*	

Plotted, each of these points would lie on the regression line going forward. It is important to remember the rule that you should only forecast forward up to one third of our data. Here, we have 11 points of data, so we should only forecast 3 years (11/3).

Other Notes on the Regression Output

Testing the slope should always be the first and primary test for linear regression. However, the regression output provides other useful information when assessing the fit and the appropriateness of the regression line. One is the F test for significance of the overall regression equation. This tests whether the variation in X helps in explaining the variation in Y. A significance of the F test below .05 is, in most cases, sufficient justification for using a regression equation. In **Table 14.5,** the F-test statistic can be seen as having a value of 144.43 with a corresponding significance of 7.60 E-07, or 0.00000076. Interpreted, this means that the model can be used. Still another is using R^2, which is the proportion of the total variance of Y explained by the regression line. In this case, our R^2 is .94, meaning that 94% of the variance in Y (births) is explained by the regression line.

LEARNING OBJECTIVE 14.4: USE REGRESSION RESIDUALS TO DEVELOP A BEST FORECAST BASED UPON MEAN FORECAST ERROR

 **VIDEO FOR LEARNING OBJECTIVE 14.4**

- Video 14.2 Calculating the MFE from Multiple *n*'s of Data

Regression forecast models are based on the assumption that the past predicts the future. The question, of course, is how far into the past does the current trend hold predictive power.

TABLE 14.7   FE Using 11 Months of Data

YEAR	YEAR	BIRTHS (y)	PREDICTED (y)	FE
2016	1	225	222.5	2.5
2017	2	236	242.2	6.2
2018	3	253	261.9	8.9
2019	4	300	281.6	18.4
2020	5	308	301.3	6.7
2021	6	325	321	4
2022	7	338	340.7	2.7
2023	8	323	360.4	37.4
2024	9	403	380.1	22.9
2025	10	390	399.8	9.8
2026	11	430	419.5	10.5
Equation: $y = 202.8 + 19.7x$			**MFE**	**11.82**

MFE, mean forecast error; FE, forecast error.

At some point, historical data are simply not useful or relevant to predicting the future. In relation to regression, this determines how much historical data is to be used in the model or, in other words, how many data points to incorporate to more accurately predict the future and how to know the difference.

The answer is the same as we used with moving averages and exponential smoothing methods in Chapter 13, "Time Series Forecasting Technique." Let us use moving averages for comparison. There, we utilized different numbers of months to average, realizing that different collections of months were either better or worse predictors of the historic data or the past. You may also recall that we forecasted the past and calculated how far we were off from what happened. From there, we took the average of the differences in absolute terms and got an MFE that could be used to compare each method.

We do the same with regression. Each time we choose a new number of x data points, our regression line changes. Examine **Tables 14.7** and **14.8** which show how reducing the historic data changes the regression output and line. In **Table 14.8,** we have removed the earliest 3 years of data, the assumption being that the more recent past is more predictive of the near future. Notice that the X variables have been renumbered so that the earliest time period is labeled as time period one.

Examining the output in **Table 14.8,** the regression line becomes $y = 259.4 + 20.03x$. Because the significance of the F statistic and p value for the t test are both <.05, we can be assured within a 95% level of confidence that the regression model has explanatory ability and also a nonzero slope. We now must determine which regression model, the one based on all 11 points of data or the one based on eight points of data, would provide the best predictive model. Essentially, the question we are asking is "which line fits the data points more closely?" The answer to this can be determined by examining the distance from each of our actual historical data points to what each line predicts. In regression terms, this is known as calculating the residuals.

A residual is defined as Y actual $- Y$ predicted, where Y actual is the historical data and Y predicted is what our regression line would have predicted for Y given that value of X (1, 2, 3, etc.). It is essentially the same as the forecast error (FE) used in previous forecasting methods. There are two ways to calculate residuals. **Table 14.9** shows the addition of predicted values using the

TABLE 14.8 FEs Using 8 Months of Data

YEAR	YEAR	BIRTHS (y)	PREDICTED (y)	FE
2019	1	300	279.43	20.57
2020	2	308	299.46	8.54
2021	3	325	319.49	5.51
2022	4	338	339.52	1.52
2023	5	323	359.55	36.55
2024	6	403	379.58	23.42
2025	7	390	399.61	9.61
2026	8	430	419.64	10.36
Equation $y = 259.4 + 20.03x$			**MFE**	**14.51**

MFE, mean forecast error; FE, forecast error.

regression formula. The residual column subtracts the predicted value for y at each x time period from the observed y value. Taking the absolute value of the residuals and then totaling those values gives the absolute deviation for the regression line. Taking the average of the residuals gives the MFE for this regression line. By calculating the MFE for each of our regression lines using different n numbers of x variables, we can assess which fits the data more closely. As expressed in previous chapters, the lower the MFE, the less the variance of the predictions around the regression line and the more accurate the line is at fitting the data.

From **Table 14.7**, the MFE is 11.82. Repeating this with the model using eight historical points of data in **Table 14.8,** we produce an MFE of 14.5. Because the MFE is lower when using eight points of historical data, we would be better served by using this regression model for prediction as it is more accurate. We could have repeated this with other n's of data, for example, using 10 months of data or 9, and compared the MFE from those if the f test and p value showed a nonzero slope.

Residuals can also be produced in Excel and many other statistical programs when using the regression function. Most, however, will not provide the total, absolute, or mean deviation of the residuals, so care should be taken to adjust the output correctly. An example of the aforementioned analysis is provided in Video 14.2, "Calculating the MFE from Multiple n's of Data."

Here, we have calculated regression models based on two proposed lines. The "best" number of regression lines, however, is a matter of judgment on the part of the manager. Choosing the number of x values can be a matter of examining historical trends in the data or having some knowledge about when a fundamental change may have occurred in the environment. It is important to realize, however, that predictions based on regression will always be linear as they proceed into the future. In reality, this is unlikely to be the case. It is important to assess how long these trends can be expected to continue. If using regression for short-term forecasting, it is also possible to calculate confidence intervals around the final forecasts.

LEARNING OBJECTIVE 14.5: CONSTRUCT CONFIDENCE INTERVALS AROUND REGRESSION FORECASTING ESTIMATES

Regardless of the type of independent variable in a regression equation, it is important that the resulting prediction be presented with a 95% confidence interval. This is because, as previously stated, a forecast is never totally accurate. Using the data from **Table 14.7**, x ranged from 1 to 8

TABLE 14.9 Regression Output for Table 14.8

SUMMARY OUTPUT								
Regression Statistics								
Multiple R	0.914851193							
R^2	0.836952706							
Adjusted R^2	0.804343247							
Standard error	20.92691363							
Observations	7							
ANOVA								
	df	**SS**	**MS**	**F**	**Significance F**			
Regression	1	11,240.03571	11,240.03571	25.66594901	0.003879685			
Residual	5	2,189.678571	437.9357143					
Total	6	13,429.71429						
	Coefficients	**Standard error**	**t stat**	**p value**	**Lower 95%**	**Upper 95%**	**Lower 95.0%**	**Upper 95.0%**
Intercept	259.3928571	21.29733024	12.17959501	6.59588E-05	204.6463269	314.1393874	204.6463269	314.1393874
1	20.03571429	3.954814942	5.066157224	0.003879685	9.869538833	30.20188974	9.869538833	30.20188974
$y = 259.4x + 20.03$								

ANOVA, analysis of variance; df, degrees of freedom; MS, mean square; SS, sum of squares.

and y ranged from 300 to 430. The calculated regression formula ($y = 259.4 + 20.03x$) is the line of best fit based upon the available data. Extending the line beyond the domain of the original data, although appropriate, has inherent risk.

The confidence we have in this line predicting the future will lessen each time period we move forward, or otherwise put, the confidence interval is not a constant width for all values of x. This is because of the way in which least squares works and the fact that the formula for regression is rooted in the values for the mean of x and mean of y. Because of this, for predictions based upon values of the x variable close to the mean, the confidence interval is the smallest. The farther away from the mean, the less precise or wider the confidence interval becomes. Thus, the confidence interval on a predicted value of y depends on the value of x that predicts it.

SUMMARY

Regression analysis is one of the more precise forecasting tools when examining a linear relationship between variables. When used correctly, it provides the line of best fit to the data. It is based on the assumptions of the past predicting the future and that an underlying linear trend exists within the data. Here, we describe a simple relationship between two variables; however, regression can be used to examine the collective effects of multiple x variables on some dependent variable, y. Doing so, however, requires further study of multiple regression techniques, which is beyond the scope of this chapter.

END-OF-CHAPTER RESOURCES

DISCUSSION QUESTIONS

1. What is the foundational assumption of regression?
   a. Does this hold in the real world typically?
2. Discuss why one might use regression when forecasting over another method.
3. How does using subsets of historical data change the use of regression when forecasting?
   a. When might having more data help or hinder a forecast?

LEARNING ACTIVITIES

CourseConnect ▶

To access self-assessment questions and interactive, competency-based learning activities for this chapter, visit www.springerpub.com/courseconnect. See inside front cover and tear-out card for CourseConnect details.

CHAPTER 15

SEASONALITY AND OTHER MODEL CONSIDERATIONS

LEARNING OBJECTIVES

15.1. Define seasonality in healthcare.
15.2. Recognize seasonality in time series data.
15.3. Break down a time series into components for forecasting.

REAL-WORLD SCENARIO

Dr. Harris, the director of operations at a busy metropolitan hospital, is reviewing patient admission data from the past 5 years. They notice a familiar pattern—every winter, the number of ED visits spikes dramatically due to flu cases, while the summer months are significantly calmer. Meanwhile, elective surgeries seem to peak every December. Despite these predictable trends, the hospital still struggles with staff shortages and resource allocation during these periods of high demand. Dr. Harris wonders how they can use historical data to improve planning and avoid last-minute crises.

LEARNING OBJECTIVE 15.1: DEFINE SEASONALITY IN HEALTHCARE

Seasonality refers to patterns that repeat at regular intervals over time. For example, flu cases tend to increase reliably during the fall and winter months, which leads to a predictable increase in patient visits for respiratory illnesses (Lofgren et al., 2006). Similarly, there is often a surge in elective surgeries near the end of the calendar year because patients who have met their insurance deductible may try to take advantage of their insurance benefits before they reset in January (Shukla et al., 2022).

Identifying and understanding these recurring patterns can give healthcare managers an advantage in planning for resource allocation, maintaining inventories, managing staff, and improving patient outcomes. For instance, a hospital ED can prepare for flu season by ensuring adequate staff levels to prevent long wait times and reduced patient satisfaction. An outpatient surgical center that anticipates the year-end increase in elective procedures can adjust budgets to account for higher demand and prevent financial hardship. This chapter gives you the tools to identify seasonality and integrate it into your forecasts so that you can plan for potential challenges proactively.

LEARNING OBJECTIVE 15.2: RECOGNIZE SEASONALITY IN TIME SERIES DATA

Seasonality often can be recognized when visually inspecting time series data. For example, let us visualize the number of weekly flu deaths in the United States from fall 2016 to fall 2024 (**Figure 15.1**).

FIGURE 15.1 Time series of weekly deaths from influenza in the United States.

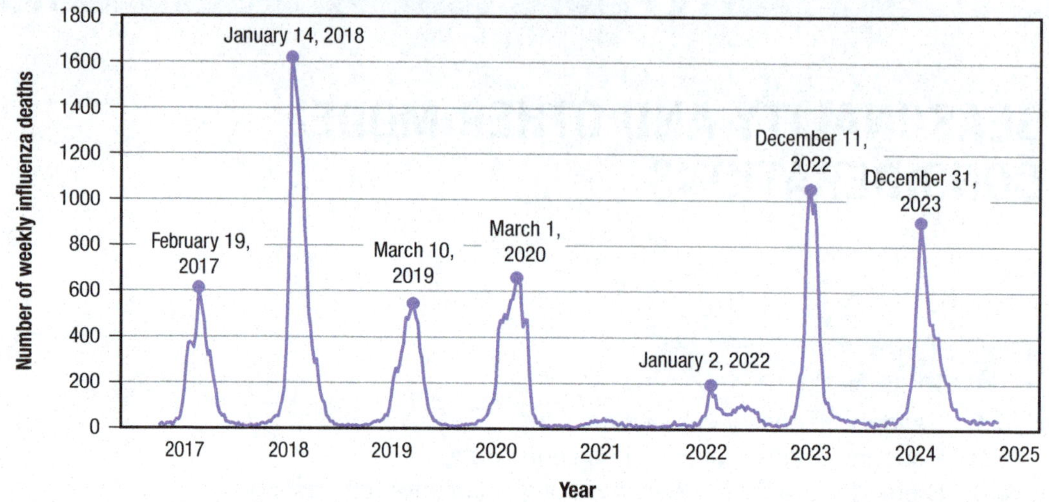

The exact timing of the peaks in influenza mortalities varies from December to March, but it is apparent that the same general pattern appears regularly: the number of weekly deaths begins to increase in late fall or early winter, it peaks sometime during the winter, and then it decreases to a very low level during the late spring or early summer.

An obvious exception to this pattern occurred in the winter of 2020 to 2021. Recall that there were widespread mask mandates and social distancing efforts throughout much of the United States during that period to prevent the spread of the COVID-19 virus. The mask mandates and social distancing proved to be highly effective at limiting the spread of other respiratory viruses like influenza as well (Rana et al., 2023). It is important to remember that, even in time series with strong seasonality, extraordinary events or unusual circumstances may cause deviations from the typical pattern.

A common misconception about seasonality is that it is limited to the timescale of meteorological seasons (spring, summer, fall, and winter). In reality, seasonality can occur at *any* timescale. For example, ED arrivals can exhibit seasonality on the scale of hours (Hertzum, 2017; Rostami-Tabar et al., 2023). Arrivals tend to be lowest between midnight and early morning, which are the hours when most people sleep. Then, arrivals increase during the daylight hours from morning until evening before decreasing again. This pattern demonstrates how seasonality can emerge from predictable hourly circadian rhythms, emphasizing the need to consider various timescales when analyzing trends in healthcare data.

Sometimes, visual inspection alone may not reveal seasonality easily. In these cases, autocorrelation analysis may help tease out seasonality from noisy data. Autocorrelation analysis measures how strongly a data point is related to past values in the same time series. If there is seasonality, the autocorrelation function (ACF) will show repeating peaks at regular intervals that correspond to the seasonal cycle. For example, if hospital admissions have a weekly pattern, the ACF plot will show peaks at lags of 7, 14, and 21 days, aligning with the weekly peaks in patient visits. Interested readers are referred to Hyndman and Athanasopoulos (2018) for more details.

LEARNING OBJECTIVE 15.3: BREAK DOWN A TIME SERIES INTO COMPONENTS FOR FORECASTING

While seasonality is a key feature of many time series in healthcare, there are other important components that should be considered when performing analyses and creating forecasts. A statistical

FIGURE 15.2 Time series decomposition.

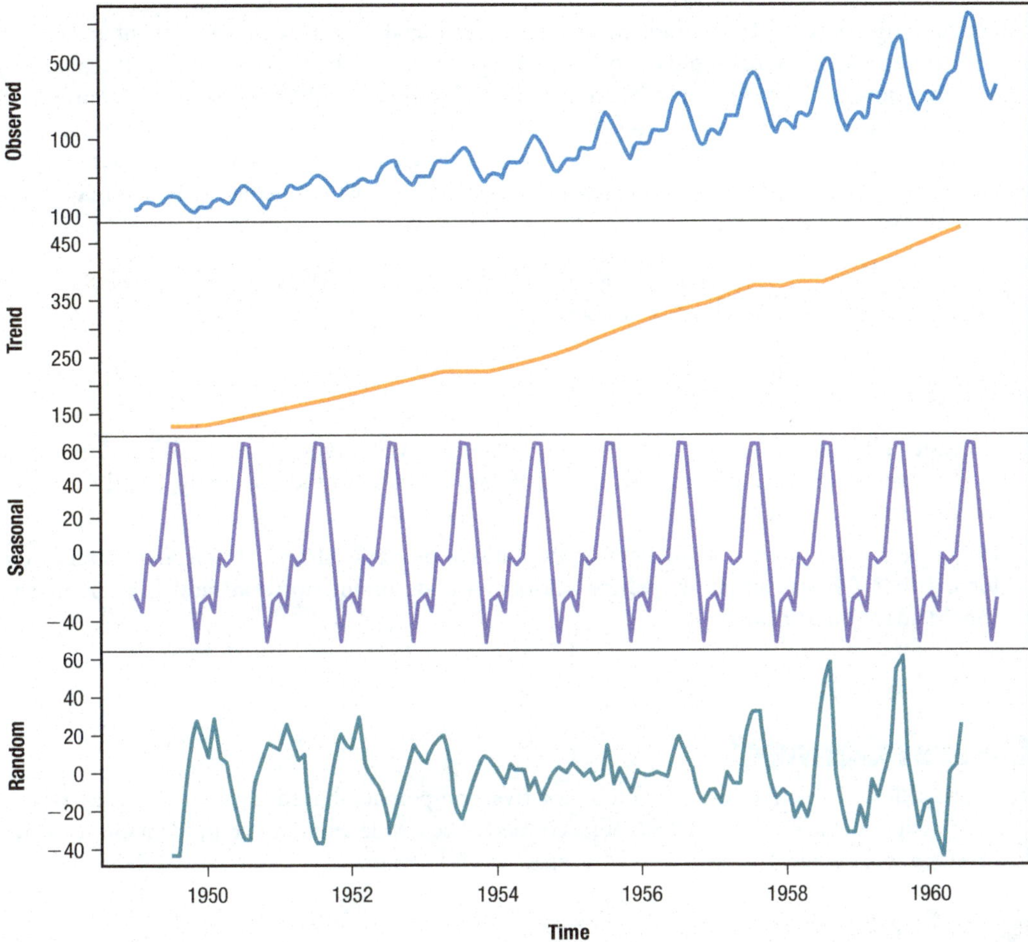

technique known as *time series decomposition* can break down a time series into its components: the overall trend of the time series, its seasonality, and the "random noise." Consider **Figure 15.2**, which is divided into four sections labeled "observed," "trend," "seasonal," and "random." The top section ("observed") displays the original time series.

Examining the observed data, we can see that the numbers generally increase over time. This gradual, long-term shift represents the trend of the time series, shown in the second section of the figure. Unlike seasonality, which involves repeating short-term fluctuations, the trend reflects sustained growth or decline. For example, a hospital in a rapidly growing urban area may observe a steady upward trend in admissions over several years due to population increases. The observed time series in **Figure 15.2** also exhibits peaks at regular intervals, though the height of these peaks changes through time. This repeating pattern represents the seasonality of the data, which is illustrated in the third section of the figure. Seasonal components reflect the predictable, time-dependent variations in the data.

If we remove the trend and the seasonality from the original time series, we are left with the final component: the random noise. Random noise refers to unpredictable variations in the time series data that do not follow a discernable pattern. Noise can result from numerous factors, including random external events. For example, a pandemic or a natural disaster can cause an unexpected spike in hospital admissions that departs significantly from historical trends.

SUMMARY

Understanding these three components—trend, seasonality, and noise—is advantageous for effective forecasting. By distinguishing between systematic patterns and random fluctuations, healthcare managers can develop more accurate predictions to enhance resource planning and operational efficiency. However, these statistical techniques should be used in conjunction with domain knowledge and contextual understanding. Healthcare managers should consider external factors, such as policy changes, disease outbreaks, or shifts in patient behavior, which may influence trends, seasonality, and noise.

END-OF-CHAPTER RESOURCES

DISCUSSION QUESTIONS

1. Consider a healthcare setting in your own community. What types of seasonal patterns might exist in patient visits, staffing needs, or supply usage? How would you analyze and use these patterns to make better decisions?

2. What are some potential challenges or limitations of using historical seasonal patterns for forecasting? Discuss situations where seasonal trends might not hold and how managers should adapt their strategies.

LEARNING ACTIVITIES

CourseConnect ➤

To access self-assessment questions and interactive, competency-based learning activities for this chapter, visit www.springerpub.com/courseconnect. See inside front cover and tear-out card for CourseConnect details.

REFERENCES

Hertzum, M. (2017). Forecasting hourly patient visits in the emergency department to counteract crowding. *The Ergonomics Open Journal, 10,* 1–13. https://doi.org/10.2174/1875934301710010001

Hyndman, R. J., & Athanasopoulos, G. (2018). *Forecasting: Principles and practice* (2nd ed.). OTexts. Retrieved January 24, 2025, from https://otexts.com/fpp2

Lofgren, E., Fefferman, N. H., Naumov, Y. N., Gorski, J., & Naumova, E. N. (2006). Influenza seasonality: Underlying causes and modeling theories. *Journal of Virology, 81*(11), 5429–5436. https://doi.org/10.1128/jvi.01680-06

Rana, V., William, M., Kewalramani, A., Daloya, J., Barnes, M., Chang, T., Miele, A. S., Haggerty, G., & Ng, J. (2023). COVID-19 mask mandates in NY and their effect on the incidence of flu. *Journal of Community Hospital Internal Medicine Perspectives, 13*(1), 1–5. https://doi.org/10.55729/2000-9666.1140

Rostami-Tabar, B., Browell, J., & Svetunkov, I. (2023). Probabilistic forecasting of hourly emergency department arrivals. *Health Systems, 13*(2), 133–149. https://doi.org/10.1080/20476965.2023.2200526

Shukla, D., Gilliland, T., Gurland, B., Patel, S., & Shanafelt, T. (2022). Mitigating the impact of the year end spike in elective surgery on surgeon and staff well-being: A surgical perspective. *Annals of Medicine and Surgery, 75,* 103370. https://doi.org/10.1016/j.amsu.2022.103370

FINANCIAL ANALYSIS

CHAPTER 16

THE TIME VALUE OF MONEY

LEARNING OBJECTIVES

16.1. Understand the concept of the time value of money.

16.2. Compute the future or present value of money (compounding and discounting).

REAL-WORLD SCENARIO

The manager of strategy for Mercy Medical Center in a Midwestern city is presented with an offer of $100,000 to purchase a new piece of laboratory equipment that the medical center has begun developing. The prospective purchaser of this equipment has offered them an option of receiving the $100,000 for the rights to the equipment immediately or in 12 months. The manager is planning to sell the rights anyway, and there is no prospect of generating any revenue from the use of the equipment in the coming 12 months. Should they accept the money now or in 12 months? This is an easy choice: they elect to receive the $100,000 now rather than waiting for 1 year. But what were the reasons behind the manager's decision?

There are at least two factors that influenced this decision. First, we must assume that some level of inflation will occur within the next 12 months. In other words, $100,000 can buy *more today* than in 12 months. With inflation, the value of money degrades over time. Second, there is always an option of investing the $100,000 today or during the next year, an option that may result in greater financial return or gain in 12 months than accepting $100,000 in 12 months. At a minimum, the $100,000 could be used to purchase a certificate of deposit or a government note of minimum risk, where it would earn interest for the period of the investment. In other words, money received today has greater value that money received in the future since it can immediately be used to earn income or interest.

LEARNING OBJECTIVE 16.1: UNDERSTAND THE CONCEPT OF THE TIME VALUE OF MONEY

The previous scenario illustrates one of the fundamental concepts of management: There is a "time" value associated with money. All other things being equal, money that you have today is worth more than the same amount of money received in the future. This concept, known as the *time value of money*, comes from the field of finance. Issues related to the time value of money become more critical as the period of time in question increases. As many accounting issues pertain to issues with relatively short time horizons (e.g., <12 months), managers may not consider the time value of money in analyzing strategic decisions. Over longer periods of time, however (and occasionally shorter as well), the relationship between time and the value of money is a critical management consideration. Given the fact that most investments or project opportunities have "lives" extending over time horizons >12 months, the importance of the time value of money is magnified.

The preceding example is simple; however, most decisions faced by managers are not as straightforward. For example, suppose the manager is offered the same $100,000 now for the equipment rights or $110,000 in 12 months. Should the manager sell the rights now or sign an agreement to sell at the later time? Is it more beneficial financially to have the $100,000 in hand now, or is it more advantageous to wait for a year and receive a larger sum of money? Issues related to the time value of money also become more critical as the period of time in question increases. As many accounting issues pertain to issues with relatively short time horizons (e.g., <12 months), managers may not consider the time value of money in analyzing strategic decisions. Over longer periods of time, however (and occasionally shorter as well), the relationship between time and the value of money is a critical management consideration. Given the fact that most investments or project opportunities have "lives" extending over time horizons >12 months, the importance of the time value of money is magnified. Effective managers take a financial perspective of projects, including considerations of the time value of money, not simply an accounting perspective (such as short-term profit or loss), although both are important.

Responding to opportunities such as this requires the ability to understand and calculate what is known as the *present value* of money received at a later time. This competency enables managers to assess opportunities on an "apples to apples" perspective financially; in other words, it considers the *time value of money*. The overall objective of this chapter is to introduce the key management methods associated with the time value of money. It must be added that although financial factors should never be the only criterion used in making management decisions, particularly in healthcare, it is also true that such factors often take precedence in decision-making.

LEARNING OBJECTIVE 16.2: COMPUTE THE FUTURE OR PRESENT VALUE OF MONEY (COMPOUNDING AND DISCOUNTING)

The fundamental concepts underlying the idea that the value of money changes in relation to time are known as compounding and discounting. *Compounding* refers to the idea that, if money is invested (e.g., put in the bank or used to buy a bond with fixed returns in the future), this amount of money grows or compounds in the future. Compounding refers to the process of going from today's value of money, known as the present value, to some future value of money.

It is useful to think of discounting as the inverse of compounding. *Discounting* is a way of looking at some future amount of money, known as the future value, and calculating its value today (i.e., calculating its present value). The following sections present the ideas of compounding and discounting and give several examples of how to compute future and present value.

Calculating the Future Value of Money: Compounding

An example of money growing over time (compounding) is a savings account at a bank. Individuals choose to deposit money in the bank for a variety of reasons, including the knowledge that money invested in the bank grows because interest is earned on the money. For example, if an initial deposit of $100 is made in a bank that promises to pay 2% interest annually, at the end of 12 months, a total of $102 is available. The original deposit has grown or compounded from $100 to $102. The additional $2 is the interest earned on the deposit. If the money is left in the bank for another year, assuming no change in the interest rate, at the end of year 2, a total of $104.04 is available in the account. The original $100 has grown or compounded by $4.04 as a result of interest earnings on the account. Thus, using conventional terminology, the future value of $100 invested for 2 years at an interest rate of 2% compounded annually is $104.04. The increase in the account in the second year is $2.04, not $2.00, as was earned in year 1. This is because the amount in the account at the end of year 1 (i.e., the amount that is compounded for an additional [second] year) was $102 (the original $100 deposit plus $2 of interest earned to that point in time).

TABLE 16.1   Compounding Timeline

Time period	0	1	2
	2%	2%	
Value	$100	$102	$104
	(Present value)		(Future value)

Thus, during year 2, 2% was earned on $102, not $100. In situations involving compounding or discounting, it may be helpful to create a "picture" or timeline of the investment scenario. A timeline is used to indicate the present and future value of money, the applicable interest rate, and the length of time involved. In fact, always beginning a time value of money analysis with a timeline may be a prerequisite for accurate calculations. Note that this example is based on interest earned annually. In some situations, interest could be earned more frequently, such as semiannually. The frequency of compounding—annually, semiannually, or monthly—will change the future value calculation since interest earned in one period will increase the basis for interest earned in the next period. **Table 16.1** depicts the situation just described. Note that time period "0" refers to the present time (i.e., now), and that the value refers to the size of account at the end of the time period indicated.

The compounding (interest) rate is shown on the timeline for the appropriate time periods. Creating a timeline is a simple yet helpful tool to organize the "facts" of the investment opportunity and to help ensure that managers will have all the information required for decision-making. In general terms, compounding is represented by the following equation. This equation assumes interest being earned annually:

Equation 16.1: Future Value

Future Value = Present Value + Interest Earned (I)

where:

Interest Earned (I) = Present Value × Interest Rate (i)

The master equation for compounding is expressed as:

$$FV_n = PV (1 + i)^n$$

where:
FV = Future value
 n = number of time periods (e.g., years)
PV = Present Value
 i = interest rate (expressed as a decimal (e.g., 2% = .02)

If the present value is $100 and the interest rate is 2%, what is the future value after 5 years?

$$
\begin{aligned}
FV &= 100 (1 + .02)^5 \\
&= 100 (1.02)^5 \\
&= 100 [(1.02)(1.02)(1.02)(1.02)(1.02)] \\
&= 100 (1.1041) \\
&= \$ 110.41
\end{aligned}
$$

Calculating the Present Value of (Future) Money: Discounting

Earlier in the chapter, a manager was presented with an opportunity to receive $100,000 now or $110,000 in 12 months. This is a typical financial management decision. The manager's choice is based on determining the present value of the amount of money to be received in the future, in this case $110,000. That is the same as asking: "How much is that future sum of money worth today?" This is essentially the reverse of the compounding question discussed in the first part of this chapter. This new problem requires solving for the present value using the following formula:

Equation 16.2: Present Value Formula

$$PV = \frac{FV_n}{(1 + i)^n}$$

where:
PV = Present Value
FV = Future value
i = interest rate (AKA discount rate)
n = number of time periods (e.g., years)

Looking at this equation, it should be apparent that, as it stands, there is not enough information to solve the problem—there is no interest/discount rate (i) provided. Therefore, a rate must be assumed. The question is how to determine an appropriate rate. One way to determine such a rate is based on the concept of opportunity cost. A manager typically has multiple options for investing money. For example, several certificates of deposit or bank savings options may be available, each paying a specified rate of return. Suppose the manager is considering two separate savings options. Option A pays 2.5% annually and option B pays 1.75% interest on savings. If the manager selects option B for investment, they are therefore foregoing the return available with option A. The rate of return on the option(s) *not* selected is known as an opportunity cost. So, in this example, selection of option A carries with it an opportunity cost of 2.5%.

Investment opportunities are rarely the same. For example, the manager could decide to take a very financially conservative approach and deposit money in a bank savings account. The financial return from this strategy is likely to be relatively modest, but the level of risk associated with this investment strategy is quite low. Alternatively, the manager might choose to invest available funds in the bonds of a highly speculative new company. Under this scenario, it is likely that the potential financial return will be higher than the bank deposit, but this investment strategy carries substantially more financial risk. Note that in (rational) financial markets, there is a direct relationship between risk and potential reward: as the level of riskiness increases, so does the level of potential reward. The key to selecting an appropriate interest (or discount) rate to use in an analysis is to use the interest rate available on an alternative investment of similar type, level of risk, and time horizon. In other words, the manager should identify an investment opportunity, with a stated interest rate that is similar to the project being considered and use that stated rate to compute the present value. For example, following thorough research, the manager concludes that investments of similar type, risk, and time horizon pay a 3% return annually; this is the discount rate that should be used. Using the stated equation, the present value of the proposed investment is computed to be $106,796. This means that all other things being equal, the manager should be willing to invest no more than $106,796 in this project. If the manager can accept this opportunity at a cost of <$106,796, it will yield a better financial return than the investment alternative; however, if the cost of this opportunity exceeds this amount, then the manager should decline this opportunity and pursue the alternative. The manager—as a prudent investor—should be willing to pay no more than $106,796 for this opportunity. Just as was the case with the compounding formula, a manager can use the discounting formula to calculate crucial variables in addition to the present value. The formula can be used to calculate either the number of time periods required to generate a specified future value given a known present value and interest rate or the discount rate given a known present value and number of periods. For example, if:

$$FV = \$4,000$$
$$n = 6 \text{ years}$$
$$i = 4\%$$

then:

$$PV = \frac{FV_n}{(1+i)^n}$$

$$= \frac{4000}{(1.04)^6}$$

$$= \frac{4000}{(1.217)}$$

$$= \$3,287$$

SUMMARY

Management decisions frequently involve the time value of money. Investments—including fixed costs—are made in anticipation of future revenue. Competencies involving compounding and discounts are essential as they provide a reasoned estimate of the actual value of anticipated current and future expenses and revenues, recognizing that the value of money changes over time. Covered here were some foundational techniques for thinking about the value of money over time. These can now be used to do more advanced analysis such as return on investment and the net present value of investments. These are explored in Chapter 17, "Economic Analysis."

END-OF-CHAPTER RESOURCES

DISCUSSION QUESTIONS

1. What criteria do you suspect organizations use when examining the viability of project investments?
2. How should the future value of investments be used when estimating investments?
3. Is it preferable to have a higher annual interest rate or a lower rate with more compounding periods?

LEARNING ACTIVITIES

CourseConnect ▶

To access self-assessment questions and interactive, competency-based learning activities for this chapter, visit www.springerpub.com/courseconnect. See inside front cover and tear-out card for CourseConnect details.

CHAPTER 17

ECONOMIC ANALYSIS

LEARNING OBJECTIVES

17.1. Describe the interests, issues, and perspectives involved in making value-based management decisions.

17.2. Define economic analysis and differentiate among the types of economic analyses.

17.3. Describe and compare the basic elements of cost-benefit analysis (CBA) and cost-effectiveness analysis (CEA).

17.4. Design and calculate CBA and CEA.

LEARNING OBJECTIVE 17.1: DESCRIBE THE INTERESTS, ISSUES, AND PERSPECTIVES INVOLVED IN MAKING VALUE-BASED MANAGEMENT DECISIONS

Based upon the goals of the organization, a health services manager makes decisions and recommendations regarding what services to provide as well as how they are provided. Changing needs, demands, and wants, along with changing organizational goals and objectives, require the manager to revise existing services, add new services, and eliminate existing services. New technology also redefines the medical care frontier. The health services manager approaches these issues with two potentially conflicting perspectives and one stark realization. The realization is that community and organization resources are scarce, and their use must be prioritized. Value or benefit is expected from every resource used in a service. Competition for resources within an organization is typically intense. Above all, patients and clients expect value. Healthcare organizations and communities also expect value. Financing sources within those organizations continue to stress how resources are used given that doing so precludes using those same resources for other purposes, such as organizational expansions; improvements and upgrades; equipment; or in the case of public funders, economic development, transportation, education, defense, and a host of other potential uses.

Being scarce, resources need to be allocated to meet prioritized goals and objectives. Personnel budgets, organizational budgets, and governmental budgets reflect how resources are allocated between and among competing needs, demands, and wants. Markets also allocate resources based upon the interplay of supply and demand. The need to allocate resources is a given; the question becomes, on what basis will resources be allocated? The health services manager, as an employee of a healthcare organization, understands the potentially competing perspectives of the "community" and the "organization." Any manager also functions in a setting surrounded by "opportunity costs." Resources devoted to address one need are not available to address other needs. Choices must be made that best support the organization's mission and goals and contribute to the ability of an organization to survive and prosper.

Based on this perspective, any decision or recommendation involving the use of (scarce) resources must be evaluated based upon its impact on its intended beneficiaries as well as the organization and the communities served by the organization. Organizational financial performance, as reflected by profits and losses, is an especially important criterion used to evaluate management decisions involving the use of available resources. From a community perspective, however, the health services manager is also challenged to use organizational resources to improve the health status of the community served by the healthcare organization. This may be reflected in the organization's definition of "population" or population health, by the incentives for quality and health improvement it faces, or both.

Thus, the health status of the community is a dominant criterion used to evaluate the management of any healthcare organization. Although these criteria can be compatible, they can also be mutually exclusive. Organizational benefit and community benefit can range from being aligned to being opposed or nuanced somewhere in between. Each is a dominant, real, and an important perspective that every health services manager must feel and consider whenever making a decision or recommendation involving new or revised projects.

This chapter is designed to assist the health services managers formulate project recommendations based on the systematic assessment of their cost, benefit or outcome, and effectiveness. This does not imply that the manager should ignore organizational profit. It merely implies that the health services manager must examine both the organizational and community benefit associated with any project recommendation. Projects represent an investment in the community. As such, the health services manager is retained to exercise reasoned judgment and make decisions that are expected to benefit their organization and the communities served by their organization. Reasoned judgment requires that the health services manager must be able to assess and evaluate project alternatives from many and often conflicting perspectives that include the value of community benefit as well as the organization's associated costs and benefits. Sometimes, however, considerations other than economic benefits will be the dominant influence on the health services manager (i.e., a larger public benefit or a political perspective based upon stakeholder interests). Given this, the health services manager must be able to assess the costs and outcomes associated with the use of resources. Assessment must be systematic and expands the ability of the health services manager to consider the multiple implications associated with any project recommendations.

LEARNING OBJECTIVES 17.2: DEFINE ECONOMIC ANALYSIS AND DIFFERENTIATE AMONG THE TYPES OF ECONOMIC ANALYSES

There are many ways to assess potential projects. For example, management decisions and recommendations can be made on the basis of anticipated "costs" compared with anticipated "benefits or outcomes" associated with the project. To evaluate project alternatives, analyses can assess the costs and benefits associated with each option or alternative, including the alternative of doing nothing. Analysis can then be used to prioritize proposed project options based on the relationship of their anticipated benefits and costs over other project alternatives. This concept is critical in managerial decision-making in the healthcare field because it incorporates into the analysis the impact the project alternatives should have upon the clientele served by the healthcare organization. As stated, healthcare organizations strive to improve the health status of the populations they serve. This commitment is typically expressed in the mission statement of the organization. This commitment also has boundaries. For example, "their" community's health status can be defined as a group of individuals with common attributes such as socioeconomic, demographic, behavioral, geographic, disease status, or many other measures. It may also be encapsulated by the organization's definition of population health (e.g., "their" served population), not always a geographic one.

Most recently, organizations and systems have focused on "value-based" care and employ a number of techniques to measure that care. These metrics are important to utilize when providers are incentivized to deliver high-quality care while managing costs effectively. Some examples are as follows:

- **Patient-centered metrics:** Cost per patient discharge, cost per preventable hospital readmissions, and patient satisfaction scores related to cost
- **Clinical process metrics:** Cost per specific procedure, cost of medication adherence, and cost of managing chronic conditions
- **Outcome-based metrics:** Cost per quality-adjusted life year (QALY) and cost per successful treatment outcome

Individual and collective health status is influenced by prevention programs and medical treatments available to the community, as well as by factors involving behavior, genetics, and the environment. For example, an immunization program typically decreases the number of infectious disease cases, thereby increasing health status. An anticholesterol drug that lowers blood cholesterol associated with cardiovascular disease typically decreases the number of heart attacks in a community of "users" compared with "nonusers," thereby increasing individual and community health status. A neonatal intensive care unit in the community hospital should enhance the likelihood of survival for low-birth-weight babies. All these programs use "scarce" healthcare resources.

As health status in a community improves due to the prevention of adverse health outcomes (i.e., a heart attack), or the effectiveness of outreach and prevention services, fewer healthcare resources should have to be used in the community for treatment of the same health outcomes. When health status decreases, it is likely that additional healthcare resources will be expended on preventing or treating avoidable adverse health events. The major question in healthcare economic analysis is how do increased expenditures on projects to improve health status compare with the decreased expenditures on healthcare resources resulting from "averted" health related events (HRE)? Another question is where do these costs accrue and do the associated benefits also accrue to the same entities in equal measure? This question is particularly relevant today. For example, it is a fundamental question used in decisions regarding health insurance coverage, especially in managed care or quality incentivized insurance plans. It is also a basic question used to evaluate the actions and community benefit of healthcare organizations. It is also a classical question from the field of public health: Would society be better served by preventing or adverting a disease or treating a disease? Given this perspective and questions, the management decision regarding the initiation of a new project or service or the evaluation of existing services must include three parts:

1. What is the cost (per unit) of a particular service or intervention?
2. What are the benefits (aka payoffs; per unit) of this service or intervention?
3. What proportion of individuals receiving this service or intervention will actually benefit?

There are three evaluation techniques for projects aka interventions: cost-benefit analysis (CBA), cost-effectiveness analysis (CEA), and cost-utility analysis (CUA). This chapter focuses on cost benefit and CEA. CBA evaluates all project inputs (i.e., costs) and outcomes (i.e., benefits) of a service in monetary terms. This means that not only are service costs calculated but that all benefits are also calculated in terms of their monetary value, including the cost of a life saved or extended. As such, estimating benefits injects a level of subjectivity into CBA. In many instances, there is no uniform consensus on the monetary value of saving a life or extending a human life. Typically, multiple methods are used. For example, the benefit of a life saved can be calculated as the present value of the individual's future income stream. This approach, however, values the lives of a young productive population and discounts the value of those either retired from productive labor or unable to be productive. While this is a limitation, it need not be a fatal flaw. CBA and CEA have similar goals and are often referred to interchangeably. Despite what these two techniques have in common, they are indeed two distinct techniques that ask different questions and have different approaches to evaluating projects and programs.

- **CEA**: Focus on a given (e.g., health status or medical) outcome and how much spending is needed to bring about that specific outcome and/or to determine which project option is "most effective." Overall, both approaches are significant analytical tools for the manager. Despite what these two techniques have in common, they are two distinct techniques that ask different questions and have different approaches to evaluating the efficiency of a program. As stated, CBA and CEA are centered on two different questions. CBA asks whether the economic benefits outweigh the economic costs of a given policy, project, or intervention.
- **CEA**: Focus on the question of how much it costs to get a certain amount or level of output from a specific program or intervention.
- **CUA**: Also compares projects' costs and benefits. Benefits, however, are expressed in terms of consumer preferences.

LEARNING OBJECTIVE 17.3: DESCRIBE AND COMPARE THE BASIC ELEMENTS OF COST-BENEFIT ANALYSIS AND COST-EFFECTIVENESS ANALYSIS

In CEA, project and service costs are calculated in monetary terms. Benefits, however, are calculated in their *natural units*, such as the number of cases of heart disease or cancer averted. CEA compares alternative interventions (i.e., project A vs. project B) whose outcomes (benefits) are measured in *identical units*.

To use CEA, a manager must be able to determine the cost of the intervention or project. In certain situations, the cost of adverse health-related events (i.e., HREs) *averted* or other benefits and the estimated proportion of current HREs averted by the intervention or project also must be determined. Every project needs resources to be implemented and maintained. As such, relevant costs include labor costs associated with services rendered and the cost of facilities and utilities, equipment and supplies, and administrative support. Direct and indirect costs specifically related to the project or intervention also must be estimated and included.

Intervention/Project Side Effects

All interventions have an effect, or one would not implement them. Some interventions, however, have adverse side effects as well as beneficial results. As for all interventions, the benefits must exceed the risks for the intervention to be implemented ethically. Costs associated with these risks must also be included. Thus, the extremely small risk of severe vaccine reactions must be included in the analysis of a mass vaccination program. Diagnostic procedures to rule out false positives in a screening intervention also must be included in a CEA.

Costs of Health-Related Events Averted

A prevention program is undertaken to avert an adverse HRE. For every adverse HRE averted, the direct costs associated with the averted event are not included. When enough HREs are averted, the cost savings may exceed the prevention intervention's cost.

Personal Costs of a Health-Related Event Averted

Personal costs are the economic impacts associated with an adverse HRE. Examples include earnings (productivity) losses to society as a whole because of the premature morbidity and mortality of persons who become ill with an adverse HRE. Thus, if one can avert adverse health outcomes, one avoids premature morbidity and mortality. Two methods of costing this morbidity and mortality are the *human capital* and the *willingness-to-pay* approaches. The human capital approach values personal loss as the income not earned by the individual who experienced the HRE. The willingness-to-pay approach values this loss as what someone might spend to avert this particular event, for example, how much an individual was willing to pay to install automobile seat belts or air bags in a car to avert death or injury.

Determining Resource Costs

Resources are those project inputs to the prevention intervention; without them, the intervention would not exist. To determine the resource costs, the following steps should be followed:

1. Choose a time period for the intervention analysis.
2. Choose the service unit of the intervention.
3. List the resources required for all activities comprising the intervention.
4. Measure or count the units of each resource used in the time period.
5. Determine the cost per unit of each resource.
6. Multiply the cost/unit by the number of units (this will equal the total cost of each resource).
7. Determine the cost of any resources not measured per unit of service.
8. Add up all total resource costs to determine the total cost for the intervention—for a specific period and based upon an anticipated level of service.
9. Divide the total cost by the number of service units to determine the *expected* cost per service unit.

Following these steps will yield an estimate of the cost per unit of service and the total cost of the project. The time period for any cost analysis, however, is important. It is recommended that at least 1 year of resource data be used to determine and/or estimate current and future costs.

The choice of the appropriate service unit(s), such as patient days or discharges, in advance of data collection, also is critical because it may drive the way in which data are collected. The cost-effectiveness (CE) calculation is predicated upon a denominator of effectiveness; thus, the unit of this denominator must be chosen in advance. The list of resources to be collected may include the following:

- Direct provider time for each type of service or activity, by provider type, and their salary and fringe benefit expenses
- The supplies and materials for each type of service provided and their costs
- The type of laboratory or other tests for each service provided and their costs
- Lab controls and so forth
- Additional facilities, including rent and utilities required for this intervention
- Additional equipment
- Maintenance of facilities and equipment
- Additional staff
- Other direct costs of providing services, such as courier services, cars and vans, uniforms or badges, additional insurance or permits, travel reimbursement, and computer database development/maintenance

Not all interventions will include all these items. A table of unit costs, however, can be constructed based upon this list. Information on the participants may also need to be collected. Participation in prevention activities may be influenced by the time it takes and the extra expenses it entails. This is a form of personal or indirect costs—costs not associated with direct use of medical or health resources but rather with participation. Participant costs include participant time (e.g., travel, wait, and actual service) and participant expenses (e.g., for travel, childcare). These costs can be determined by a survey of the participants as they enter the facility and by collecting time information about arrival and service time.

Measuring Resources Consumed and Provider Time and Costs

There are numerous methods of estimating provider time including direct observation of services, random observations of activities, time records, patient records, and provider surveys. Because of the variable nature of service times, many observations may have to be collected. Regardless of the technique chosen, a histogram of service times should be produced. If service times are clustered and look symmetric, a sample of 30 may be sufficient as a basis for estimating mean service time. However, if the times are highly variable and asymmetric, a larger sample (e.g., $n = 100$) may be needed. The Poisson distribution has a mean equal to the standard deviation. This is the most conservative case and yields a sample size calculation of $n = 96$ for a 95% confidence level.

Direct Observation

Direct observation of services requires a trained observer who can determine what type of service is happening at a particular time. Data would be collected on each type of service included in the intervention. For example, in breast cancer screening, the time for counseling, the mammogram, the radiologist's interpretation, and the clinical breast examination would be collected. Some of these data may be available or estimated using existing data systems, for example, measuring time stamps at check in; at check out; and, if available, during the visit. Often, however, only time in and time out are available. In this case, the analyst would need to collect data on time to service, wait times, and the like.

Random Observation

Random observation is a technique based upon the proposition that the proportion of time spent on an activity is equal to the proportion of observations made of that particular activity during the workday. To do this, each provider is assigned a code number. Before the beginning of the observation period, a schedule of observations is drawn up. A random number table is used to determine which provider is to be observed every t minutes. Time interval t is based on how far apart these providers are—that is, how long it will take to go from one to another. When a particular provider's code number comes up on the schedule, the observer goes to find them and notes what the provider is doing at that instant. This technique typically requires at least 100 observations of each type of service to obtain a confident estimate of the proportion of time spent on each activity. To determine the time for each activity, the frequency of each activity is noted. Each activity frequency is a proportion of the total observations taken during the workday. Thus, that proportion equals the proportion of time spent in that activity during the workday.

Time Diaries

Diaries are a provider-based technique. Each provider is given a sheet to fill out during their workday that requires the notation of the time used for specific activities. Because this is an intrusive method for the provider, it is important to study the types of activities the provider is usually engaged in and to construct a checklist on the form for the provider. Personal time should always be a choice to be checked. If the time diary option is used, the providers need to be assured of the confidentiality of the diaries. The diaries should be collected in sealed envelopes and analyzed offsite. Note that time diaries are often not feasible given the busy and often variable nature of providing care and the demands on provider's time. In these cases, it may be more feasible to use a secondary observer/recorder to estimate times.

The Patient *Record* Method

This requires that each patient be tracked through the intervention. The exact time the patient enters a new service and leaves an old service must be noted. This type of following can yield information about patient flow and patient waiting time. Each patient carries a form upon which each provider can note the time the patient begins and ends the service by that provider. Many current and operational data systems have the ability to track a number of variables that can extend to previsit registration all the way through follow-up appointments. It is important that a list of potential and available data points be assessed. For more on this, refer to Chapter 2, "Data, Data Sources, Data Quality, and Foundations."

A Survey of Providers

Surveys can be the least accurate data collection method. Individuals do not remember how long they spent on activities throughout a day, especially in retrospect. Contemporaneous collection—that is, collection of data each day— may work, but asking a provider how much time they spent immunizing a child during a routine visit will not elicit an accurate response. In addition, many providers dislike additional time requests for administrative functions, so data completeness is often an issue when evaluating responses.

Challenges to Accurate Measurement

As discussed in Chapter 2, "Data, Data Sources, Data Quality, and Foundations," analysis is only as accurate as the data that informs it. Beyond measuring provider time, there are a number of considerations that could impact a CBA or CEA. Some are as follows:

- **Data complexity:** Gathering accurate and comprehensive data on costs and quality measures across different healthcare settings can be complex. Specificity about what is needed and who/what that includes over what time period needs to be transparent and available.

- **Variation in pricing:** Different healthcare providers may have different costs for the same service, making comparisons difficult. Doing so should be noted, or some type of parity or weighting adjustment should be used.

- **Attribution issues:** Assigning costs to specific quality outcomes can be challenging, especially when multiple factors contribute to patient results. For example, it is hard to know what actually led to a readmission if there is no direct knowledge of other factors (e.g., behavior, home environment, and other withheld conditions). In these cases, providing some sensitivity estimates or confidence intervals for measure could be useful.

LEARNING OBJECTIVE 17.4: DESIGN AND CALCULATE COST-BENEFIT ANALYSISEFFECTIVENESS ANALYSIS AND COST-EFFECTIVENESS ANALYSIS

Scenario: An international health agency needs to determine the most cost-effective means to attract pregnant women to seek and avail themselves to prenatal care services. Existing and new methods need to be evaluated.

Cost-Effectiveness Analysis

CEA compares the cost of achieving a specific project outcome using different recruitment options. It begins with the identification of a specific question which focuses on the selected outcome. If you are comparing two or more outcomes, each outcome needs to be identified. The second step involves measuring the outcome. For example, given our cited scenario, the selected outcome is "attendance." In prenatal programs, this outcome can be measured using attendance or patient records. A CEA is being performed to assess the CE of current and new methods to publicize the availability of prenatal services to pregnant women based on the premise that increased awareness of the rationale and availability of prenatal care will lead to increased attendance. As stated, the measurable outcome is attendance and participation in formal prenatal care programs and services.

Table 17.1 shows that 300 pregnant women were identified and randomly grouped into three groups of 100 each. All women were provided a traditional medical referral for prenatal care once their pregnancy had been confirmed in the clinic. This has been standard practice. In Group A, no other approach was used to inform the women of the availability of prenatal services. In other words, this group did not experience any *new* intervention to seek prenatal services. For Group B, each woman also received a one-on-one outreach home visit from staff and was informed of the availability and benefits of prenatal care. Group C received the same information as Group B using an email or text message. The question is which contact strategy—home visit or text messaging—is the most cost-effective motivation to seek prenatal care?

TABLE 17.1 CE Program Participation Interventions

INTERVENTION:	GROUP A: NO NEW INTERVENTION	GROUP B: INDIVIDUAL HOME VISIT	GROUP C: TEXT MESSAGE
Number of participants	100	100	100
Number attending prenatal care	23	44	30
Increased number of participants	NA	21	7
Additional costs:			
Personnel	$0	$2,000	$140
Travel expenses	$	$400	$0
Equipment and supplies	$0	$100	$500
Administration	$0	$400	$100
Total cost	$0	$2,900	$740
CE ratio	NA	$138.10	$105.71

CE, cost-effectiveness.

Study Results

The data in **Table 17.1** indicates that without any new intervention, 23 of the 100 women in Group A participated in prenatal services. As such, we can conclude that if we do nothing new, approximately 23 out of every 100 women will continue to participate in prenatal service. Given this finding and our goal to determine the CE of two new recruitment approaches, we need to focus the analysis on the "extra participants" attracted to participate using the two potential new recruitment options reflected in Groups B and C. Note that "individual home visits" attracted a total of 44 participants, indicating that this approach (Group B) attracted 21 more women than current practices (Group A). Data in **Table 17.1** also indicate that the "individual home visit" intervention cost for 100 women was $2,900. Similarly, the "text message option" (Group C) had an additional cost of $740 and attracted 7 more participants than those reached by existing practices (Group A).

The CE ratio is calculated by dividing the project/intervention cost for Groups B and C by the measure of effectiveness. In this case—given the intent of the study—the measure of effectiveness is the number of additional women associated with Groups B and C.

$$\textbf{Cost-Effectiveness} = \frac{\textbf{Cost}}{\textbf{Measure of Effectiveness}}$$

$$\text{Cost-Effectiveness Individual Home Visit} = \frac{\$2,900}{21}$$

$$= \textbf{\$138.10 per prenatal program attendence}$$

$$\text{Cost-Effectiveness of Text Messaging} = \frac{\$740}{7}$$

$$= \textbf{105.71 per prenatal program attendence}$$

From this study, we can conclude that the option to use text messaging to inform pregnant women of the availability and benefit of prenatal service is—in this context—the more cost-effective option. The finding indicates that text messaging costs $105.71 per additional participant, whereas individual home visits cost $138.10 per additional participant. The text messaging option to enhance attendance was the most "cost-effective" project option.

Cost-Benefit Analysis

Scenario: The Metropolitan County School District owns and operates 850 schools (K–12) that currently serve 423,886 students. It is totally supported by state and local taxes. The district is organized into 34 administrative units. Each unit within the district operates multiple elementary schools and at least two high schools. All schools provide school health services using full-time RNs. The district employs 1,045 school nurses and 12,055 teachers. State legislation requires each school district to annually select and assess one nonteaching district activity that could be potentially eliminated in order to expand funding for direct instruction and/or reduce additional taxes. This year, the focus of evaluation is school health services provided by an RN.

Table 17.2 indicates the costs associated with providing (WITH) and not providing (WITHOUT) the district-wide school health programs (SHP) using RNs. If the SHP is canceled, however, ill or injured students cannot just be ignored. As such, residual responsibility for attending to students' illnesses or injuries shifts to teachers and parents. Program cancelation leads to the elimination of specific direct costs but also increases other external costs. These other costs include the costs that would be borne by parents due to a school dismissing a student early due to illness or injury. This estimate includes a parent's potential lost wages and travel expenses to and from the school to retrieve the ill or injured child and the expense of providing a student needing medications or care during school hours.

Other program cancellation costs also include the estimated cost of time teachers would devote to addressing the needs of ill or injured students. Note that when a teacher is caring for an ill or

TABLE 17.2   Cost Analysis District School Nursing Program

SCHOOL NURSING PROGRAM COSTS	WITH PROGRAM	WITHOUT PROGRAM
Annual (direct) program costs:		
Salaries and benefits	73,678,332	0
Equipment and supplies	2,858,335	0
Program costs subtotal	76,536,667	0
Other costs		
Parent productivity loss costs:		
Due to early dismissal of students	16,398,550	30,783,267
Due to giving medication at school	0	9,453,112
Teacher productivity loss costs:		
Due to dealing with student illness or injury	32,875,995	157,493,965
Medical costs if performed by other medical providers	0	16,343,994
Other costs: subtotal	49,274,545	214,074,338
Total costs	**125,811,212**	**214,074,338**

TABLE 17.3 Averted Cost Tabulation

SHP COSTS	COST WITH PROGRAM	COST WITHOUT PROGRAM	AVERTED COST	
SHP direct costs	76,536,667	0	76,536,667	
Parent productivity loss:				
Due to early dismissal	16,398,550	30,783,267	14,384,717	
Due to giving medication in school	0	9,453,112	9,453,112	
Teacher productivity loss:				
Due to student illness or injury	32,875,995	157,493,965	124,617,970	
Medical costs by other providers	0	16,343,994	16,343,994	
Total	**125,811,212**	**214,074,338**	**164,799,793**	
	Cost		Benefit	B/C ratio
Benefit-cost ratio	125,811,212		164,799,793	1.31

SHP, school health program.

injured student, the teacher is not teaching. Parental, teacher, and additional medical care costs were estimated based on local data, interviews, and national statistics.

The Cost-Benefit Ratio

As listed on **Table 17.2**, the total costs SHPs offered by RN is estimated at $125,811,212. If these programs were eliminated, certain additional responsibilities would be shifted to teachers, parents, and off-site medical professionals. This cost is estimated as $214,074,338. The estimated cost of having these programs ($125,811,212) and not having them ($214,074,338) results in the estimated cost benefit of having the program at $88,263,126. Note that the SHP offered by the RN has costs that would need to be borne by parents, teachers, and other medical providers. In this situation, these "averted costs" are the monetary benefit associated with retaining the SHP offered by the RN.

The averted cost tabulation indicates the total value of the averted costs associated with elimination of the SHP provided by an RN (**Table 17.3**). The formula for the Benefit-Cost ratio is $\frac{\text{Total Benefits}}{\text{Total Cost}}$. Any value >1.00 indicates that estimated benefits exceed estimated costs. The higher the value, the better. Given the actual formula, some refer to CBA as benefit-cost analysis.

SUMMARY

This chapter presents two management tools: CEA and CBA. Each provides an approach to define and assess decisions related to the prudent utilization of resources. Each also has its strengths and limitations. As tools, knowing when and how to use them is implied throughout this chapter. Also, neither is presented as a receipt—a detailed and exact workplan that must be followed to achieve a specific result. Instead, both of these tools are frameworks that need to be fitted to the question or issue being considered. Both tools require an estimate of costs—both direct and indirect. The rationale for including specific indirect costs and their monetary value must be consistent and explicit. The rationale provided for the methodology is as important as the calculated values derived using either of these tools.

Benefits also must be expressed in monetary terms. This presents challenges. For example, the benefit of a longer life due to a specific intervention must be monetarized when there is no consensus as to the monetary value of additional years of life as well as the value differences when the patient 91 years of instead of 21 years of years of age. As shown in our example, "benefits" also can be costs that have been averted—either avoided, eliminated, or minimized—as a result of a specific project or intervention.

CEA and CBA each have an explicit purpose. Consistency and transparency of methods and measures is important when conducting these given the limitations presented earlier. Novice analysts may want to consider CEA and CBA examples readily available either in published works or electronically for reference before starting out anew. These are but two examples of conducting value-based quality and outcomes assessment.

When presenting results, such as specific benefit/cost ratios, you address the question or issue being considered explicitly, define your measures openly and fully, and explain your analysis within the context of the patient or population being addressed. You should also explicitly explain all assumptions used and discuss the findings and recommendations with as much transparency and clarity as possible.

END-OF-CHAPTER RESOURCES

DISCUSSION QUESTIONS

1. Consider the variety and types of reimbursement health organizations receive. How do each of them influence what types of services are offered to both patients and in the community?

2. Assume your organization wished to improve the outcomes for patients with type 2 diabetes with a new program and then assess the benefit and effectiveness of that program. Typical diabetes outcome measures include hemoglobin (H1C), body mass index (BMI), the number of related prescriptions taken, diet and exercise, and other health behaviors.

   a. What types of interventions would you recommend? Would these be administered in the facility or in the community?

   b. Would these require existing staff and resources or new ones?

   c. List some challenges you could foresee in collecting the information required to conduct a CBA or CEA.

LEARNING ACTIVITIES

CourseConnect ▸

To access self-assessment questions and interactive, competency-based learning activities for this chapter, visit www.springerpub.com/courseconnect. See inside front cover and tear-out card for CourseConnect details.

PROJECTS AND STRATEGY

PROJECT MANAGEMENT

REAL-WORLD SCENARIO

As a new manager in the planning division of a behavioral health start up, you have been tasked with the migration of some of its current in-person treatment options to telehealth. You are charged with determining the scope of this undertaking as well as the timeframe it will take to be able to coordinate with patients, providers, and the marketing department for effective communication of the change and the new services. This requires that you have tools to effectively understand what is currently done within those service lines and types, what will change, and what new capabilities will be required. You also need to ensure you meet all regulatory standards for telehealth and telehealth billing.

LEARNING OBJECTIVE 18.1: DESCRIBE THE ATTRIBUTES, ISSUES, AND TOOLS ASSOCIATED WITH PROJECT MANAGEMENT

A project is an activity done once. The scale and complexity of a project influences the selection of specific management tools. For example, constructing and opening a new nursing home or modernizing and expanding an existing hospital is an example of a large, complex project perhaps best supported by using the program evaluation and review technique (PERT). Installing a new labor and delivery room in a hospital, however, may be supported by using Gantt charts to schedule needed activities. Both management tools provide a schedule of project activities.

Projects also have specific objectives that, when achieved, indicate that the project has been completed. Typically, the time between when a project is begun and completed reflects the complexity of a specific project. Project time is typically expressed in days, weeks, or months. Any project also has a formal beginning (i.e., start) and an ending (i.e., finish). Also, *project* and *program* are terms that are both antonyms and related cousins. Unlike a project, a program is a repeated activity. Developing and installing the resources for mothers to birth in the same hospital room that they will use for the duration of their maternity stay is a project. Using this new capability over and over again for many mothers is a program. In other words, projects create, and programs provide services and opportunities.

Defining Characteristics of Projects

A project seeks to achieve a desired performance capability such as "an ability to evaluate and treat on an expanded number or type of patients in an outpatient clinic." As such, every project has a defined performance goal. It also has an estimated time to completion and financial cost. Project performance, time, and the cost are all related. For example, if the time required for project completion is compressed by hiring additional staff to complete the project, project costs (defined as compression costs) will increase. Also, doing certain project activities concurrently instead of sequentially can shorten the estimated time to project completion. This approach, however, potentially increases the risk of unanticipated delays and performance objectives. Modifying one project parameter (time, cost, or performance goals) typically changes one or both of the other attributes. This three-way relationship, however, also provides unique opportunities to manage projects as they are both being designed and implemented. It also provides the project manager with the opportunity to manage and adjust project plans and schedules to meet changing priorities and circumstances.

In project management terms, *crash time* is the absolute minimum time between when a project is begun and when the project can be completed. Costs associated with a crash time schedule can involve compensating staff for overtime, hiring additional staff, purchasing new equipment, the increased use of subcontractors, and increased fixed costs.

Project Phases

All projects evolve, whether they require hours or days, months, or years to complete. The first project phase is the concept phase. During this phase, different options to achieve the intended performance goals are considered and evaluated. For example, could an off-campus urgent care center reduce demand on the local hospital's emergency department? Could additional staff alone alleviate any need for additional treatment rooms? Should the emergency department establish a fixed number of dedicated treatment rooms only for nonemergency care? During this initial project phase, broadly defined project options (called concepts) are identified. Management selects one or more of these conceptual options that are then taken to the next phase of project management. Some projects spend hours in this initial phase, whereas others spend months or years studying different concepts to achieve the desired performance objectives. Formal research and consultants are often used. This phase ends when the organization selects one or a few conceptual options that potentially could meet project expectations.

During the second, or definition phase, managers define and refine the project "concept(s)" previously identified. "Definition" includes developing detailed project workplans, specifications, schedules, and estimated development and operational costs. Typically, a formal business plan or a similar type of formal report is also developed. Detailed plans defined during the definition project phase are reviewed and approved by senior management and other stakeholders. At this point in the evolution of a project, the project also may seek regulatory approvals, such as approval granted in the form of a certificate of need issued by state government or zoning approvals provided by local government. Based on the information developed during this definition phase, organizational approval is sought to implement the project, which begins the next phase, the project implementation phase. Formal approval typically requires a detailed description of the project as well as its anticipated total cost and the anticipated time required to complete the project once it has been approved for implementation.

For example, the local hospital, after considering numerous options, decided that it would increase the number of the emergency department beds/treatment rooms from 9 to 15 and add the needed additional staff. The implementation phase of project development implements the project plans developed during the definition phase. In other words, resources and capabilities are installed in the organization in accordance with the approved project plans developed during the definition phase. During this implementation phase, the actual project can involve new construction, buying new equipment, hiring and training staff, revising job descriptions, establishing policies and procedures, and any other activities needed to implement the desired capability. During all phases of project development, from concept to implementation, project managers face specific challenges.

LEARNING OBJECTIVE 18.2: APPLY SPECIFIC PROJECT MANAGEMENT TOOLS

Project Planning and Management Tools

Total System Performance Responsibility

Projects alter the existing capabilities of an organization. To effectively and efficiently meet expectations, managers must identify and install the "total package" of capabilities necessary to operationalize the specific project. For example, installing a new computer system that exceeds the capability of existing electrical circuits violates total system performance responsibility (TSPR). Installing the equipment to do laser surgery without training the operating room staff to use or service the equipment violates TSPR. Expanding the emergency department's service capabilities also may necessitate expanding parking and other organizational capabilities.

Consider an example: A hospital has decided to add smart room technology to some of its patient stay rooms. The technology is provided, on contract, for in-room screens that have tabs for things like patient name and information, care, meals, and entertainment. Patients can interact with the technology via remote and it integrates with intake and other data for both patients and providers. The technology is provided through a contract with a private company that will install, troubleshoot, maintain, and train staff on the equipment. The manager is responsible for identifying the steps involved and ensuring the items in the contract are met and maintained. Failing to do so would impede both patient and provider satisfaction with the devices but could also create additional manual care steps such as vital signs monitoring or meal delivery.

Having TSPR means defining the project to include all the capabilities needed to fully operationalize the project. This often entails the effective integration of the project into existing workflows and capacities of the organization. What may appear as a minor or trivial detail can be a major flaw in project performance with significant impacts on successful completion. And even though some services may have third parties or vendors contractually responsible, it is imperative in care environments that all functions operate smoothly.

Work Breakdown Structure

The foundation for the efficient and effective management of projects is the work breakdown structure (WBS). It is a hierarchical listing of all required work activities. It categorizes and defines the *activities* that need to be completed to achieve the project's intended outcomes. Using the previous example involving the local hospital's goal to increase the service capacity of its emergency department, the following is an example of a high-level WBS for this project. It begins with a categorized listing of project activities such as this simplified example:

1.0	Regulatory Approvals
2.0	Physical Plant Expansion and Construction
3.0	Equipment
4.0	Staffing

Note that *activities* require time to be completed. In contrast, an *event* is a moment in time. For example, the start, stop, or finish of a project are events, not activities. *Preparing a report* is an activity, given it requires time as well as other resources. All project activities also have *predecessor* and *successor* activities. A *predecessor* activity is one or more activities that must be completed immediately before another activity can be begun. As such, a *successor* is one or more activities that can only start after one or more specific predecessor activities have been completed.

For the WBS, each "first-level" macro category of activities is then divided into more detailed required activities. For example, 2.0 Physical Plant Expansion and Construction could be divided into:

2.1	Develop architectural plans
2.2	Identify qualified construction contractors
2.3	Develop request for proposals (RFPs) with time and cost estimates

2.4   Distribute RFP to qualified contractors

2.5   Host interested contractors to tour current facility and answer their specific questions

2.6   Evaluate all contractor plans and proposals

2.7   Select a specific contractor

2.8   Secure all needed regulatory approvals

2.9   Construct and modify physical plant

Based on this listing of project activities, activity 2.4, *Distribute RFP to qualified contractors,* has as a predecessor activity, *Identify qualified construction contractors (2.2)*. Again, each of these second-level project activities can then be divided into third-level activities.

For example, 2.1 Develop architectural plan could be divided into:

2.1.1   Identify qualified architects to develop plans with cost and time estimates

2.1.2   Select project architect and sign contract

2.1.3   Architect develops formal construction plan

This process of defining the work activities needed to complete the project continues until the project team has sufficient detail in the WBS so that it can plan, monitor, and adjust resources as needed as the project develops from plans to reality. For example, activity 2.1.2, *Select project architect and sign contract*, could be divided into:

2.1.2.1   Develop criteria to evaluate all proposals

2.1.2.2   Review all proposal and contracts

2.1.2.3   CEO review of architect recommendation

Note that the sequential numbering system used in a WBS also divides the project into appropriate and logical categories of required project activities. As illustrated, a WBS is a categorized and hierarchical listing of the activities that need to be accomplished in order to meet project objectives. The level of detail in a WBS also reflects the complexity, duration, and/or cost of the project. The level of project complexity also influences the selection and use of specific project management techniques and tools.

An important note here is that defining all the steps necessary for a WBS does not typically rest with one person. Many of these steps might be provided by a contractor or outside vendor by way of a project plan. What is important for the manager is to understand how these plans, activities, and events intersect and interact with existing functions. This also often requires talking to those individuals and departments involved.

Key performance indicators (KPIs) can also be used to manage and monitor project development and are significant derivatives of the WBS. Specific events associated with the completion of activities can be identified as a KPI. For example, in the WBS example, step 2.7, *Select a specific contractor,* is an activity that, when completed, implies a formal event (e.g., a contactor is selected) and could be used as a KPI for this specific project. This differs slightly from KPIs as previously mentioned which are measures routinely used to monitor some level of system or function performance over time.

General Systems Flowcharts

This management tool is a graphical technique used to create a descriptive picture of a process. It is often also referred to as "process mapping." Flowcharting is used to plan and design new work processes as well as to evaluate existing practices. As noted, administrative operations and processes within any organization are complex. Any work process, such as preparing a meal, sending a letter, admitting a patient to a hospital, or developing a budget can be a complex process that requires the systematic interplay of numerous people doing different "activities" in some predetermined order or sequence. Just because a process is complex, however, does not mean it is random array of activities. Consider the example of making coffee:

1. Select coffee.

2. Grind if necessary.

3. Place coffee into a machine or filter.

4. Turn on the machine.

5. Press the brew button.

6. Pour the finished coffee.

7. Add any desired ingredients.

As depicted, making coffee can be described as a seven-step activity-based process. Because it is a commonly done process, the steps may seem as a natural and/or implicit sequence of activities. Note that specific duties and responsibilities associated with specific activities are usually set by job descriptions. Of course, this would not be true for our example but could for many other work-related ones.

Typically, efficient systems seek routine and stability. They also adhere to precedents. How a process was done yesterday is an accurate predictor of how that process will be done tomorrow. When systems and the people who function in them confront uncertainty and ambiguous expectations, "systems" attempt to drive out uncertainty and replace it with explicit (or implicit) direction. Managers also make systems (e.g., work processes) more efficient by establishing explicit expectations involving roles and functions. So, while making coffee at home may be a process that varies every time we do it, doing it in a coffee shop requires consistency so that the costs of coffee, sugar, milk, and so forth can be anticipated and budgeted and thus controlled.

General systems flowcharting provides the manager with a technique able to capture both the micro and macro elements of a system. It can be used to plan, describe, and/or analyze and evaluate any type of processes used to convert inputs (e.g., staff time) into desired outcomes at the system and subsystem levels. Using flowcharting requires two conditions. First, the work process should be complex, typically meaning it involves multiple steps and decisions. It also should involve multiple workers or workstations contributing to accomplishing some predetermined objective. Also, the work process being diagramed must have a formal starting and stopping point (i.e., an event). As such, general systems flowcharting requires the ability to define when a complex process starts and stops, even if the process or operation is continuous or repetitive. General systems flowcharting also has specific rules and conventions:

- Charts flow from top (start) to bottom (stop) and from left to right.
- Any decision included in a chart must be able to be answered as either *yes* or *no*.
- If possible, the "routine or most common" work process flows downward while other work processes flow horizontally.
- Lines on charts have arrowheads that indicate flow and sequence.
- Specific symbols are used and vary by industry.

Many of these symbols can be found as subsets of office spreadsheets or word-processing tools or there are more elaborate programs dedicated to only making flowcharts. Using these symbols with appropriate labels, charts are constructed that describe the operation of a work process. Managers create charts that describe how a current process works or should work. In the development of these charts, the manager also must ensure that all logical possibilities are included in the chart.

Scheduling Work Activities: Gantt Charts and Program Evaluation and Review Technique

The WBS is the foundation for project planning and scheduling using either Gantt charts or PERT. Both use "activities" identified in a WBS, either individually or collectively, to develop, plan, schedule, monitor, and manage a project. The Gantt chart was developed during the classical era of management and is typically used for simple and short-duration projects. The project activity listing identified in **Table 18.1** are shown in the following examples of both a Gantt chart and PERT (**Figure 18.1** and **Table 18.2**). This allows for a side-by-side comparison of these

TABLE 18.1 Project Activity Listing Corner General Hospital Emergency Department Expansion

LETTER	ACTIVITY	TIME (WEEKS)
A	Board of trustees project approval	2
B	Develop and issue press release	1
C	Develop architectural plans	9
D	Identify qualified construction contractors	3
E	Develop RFP	4
F	Distribute RFP to qualified bidders	1
G	Arrange and host bidders' conference	3
H	Provide record of all questions and answers to all bidders	1
I	Evaluate all contractor plans and proposals	4
J	Select a specific contractor	2
K	Legal review of proposed contract	2
L	Contract negotiations with selected general contractor	2
M	Secure all necessary permits and licenses	3
N	Contract implemented, modify physical plant	14
O	Final review & inspections of new construction	2
P	Order/receive/install new equipment	8
Q	Advertise, interview, and hire new staff	9
R	Expand parking area	4
S	Train new staff	3
T	Complete all required final inspection	2
U	Final report prepared	2
V	Final review by board of trustees	1
W	Develop and issue press release	1

RFP, request for proposal.

management tools. Also note that the scheduled beginning and end of each cited activity is an event which could be classified as KPIs.

A Gantt chart is a schedule of project activities presented sequentially. Its sequential display of individual activities implicitly suggests successor and predecessor relationships between activities. As stated, its simplicity may be its most attractive attribute, especially for simple projects.

Program Evaluation Review Technique

PERT identifies all project activities land the explicit relationship (i.e., successor/predecessor) between and among all the project's activities. It creates a network illustrating the relationship between and among project activities. A similar approach in the critical path method (CPM), PERT requires and illustrates the identification of project activities, the estimated time associated

FIGURE 18.1 Gantt chart example Corner General Hospital's emergency department expansion.

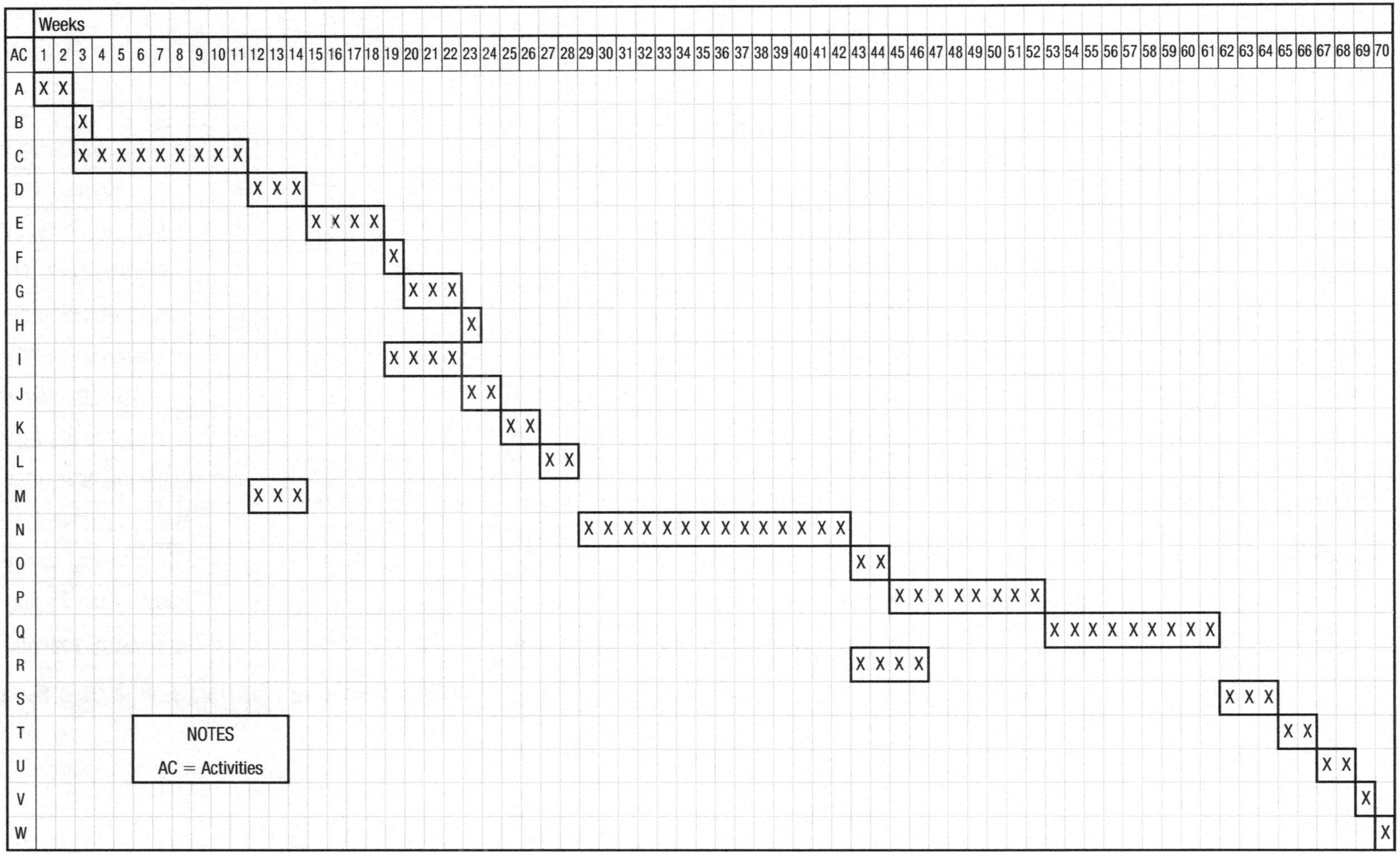

Weeks

AC	1	2	3	4	5	6	7	8	9	10	11	12	13	14	15	16	17	18	19	20	21	22	23	24	25	26	27	28	29	30	31	32	33	34	35	36	37	38	39	40	41	42	43	44	45	46	47	48	49	50	51	52	53	54	55	56	57	58	59	60	61	62	63	64	65	66	67	68	69	70
A	X	X																																																																				
B			X																																																																			
C				X	X	X	X	X	X	X	X	X																																																										
D													X	X	X																																																							
E																X	X	X	X																																																			
F																				X																																																		
G																					X	X	X																																															
H																								X																																														
I																				X	X	X	X																																															
J																								X	X																																													
K																										X	X																																											
L																												X	X																																									
M												X	X	X																																																								
N																												X	X	X	X	X	X	X	X	X	X	X	X	X																														
O																																									X	X																												
P																																											X	X	X	X	X	X	X	X																				
Q																																																			X	X	X	X	X	X	X	X	X	X										
R																																												X	X	X	X																						
S																																																														X	X	X						
T																																																																	X	X				
U																																																																			X	X		
V																																																																					X	
W																																																																						X

NOTES

AC = Activities

TABLE 18.2 PERT Critical Path Calculations

PROJECT ACTIVITIES	A	B	C	D	E	F	G	H	I	J	K	L	M	N	O	P	Q	R	S	T	U	V	W		
Time Estimate (weeks)	2	1	9	3	4	1	3	1	4	2	2	2	3	14	2	8	9	4	3	2	2	1	1		
Activity Pathways:																								Total WKS	
ACDEIJKLNOPQSTUVW	2		9	3	4				4	2	2	2		14	2	8	9		3	2	5	1	1	73	Critical Path
ABDFGHLNOPQSTUVW	2	1	9			1	3	1				2		14	2	8	9		3	2	5	1	1	64	
ACDFGHLNOPQSTUVW	2		9	3		1	3	1						14	2	8	9		3	2	5	1	1	64	
ACMNOPQSTUVW	2		9										3	14	2	8	9		3	2	5	1	1	59	
ACMNOPQSTUVW	2		9										3	14	2	8	9		3	2	5	1	1	59	
ACDEIJKLNOPTUVW	2		9	3	4				4	2	2	2		14	2	8				2	5	1	1	61	
ACDEIJKLNRSTUVW	2		9	3	4				4	2	2	2		14				4	3	2	5	1	1	58	
ACDEIJKLNOPTUVW	2		9	3	4				4	2	2	2		14				4	3	2	5	1	1	58	
ACMNRSTUVW	2		9										3	14				4	3	2	5	1	1	44	
ACMNOTUVW	2		9										3	14	2					2	5	1	1	39	

PERT, program evaluation and review technique.

with each activity, and the explicit identification of predecessor and successor activities associated with each activity.

Traditional PERT was originally developed to manage large-scale projects (e.g., ballistic missile systems) and used probabilistic time estimates for each project activity based on the estimate of the pessimistic (worst case) and optimistic (best case) time estimate for each activity. Other PERT models added specific cost estimates for each activity. The common approach presented uses a hybrid model of PERT and CPM. It is based on the project team's single estimate of the "most likely amount of time" required for each activity and the explicit identification of each activity's predecessor and successor activities. Based on this data, specific project activities are identified for continued scrutiny by project managers. For example, **Table 18.1** illustrates the critical aspects of PERT and Gantt charts as tools to manage projects. **Table 18.2** is derived from the WBS involving the expansion of Corner General Hospital's emergency department. It identifies predecessor and successor activities for all activities.

PERT introduces unique concepts and capabilities, such as a project's *critical path* and the *slack time,* associated with each individual project activity. Note there are 28 different activity paths through this PERT, as seen in **Table 18.2**. The *critical* path represents the one specific pathway through the PERT network with no slack time. Of all the "paths" through a PERT network, the *critical* path requires the longest amount of time to be completed. If any of the activities on this longest pathway—aka the critical path—are delayed, the entire project is delayed. There is no—meaning zero—"slack" on the critical path.

Slack is the amount of time a specific activity (not on the critical path) can be delayed or extended without lengthening the scheduled completion time of the entire project. Knowing the slack associated with each of the project activities in a PERT chart provides the manager with time cushions that can also be used if scheduling changes become necessary. Note that for any project activity of the project's critical path, the time cushion is zero. Knowing a project's critical path and the slack associated with project activities not on the critical path provides the manager with the ability to adjust and modify plans as the project develops and/or when the project encounters unanticipated circumstances. Examples of unanticipated circumstances include a supply shortage, worker labor actions, natural disasters, and any other change with project implications.

Table 18.3 shows the variety of times associated with each project step based on the project activities listed on **Table 18.2**. For this PERT example, selected project activities have estimated completion times expressed in weeks. Other projects could use other time denominations. For example, activity N, "contract implemented, modify physical plant," is estimated to require 14 weeks. This estimate would usually be derived using a formal contract with the selected general contractor and thereby is outside the direct control of the project manager.

Based on this information, multiple project paths from start to finish can be identified and the time to complete each path also can be calculated. The longest (in time duration) path from project start to finish is designated "the critical path." By definition, all project activities on the critical path have zero slack time. All the other activities (on the noncritical paths) have slack time. This means that their actual time durations can increase a certain amount—defined by the slack—without impacting the overall project completion time. Note that there are 28 individual paths through this PERT network, the longest is this project's "critical path."

It is interesting to note that the total time estimated to complete the Corner Hospital emergency department expansion would be 83 weeks if all activities were done sequentially. Although some activities were done concurrently, the critical path for this project is 70 weeks. Once a project begins, based on actual and/or revised activity times for remaining activities, the original critical path designation and slack calculations also change. Note that Figure 18.1 depicts this same project's activities using a Gantt chart. This chart also indicates 70 weeks between the start and finish of the project but lacks the ability to identify a critical path and evaluate the impact of changes as they occur. As such, both PERT and Gantt depict the duration of a project based on time estimates of required activities. PERT also identifies the relationships between and among all project activities. At best, a Gantt chart only infers these relationships. PERT makes these

TABLE 18.3 PERT Estimated Slack Time by Activity

LETTER	ACTIVITY	TIME (WEEKS)	CP	CUM	ES (WEEKS)	LS (WEEKS)	SLACK (WEEKS)
A	Board of trustees project approval	2	2	2	0	0	NA
B	Develop and issue press release	1			2	10	8
C	Develop architectural plans	9	9	11	2	2	0
D	Identify qualified construction contractors	3	3	14	11	11	0
E	Develop RFP	4	4	18	14	14	0
F	Distribute RFP to qualified bidders	1			12	20	8
G	Arrange and host bidders conference	3			13	21	8
H	Provide record of all questions and answers to all bidders	1			16	24	8
I	Evaluate all contractor plans and proposals	4	4	22	18	18	0
J	Select a specific contractor	2	2	24	22	22	0
K	Legal review of proposed contract	2	2	26	24	24	0
L	Contract negotiations with selected general contractor	2	2	28	26	26	0
M	Secure all necessary permits and licenses	3			11	25	14
N	Contract implemented, modify physical plant	14	14	42	28	28	0
O	Final review & inspections of new construction	2	2	44	42	42	0
P	Order/receive/install new equipment	8	8	52	44	44	0
Q	Advertise, interview, and hire new staff	9	9	61	52	52	0
R	Expand parking area	4			42	62	20
S	Train new staff	3	3	64	64	64	0
T	Complete all required final inspection	2	2	66	66	66	0
U	Final report prepared	2	2	68	68	68	0
V	Final review by board of trustees	1	1	69	69	69	0
W	Develop and issue press release	1	1	70	70	70	0

Note: Slack = LS − ES.

CP, critical path; CUM, cumulative; ES, earliest start; LS, latest start; PERT, program evaluation and review technique; RFP, request for proposal.

relationships explicit. When the time estimated change for a specific activity, the PERT model allows the manager to evaluate the impact of the change on all project activities. PERT also provides the ability to evaluate a project from start to finish. For example, the scheduled amount time estimated to complete an activity can be compared with the activity's actual activity time. Variances between estimated and actual are monitored and analyzed and become the basis for potentially changing future project plans.

Project management tools such as WBS, PERT, and Gantt charts are means to facilitate the appropriate definition and completion of any project. The WBS identifies the specific activities associated with a project. TSPR defines a project manager's responsibilities to include all activities and factors that contribute to project goals—performance capabilities, time duration, and project costs. PERT and Gantt charts emphasize the management of the time required to complete a project. Time is also a leading indicator of project cost. For example, if time is increased, it is likely that costs will increase.

As such, monitoring and managing activity-specific times (estimated vs. experienced) is a valuable management capability. For example, since a project's critical path represents the activity path with the longest amount of time to completion, once the project is underway, an activity time change/variance can impact the identification of the project's critical path and anticipated overall finish date. PERT provides the project manager with highly detailed and relevant information not readily available using Gantt charts. For example, PERT empowers the project manager to monitor and manage based on the actual versus estimated time to complete each activity cited in the PERT network. Also, based on actual experience, once the project starts, the project's critical path can influence a manger's priorities. Any project manager is expected to have a repertoire of tools and techniques, and PERT may be a basic skill expectation. Project management presents specific management challenges and issues and requires proficiency to use specific tools and techniques.

SUMMARY

Project management is a useful set of tools that analysts can use to assess the real scope of projects, including their impact on either a narrow or more broad set of organizational functions. Using TSPR with WBS allows for project impact estimations beyond the project itself. Using general systems flowcharts allows for an understanding of not only project step dependency but also those substeps that may occur simultaneously with others. Using PERT provides critical path analysis and estimates of slack time, which can be directly tied to cost and revenue estimates and allow for project modifications.

END-OF-CHAPTER RESOURCES

DISCUSSION QUESTIONS

1. Using the telehealth example at the beginning of the chapter, how would you begin your planning work?
2. Using the same example from telehealth, what internal and external points of information individuals or offices might want to include in your time estimates?
3. If a project's time to completion has high unknown variability, what would be your approach?
4. Develop a WBS for making a sandwich (your choice of type).
   a. What steps surprised you?
   b. What assumptions did you need to make beforehand?

LEARNING ACTIVITIES

CourseConnect ›

To access self-assessment questions and interactive, competency-based learning activities for this chapter, visit www.springerpub.com/courseconnect. See inside front cover and tear-out card for CourseConnect details.

STRATEGY AND APPLICATIONS

CHAPTER 19

POSTSCRIPT: STRATEGY AND APPLICATIONS

The preceding chapters emphasize specific management tools and techniques. Each presents methods to address specific types of management problems. For example, queuing focuses on waiting lines and program evaluation and review technique (PERT) focuses on project definition and management. In practice, however, the problems faced by managers do not always exactly fit the standards and parameters associated with a specific tool or technique or may span across many simultaneously. This may be one of the reasons that management is referred to as both an art and a science.

Professional managers are retained to analyze, anticipate, alleviate, and prevent impediments related to operational *effectiveness* and *efficiency*, thereby assisting their organization to meet specific performance goals and objectives. Recall Chapter 1, "Using Quantitative and Analytic Methods for Managing Healthcare Services," where we define managerial effectiveness as meeting specific strategic operational goals and objectives derived from the organization's mission statement, such as performing and providing available, accessible, affordable, and high-quality medical care. In contrast, efficiency is the ratio measure of work results divided by the resources needed to achieve the specific results. While it may be more "efficient" to feed hospital patients only once a day, it would not be effective given the role, function, and mission of the contemporary hospital. While efficiency and effectiveness have their distinct definitions, in practice they are inseparable.

We must also consider the manager's role in developing and implementing the organization's business strategy in potentially turbulent and competitive environments, often referred to as the organization's markets and/or service area, in times that are characterized by near-continuous change. Thus, we are reminded to call attention to the difference and relationship between "doing the right thing" and "doing things right." Doing the right things focuses on the *effectiveness* of meeting specific operational goals and objectives derived from the organization's statement of mission. For example, some essential hospital services generate more expenses than revenues but are considered essential given the hospital's role, function, and the needs of its clientele. In contrast, "doing things right" focuses attention on *efficiency*, typically meaning achieving maximum output based on the minimum use of organizational resources. For example, adjusting staffing based on actual utilization demonstrates the importance of "efficiency." We note that managers individually and collectively are both accountable and responsible for the "management" of the organization and the prudent use of its resources. Balancing between these concepts is a continuous function of the art and science of navigating healthcare and why the management sciences in healthcare can be far more difficult than other forms of production management given the ethical imperatives involved.

STRATEGY: THE MANAGER'S FRAMEWORK

Strategy is an action framework (i.e., plan) designed to achieve organizational priorities. Experts argue that any business strategy is specific to the organization's industrial sector (e.g., healthcare). For example, they argue that the business strategies of community hospitals are fundamentally different than the business strategies of large "big box" stores or supermarkets, which are also different than the business strategies of automobile manufacturers. In this context, "difference" means intent, substance, and form. This is a logical conclusion given that the factors that influence the design and definition of strategy of a long-term care facility (e.g., nursing home), an ambulatory care clinic, a community hospital, and a teaching hospital are related and also different. Similarly, while all private organizations, in contrast to divisions of government, prioritize financial performance such as return on investment (ROI) and profit, the strategy used to achieve specific goals is influenced by both the type of healthcare organization (e.g., community hospital vs. an urgent care clinic) and how the organization uses its resources to meet the needs and demands of its clientele.

Theorists also argue that every "industry" (i.e., economic sector) has unique and defining characteristics, practices, and parameters that influence how its organizations compete and act—in other words, its business strategy. Some refer to these as the "rules" of the "business competition game" for each specific industry. For example, in the health industry, many hospitals face unique state regulations such as certificate of need. All healthcare organizations also face the intricacies of the rules and regulations unique to national and state-specific financing (e.g., Medicare and Medicaid). In this context, the "rules of the competition" are defined by the type of organization (e.g., community hospital vs. nursing home) as well as many other, typically local, parameters. In the industrial sector, it is also common to find healthcare organizations owned and operated by government agencies and others that are privately owned and incorporated as either nonprofit, tax-exempt organizations or for-profit, tax-paying organizations. Some healthcare organizations are part of regional or national corporate or charitable organizations. In other words, the "rules" of the business strategy "game" are defined by the type of organization (e.g., community hospital), its specific location, and its ownership. Location also defines an organization's competition; the demographics in its services area/markets; and the associated health and medical needs, demands, and wants that could be prioritized.

The organization's service area/markets reflect its mission. Most healthcare organizations focus on proximate needs and demands. Some larger health systems, however, prioritize serving regional or national priorities and needs. Still others use different definitions of the scope and breath of "their" markets based on the specific services provided.

PROBLEM-BASED MANAGEMENT

The term "problem" denotes special meaning for a manager. When something is labeled a problem, developing and implementing its solution becomes a priority. By design, many of the tools and techniques addressed in this book are designed to assist managers define and solve specific "problems." By definition, problems have solutions. As such, problem-based management must define and prioritize the specific "problems." Multiple steps include defining and describing the problems to be addressed and the contributing factors related to the problem. Problem-based management also recognizes that how a problem is defined also defines the parameters associated with its solution. As such, the central question is "what is the problem?"

Theorists call attention to the significance of how a problem is defined and argue that its solution is dependent upon the characteristics of the problem. Using these characteristics, Cartwright, for example, presents a typology of problems (Cartwright, 1973). He calls attention to four types of problems: simple, compound, complex, and meta problems. As these labels imply, a simple problem could be a vitamin E deficiency caused by diet versus the meta problem of "poverty." Simple problems have simple solutions and meta problems have no clear-cut solution. Compound and complex problems are simple problems that also acknowledge other variables (e.g., rural vs. urban location, education, and income) and the relationships between and among them. Coetzee advocates three types of problems: simple, complex, and wicked (Coetzee, 1999). This perspective suggests the breadth and potential challenges associated with "problem-based management." Consider the question: "what is the problem?" Addressing and answering this question may be the most challenging aspect of problem-based management. Herein also lies the challenge. The tools and technique presented in this book are designed to address "simple" problems, not meta or wicked problems. Yet healthcare organizations typically face meta or wicked problems—frequently embedded in their mission statements—such as the challenge to enhance the health status of the communities it serves. This is both the paradox and challenge of problem-based management.

Professional success as a manager of organized health sector services and resources requires the competency to solve "simple" problems, in some instances using specific tools and protocols such as queuing, PERT, flowcharting, forecasting, and so forth. The actual problems faced by managers, however, typically have multiple causes often hidden in ambiguity. As such, problem-based management requires that managers analyze and define their problem based on the problem's multiple parts and dimensions and the relationships between its many interconnected parts. Some find it helpful to draw a sketch of the "problem" and its multiple parts and their interrelationships or use teams to define the problem and its component parts and then to craft strategies to "solve it" issuing available resources.

This postscript presents a framework for defining, analyzing, and solving managerial problems. The quantitative methods presented in this work are the manager's tools and techniques to support this process. This concluding statement also calls attention to the both the science and art of management—with the core being "what is the problem and how should it be addressed?"

LEARNING ACTIVITIES

CourseConnect ▶

To access self-assessment questions and interactive, competency-based learning activities for this chapter, visit www.springerpub.com/courseconnect. See inside front cover and tear-out card for CourseConnect details.

REFERENCES

Cartwright, T. J. (1973). Problems, solutions and strategies: A contribution to the theory and practice of planning. *Journal of the American Institute of Planners, 39*(3), 179–187. https://doi.org/10.1080/01944367308977852

Coetzee, J. L. (1999). A holistic approach to the maintenance "problem." *Journal of Quality in Maintenance Engineering, 5*(3), 276–281. https://doi.org/10.1108/13552519910282737